Human Diseases

by

John H. Dirckx, M.D.

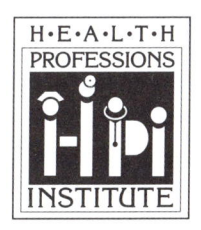

Health Professions Institute • Modesto, California • 1997

Human Diseases
by John H. Dirckx, M.D.

©1997 by Health Professions Institute

All rights reserved. No portion of this book may be reproduced or transmitted in any form or by any means, electronic or mechanical, including photocopy, recording, or any information storage and retrieval system, without written permission from the publisher.

Published by

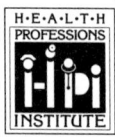

Health Professions Institute
Sally C. Pitman, Editor & Publisher
P. O. Box 801
Modesto, CA 95353-0801
Phone 209-551-2112
Fax 209-551-0404
Web site: http://www.hpisum.com
E-mail: hpi@hpisum.com

Printed by
Parks Printing & Lithograph
Modesto, California

ISBN 0-934385-03-3

Last digit is the print number: 9 8 7 6 5 4

*For my
daughter Patricia
with love*

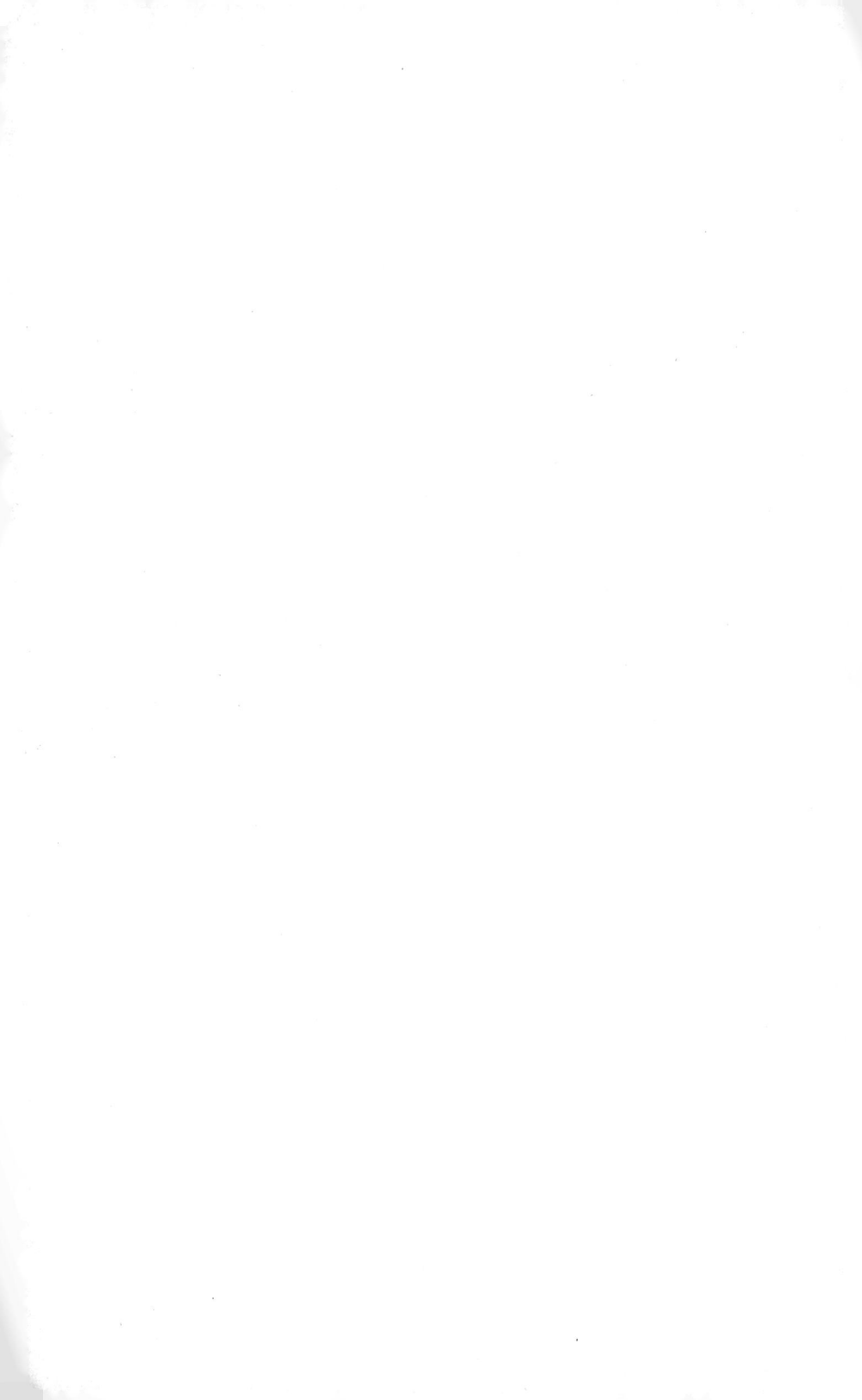

Preface

Human Diseases is intended to provide students and practitioners of the allied health professions with a grasp of basic information about the cause, symptoms, diagnosis, and treatment of common diseases. The earlier chapters set forth basic principles, and the later ones discuss, one by one, the bodily systems and important disorders to which they are subject. Rare diseases and arcane, trivial, and controversial issues have been carefully avoided throughout.

The order in which the material is presented (proceeding from the general to the particular and from the known to the unknown) renders *Human Diseases* ideal for use as a textbook. Preliminary discussions in each of the later chapters review relevant anatomy and physiology and describe symptoms, signs, and diagnostic measures. Particulars are then given about selected common diseases affecting the system in question.

The book can also serve as a quick and convenient reference source. Discussions of specific diseases are self-contained, and can be profitably consulted in isolation from adjacent material. For concise, clear definitions of terms pertaining to disease, a glance at the index will direct the user to the page on which the term is explained, either in context or in one of several specialized glossaries.

Contents

Chapter	Page

1. The Nature of Disease and the Diagnostic Process 1
2. Genetic Disease 19
3. Infectious Disease 35
4. The Immune System 55
5. Neoplasia 71
6. Trauma and Poisoning 85
7. Diseases of the Skin 101
8. Diseases of the Cardiovascular System 123
9. Diseases of the Ear, Nose, and Throat 147
10. Diseases of the Respiratory System 161
11. Diseases of the Digestive System 175
12. The Excretory System, the Male Reproductive System, and Sexually Transmitted Diseases 197
13. Disorders of the Female Reproductive System 213
14. Disorders of the Metabolism, Nutrition, and Endocrine Function 229
15. Disorders of Blood Cells, Blood-Forming Tissues, and Blood Coagulation 245
16. Musculoskeletal Disorders 263
17. Diseases of the Eye 277
18. Diseases of the Nervous System 293
19. Mental Disorders 319

Index 337

Author 350

Chapter 1

The Nature of Disease and the Diagnostic Process

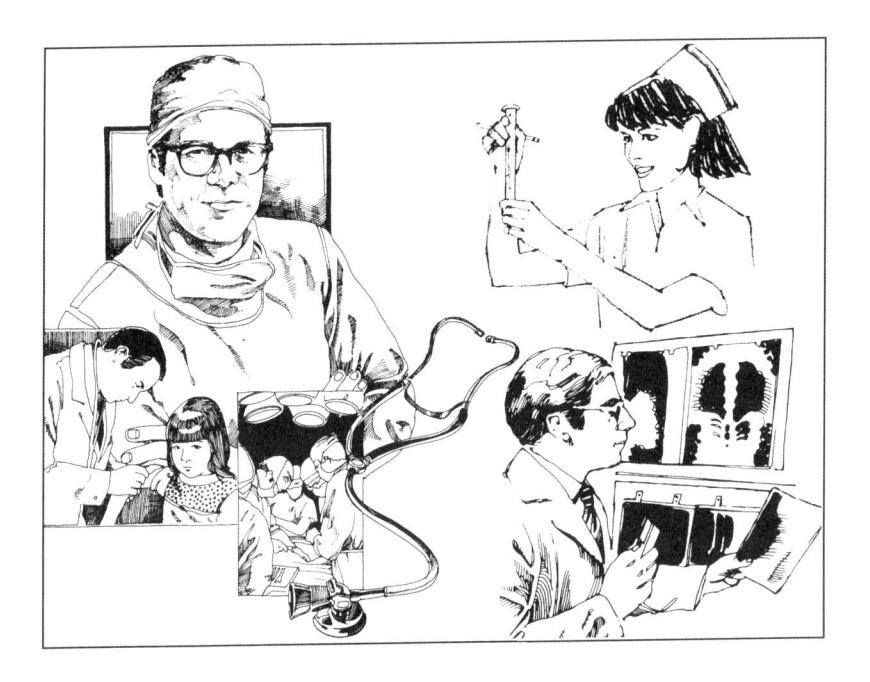

Learning Objectives

On completion of this chapter, the student should

- have an awareness of the range of human disease and of some of the ways in which diseases are named and classified;

- know the meanings of terms referring to various features of diseases;

- understand how diseases are diagnosed and treated, and be familiar with some of the basic terminology of diagnosis and treatment.

The Nature of Disease

Disease is a broad general concept, encompassing every imaginable impairment of normal bodily structure and function, and every imaginable threat to health and well-being, from genetic disorders affecting all of the cells in the body to highly localized, even microscopic, lesions; from conditions causing lifelong symptoms to mere passing indispositions; from severely disabling conditions to trivial aberrations detectable only by laboratory testing or statistical measurement.

A disease is not a "thing." Even though physicians and laity alike find it convenient to talk about diseases as if they were self-subsisting entities, a disease is actually just a state, condition, or process occurring in a living body.

Hence every case of disease is unique. No two persons with pneumococcal pneumonia or myocardial infarction have exactly the same symptoms, signs, and outcomes. On the other hand, all cases of these diseases have enough in common that it is reasonable and expedient to group them together under a single concept and a single name.

When we speak of the transmission of a disease from one person to another, we really mean the transmission of the germs that cause that disease. Similarly, expressions about diseases "going away" or "coming back" are purely metaphorical.

Disease is a complex notion, including not only biological alterations of normal structure and function but also psychological, social, and economic factors. In addition, in our culture disease is regarded as something to be treated and perhaps cured by a physician.

The discussion of diseases that follows is based on the beliefs and traditions of Western scientific medicine. Although this system of medicine is rational and coherent, and gives satisfactory explanations or interpretations of facts, and acceptable results in treatment, it is far from perfect. In our understanding of the causes of various diseases, their prevention, diagnosis, and treatment, we have a long way to go.

Radically different views on the cause, nature, and treatment of disease are held by adherents of some religions or philosophies, by members of other cultures, and by some within our own culture. Many of these alternative systems—Christian Science, the folk medicine of various ethnic groups, chiropractic, acupuncture—contain valid and useful elements, as well as others that conflict with basic facts and principles of scientific medicine.

The Nature of Disease • 3

A **disease** is a recognizable pattern of symptoms or abnormalities. What constitutes a disease? A single migraine headache is not a disease, but a lifelong tendency to get migraine headaches is considered a disease state. Is a sprained ankle a disease? A hangover? Pregnancy? There can be no precise or "official" answer to these questions. Some physicians and psychologists have objected to the classification of alcoholism as a disease on the grounds that this diminishes patients' sense of personal accountability and responsiveness to counseling. Fibrocystic disease of the breast has been renamed fibrocystic condition of the breast because the word "disease" was perceived as having negative and ominous connotations in this context. Legislation or regulations regarding health insurance coverage often require that pregnancy be treated "the same as any other disease."

Naming and Classifying Diseases

Diseases can be, and have been, named and classified in many different ways, but no system of naming or classification in present use is entirely consistent or satisfactory. Many names attached to diseases long ago remain in use even though they have been shown to be inaccurate or misleading (see box).

Influenza, a disease causing fever, headache, muscle aches, and cough, was so named because it was blamed on the influence (Italian *influenza*) of the stars and planets. We retain the name even though we now know that the disease is caused by a virus.

Malaria got its name because it was more prevalent in swampy areas, and was believed to be due to the damp, malodorous air in such places (Italian *mal'aria* 'bad air'). We now know that it is caused by a parasite, which is transmitted by mosquitoes that breed in shallow, stagnant water, but we still retain the old name.

Cholera, a bacterial infection of the intestine, was formerly thought to be due to an excess of bile (Greek *chole*).

Some disease names go back to classical Greek (asthma, coryza, dysentery, nephritis) or Latin (fistula, impetigo, scabies, vertigo). Before the era of modern science, diseases were often named for some obvious symptom or characteristic (diabetes 'a flowing through [of urine]', chlorosis 'greenness', jaundice 'yellowness'). Many disease names are metaphorical in origin: cancer 'crab', chalazion 'hailstone', lupus 'wolf', tinea 'moth'. Nowadays we are more likely to apply names referring to causes (ehrlichiosis, trichomoniasis). Numerous disease names are eponymic (based on proper names), usually honoring the person or persons who first discovered or described them (Hodgkin disease, Osgood-Schlatter disease, parkinsonism), but sometimes referring to persons so afflicted (Christmas disease, Hartnup disease, Lou Gehrig disease) or geographic areas where they were first noted or where they are endemic (California encephalitis, Lyme disease, Rocky Mountain spotted fever).

A disease name may denote a single, very specific disorder, such as otitis media or typhoid fever, or it may stand for a whole group of different conditions with one thing in common, such as anemia or salmonellosis. The term hyperthyroidism means a condition in which excessive thyroid hormone causes symptoms. This is not one single disease, but an abnormal state that can have various causes. It may be appropriate for a physician to diagnose hyperthyroidism on the basis of an initial evaluation of the patient, but with further investigation a more precise diagnosis, such as Graves disease, will usually be possible.

A **syndrome** is a combination of symptoms that consistently occur together (Cushing syndrome, irritable bowel syndrome, toxic shock syndrome). For some syndromes there are several known causes; for others, no cause has been identified. Disease names formed with Greek suffixes have fairly rigid patterns of meaning: *-ia* denotes an abnormal condition (ophthalmia, pneumonia); *-itis* means inflammation (appendicitis, dermatitis); *-osis*, an abnormal condition (cyanosis, nephrosis); *–ism*, intoxication or habituation (alcoholism, atropinism).

Textbooks of medicine contain elaborate classifications of disease. In addition, official systems of naming and classification, particularly the ***International Classification of Diseases*, 9th edition (*ICD-9*)**, are in wide use to standardize the statistical reporting of diseases and billing for medical services. Some of these classificatory systems, such as the ***Diagnostic and Statistical Manual*, 4th edition (*DSM-IV*)**, published by the American Psychiatric Association, include precise definitions of diseases.

The classification of diseases must constantly change as scientific information increases. What was formerly considered a single disease may come to be recognized as a group of diseases with similar symptoms but different causes, while diseases that were formerly thought to be different may eventually be recognized as just different forms or stages of the same disease.

One classification may be appropriate in one setting, and another classification in another setting. For example, anemia (deficiency of red blood cells) can be classified on the basis of its cause as due to:
Deficient formation of red blood cells.
Excessive hemolysis (destruction of red blood cells in the body).
Blood loss.
But for the diagnostician, a more useful classification may be on the basis of the size of the red blood cells:
Normocytic, with normal-sized cells.
Macrocytic, with cells larger than normal.
Microcytic, with cells smaller than normal.
These two classifications overlap but do not match; they cannot be meaningfully combined, and yet each has its place in the theory and practice of medicine.

The discussion of diseases presented in the following chapters is not exhaustive, and the classification used does not necessarily match those used in textbooks of medicine or in *ICD-9*. The purpose of these chapters is not to impart a medical education but to give the student an awareness of the range of disorders, diagnostic measures, and treatments, with emphasis on conditions that are encountered daily in transcription practice. Material has been selected and arranged so as to be maximally useful for study, review, and reference.

The following are some common ways of describing, characterizing, or classifying diseases. Under each basis of **classification**, some of the more common terms are defined or explained, and examples are given.

Temporal Classification (according to time of onset, duration, severity, and rapidity of evolution and resolution):
   acquired: not congenital (acquired hemolytic anemia, acquired immunodeficiency syndrome).
   acute: developing relatively suddenly and running its course in a few days or weeks (acute pharyngitis, acute glomerulonephritis).
   asymptomatic: causing no symptoms, often referring to a disease or condition that is discovered during a routine or screening examination, or in the evaluation of another condition.

chronic: having a protracted course, often lifelong (chronic bronchitis, chronic pancreatitis).

congenital: present at birth, though not necessarily inherited (congenital cataract, congenital adrenal hyperplasia).

disabling: causing impairment of normal functions or capabilities, such as the ability to see, stand, and walk, or earn a living.

end-stage: referring to a progressively deteriorating condition that has reached the point of lethal (terminal) functional impairment of an organ or organ system (end-stage renal failure, end-stage lung disease).

fulminant or fulminating: rapidly progressive and severe (fulminant hepatitis, fulminating dysentery).

hyperacute: having a very abrupt onset or very brief course (hyperacute purulent conjunctivitis, hyperacute graft rejection).

infantile: occurring or becoming evident during infancy (infantile autism, infantile cataract).

intermittent: causing symptoms at intervals, with intervening periods without symptoms (intermittent claudication, intermittent acute porphyria).

juvenile: occurring in early life (juvenile rheumatoid arthritis, juvenile kyphosis).

life-threatening: referring to a disease or injury that may prove lethal, even with aggressive treatment.

malignant: tending to cause death (malignant tumor, malignant hypertension).

neonatal: affecting newborn infants (neonatal anemia, neonatal hypoglycemia).

paroxysmal: occurring in sudden attacks (paroxysmal cold hemoglobinuria, paroxysmal atrial tachycardia).

progressive: characterized by increasingly extensive or severe symptoms or signs (progressive cataract, progressive muscular atrophy).

recurrent: referring to a condition that reappears after symptoms had largely or entirely resolved (recurrent corneal erosion, recurrent ulcerative stomatitis).

relapsing: essentially the same as the preceding (relapsing fever, relapsing polychondritis).

remissive, remittent: referring to a condition of which most or all signs and symptoms have resolved, either naturally or as a result of treatment; remission may be temporary or permanent.

self-limiting (-ed): said of a disease such as the common cold that typically runs its course and resolves spontaneously without complications or sequelae, even when left untreated.

senile: occurring as a result of aging (senile cataract, senile dementia).

silent: asymptomatic; referring to a disease or medical event discovered only by chance (silent gallstones, silent myocardial infarction).

subacute: lasting somewhat longer than an acute illness (subacute bacterial endocarditis, subacute granulomatous thyroiditis).

subclinical: causing no symptoms or signs; essentially the same as silent.

terminal: a disease that is expected to cause death within the near future, regardless of treatment.

Etiologic Classification (by cause)

deficiency: due to a lack or insufficiency of some essential chemical substance or property (leukocyte adhesion deficiency, iron deficiency anemia).

degenerative: caused by deterioration in the structure or function of cells or tissues (degenerative joint disease, degenerative myopia).

developmental: characterized by some abnormality in the development of a tissue, organ, or body part, either before or after birth (rickets, ventricular septal defect).

essential: of unknown cause; apparently arising spontaneously (essential hypertension, benign essential tremor).

familial (heredofamilial): due to an inherited abnormality expressed in other members of the patient's family (familial hypertrophic cardiomyopathy, heredofamilial tremor).

functional: due to a disturbance of function without evidence of structural or chemical abnormality (functional dysmenorrhea, functional heart murmur).

hereditary: due to an inherited abnormality or tendency (hereditary cerebellar ataxia, hereditary multiple exostoses).

idiopathic: of unknown cause; apparently arising spontaneously (idiopathic cardiomyopathy, idiopathic hypertrophic subaortic stenosis).

infectious (infective): caused by the adverse biologic, chemical, or immunologic effects of the growth of microorganisms in the body (infectious mononucleosis, infective embolism).

molecular: a disease caused by abnormality in the chemical structure or concentration of a single molecule, usually a protein or enzyme; virtually all molecular diseases are inherited (congenital adrenal hyperplasia, sickle cell anemia).

neoplastic: involving the formation of one or more growths or tumors, which may be benign or malignant.

nutritional: due to insufficient or excessive dietary intake of some nutrient (nutritional anemia, nutritional hemosiderosis).

organic: due to some demonstrable abnormality in a bodily structure (organic dementia, organic heart murmur).

traumatic: due to injury—physical, chemical, thermal, or psychological (traumatic amnesia, traumatic neuroma).

Diseases can also be classified **anatomically**, by the organs or tissues principally involved; **physiologically**, by the body system or function affected; or by the medical **specialties** concerned with their treatment.

In the following chapters, each disease or category of disease chosen for inclusion is treated in a separate section. The more elaborate discussions are divided under some or all of the following headings:

Disease Name and Synonyms
Brief Description
Cause(s)
History
Physical Examination
Diagnostic Tests
Course
Treatment

In the following section, crucial terms and concepts relating to some of these divisions of the material are defined or explained.

Cause

etiology: strictly speaking, the study of the causes of disease; universally used by physicians to mean the cause itself.

multifactorial etiology: indicates that a given disease has more than one cause operating together (lung cancer may develop because of a genetic predisposition *and* exposure to carcinogens in cigarette smoke; *Pneumocystis carinii* pneumonia is due to the parasite, *Pneumocystis carinii*, but usually does not develop unless the immune system is impaired, as in AIDS).

primary: said of a disease or condition that does not result from some other disease (primary aldosteronism, primary malignancy).

secondary: said of a disease or condition that results from some other disease (secondary hypertension, secondary malignancy; tachycardia secondary to congestive heart failure).

History

The medical history is a detailed record of the course of an illness, as perceived and recalled by the patient.

noncontributory: of no help in arriving at a diagnosis; said principally of elements of the patient's history, such as family medical history.

symptom: any distress, abnormality, or malfunction experienced by the patient as a result of illness; a symptom may be entirely subjective (headache, vertigo) or it may be partly or entirely evident to others (paralysis, vomiting).

Physical Examination

A formal assessment of bodily structure and function by the physician in an effort to establish a complete clinical picture of the patient's illness. Traditionally, physical examination includes four basic techniques: inspection, palpation, percussion, and auscultation.

auscultation: listening to selected body regions with a stethoscope; principally to assess heart sounds, breath sounds, and bowel sounds.

inspection: visual examination of the external body surface and of the mouth and pharynx, the external ear, the nares, and other orifices and cavities accessible to direct examination without a surgical incision.

palpation: feeling superficial and deep structures with the fingers or palm to detect tenderness, spasm, abnormal masses, abnormal texture of tissues, enlargement of abdominal organs, and other departures from the normal or expected.

percussion: tapping with a finger on the body wall, usually with a finger of the other hand interposed, to detect variations in sound quality over abnormal cavities, masses, accumulations of gas or air, or effusions of fluid (see box).

> The technique of **percussion**, which has been rendered largely superfluous by x-ray, fluoroscopy, ultrasound, and MRI, is now the least used of the four basic methods of physical diagnosis. Before these imaging procedures became available, however, percussion was at least as important as auscultation in the examination of the chest.
>
> This technique was first described by the Austrian physician Leopold Auenbrugger (1722-1809), who translated to clinical medicine the common practice of tapping on a wine barrel to determine the level of the fluid inside. Auenbrugger made extensive experiments with the method and confirmed its validity by comparing his findings in the living patient with autopsy results.
>
> He published his method in a small book in 1861, which was largely ignored by the medical profession until Corvisart, Napoleon's personal physician, issued a French version in 1808. Auenbrugger was a man of wide interests and broad culture. He played an important role in Viennese society for several decades, and wrote the libretto for an opera, *Der Rauchfangkehrer* (*The Chimney Sweep*, 1781) for which the music was composed by Mozart's rival, Antonio Salieri.

sign: any abnormality of bodily structure or function that is observable by the physician, whether evident to the patient or not.

Space limitations do not permit a full general discussion of the physical examination. The student is advised to supplement material given here by reading or referring to *H & P: A Nonphysician's Guide to the Medical History and Physical Examination* by John H. Dirckx, M.D. (Modesto, Ca.: Health Professions Institute, 1991).

Diagnostic Tests

Under this heading are included all diagnostic procedures not included in the basic physical examination. These include laboratory tests, diagnostic imaging, electrophysiologic measurements, endoscopy, radionuclide procedures, and others.

culture: the growth of microorganisms from a specimen (blood or other body fluid, secretions, tissue) under controlled laboratory conditions.

cytology: microscopic examination of stained cells, usually cells brushed or scraped from a surface such as the uterine cervix or the interior of the stomach; the principal use of cytology is in detecting any malignant or premalignant cellular changes.

electrodiagnostic procedures: methods for recording the electrical activity accompanying the function of certain organs or tissues (electrocardiogram, electroencephalogram, electromyogram, and others).

endoscopy: examination of the interior of a cavity or hollow organ with an instrument introduced through a natural orifice (cystoscopy, colonoscopy) or a small incision (laparoscopy, arthroscopy).

histology: microscopic examination of stained, very thin sections of tissue obtained by biopsy or surgical excision, or at autopsy.

imaging (diagnostic): any procedure used to study or visualize internal organs or tissues by application of irradiation or other physical energy: x-ray, CT scan, fluoroscopy, ultrasound, magnetic resonance imaging, and others.

invasive: refers to a procedure requiring the introduction of a needle, catheter, or other instrument into the body through a puncture or incision.

laboratory test: any test performed in a laboratory on a specimen of tissue or body fluids removed from the patient; includes physical, chemical, microscopic, microbiologic, immunologic, and other examinations.

microbiology: the branch of biology and medical laboratory technology concerned with the study of microorganisms (bacteria, fungi), particularly those that are pathogenic for human beings.

noninvasive: referring to a diagnostic procedure such as an x-ray examination or electrocardiogram that does not require introduction of instruments into the patient's body.

radiography: the branch of medical technology concerned with the performance of x-ray and other imaging procedures.

radiology: the branch of medicine concerned with the diagnosis and treatment of disease through the application of x-rays, ultrasound, magnetic resonance imaging, radioactive materials, and related methods.

scan: examination of part or all of the body by a radiographic procedure, particularly one involving radioactive substances, to identify or localize an abnormal condition.

serology: the branch of medical laboratory technology that employs antigen-antibody reactions to diagnose infections and other diseases, particularly autoimmune diseases.

smear: a thin film of fluid or semisolid material (blood, stool, nasal secretions, cells scraped from a surface), usually stained, that is examined microscopically for diagnostic purposes.

Space will not permit a full discussion of diagnostic laboratory procedures. The student is advised to supplement information given here and in the following chapters by reading or referring to *Laboratory Medicine: Essentials of Anatomic and Clinical Pathology,* 2nd ed., by John H. Dirckx, M.D. (Modesto, Ca.: Health Professions Institute, 1995).

Course

The course of a disease is the sequence of events from the first appearance of symptoms to the final resolution of all abnormalities. Diseases evolve. The signs and symptoms noted at the beginning of an illness are often entirely different from those noted a few hours, days, or weeks later. In diagnosis and prognosis, the pattern according to which the manifestations of disease change is almost as important as the manifestations themselves.

complication: a disease or abnormal condition induced by a pre-existing condition, which renders treatment more difficult, recovery more protracted, or death more likely.

form: any of several clinical patterns that a disease may manifest (the discoid and systemic forms of lupus erythematosus).

grade: a measure of the severity of a disease or abnormal condition, particularly a malignant disease.

life-threatening: a prognostic indication that a disease or injury may prove lethal in spite of aggressive treatment.

onset: the first appearance of signs or symptoms of a disease.

present [verb]: refers to the symptoms or signs that are evident when the patient first seeks medical attention. ("Mrs. Jones presented to the emergency department at 1:00 a.m. today with acute, diffuse chest pain and dyspnea." "Infectious mononucleosis occasionally presents as painless jaundice or a nonspecific rash.")

prodrome: a period during which (usually nonspecific) symptoms such as fever or malaise precede the appearance of typical signs and symptoms of a disease.

prognosis: the probable outcome of a disease, as predicted on the basis of diagnosis and course.

sequela [plural, **sequelae**]: an abnormality or impairment, such as scarring or weakness, that persists after a disease has resolved.

stage: a measure of the extent to which a disease, particularly a malignant disease, has developed.

T-N-M classification: a formal mode of staging that is used for many malignant diseases; T, tumor; N, (lymph) nodes; M, metastases. Subscript numbers are used to indicate the extent of involvement; for example, $T_1 N_2 M_0$ for a given tumor might mean a tumor that is not locally invasive, with extension to two groups of regional lymph nodes, but no apparent metastases.

Treatment

Under this heading are included all measures undertaken to reduce symptoms, maintain or restore function, eradicate the cause of a disease, and prevent recurrence.

aggressive: referring to a prompt, energetic program of treatment.

benign neglect: a program of doing essentially nothing when a disease is either beyond hope of cure by even the most radical methods, or is expected to resolve without any specific treatment.

conservative: a mode of treatment, medical or surgical, that has a low risk of causing serious adverse effects, but also less likelihood of effecting a cure than other available methods.

cosmetic: referring to physical appearance; said of surgical procedures designed primarily to improve the patient's appearance, such as breast augmentation, revision of scars, and excision of benign skin lesions.

cure: complete extinction of a disease, usually by arresting the basic process or removing the cause.

elective: referring to a treatment or therapeutic procedure, usually a surgical operation, that is not absolutely required to save the patient's life or restore health, but that is, or may be, performed to improve the prognosis or to correct a minor problem; also, a procedure that is necessary but that is deferred until it is convenient for the patient.

heroic: referring to radical or extreme therapeutic measures that are only justified by the desperate condition of the patient.

inoperable: referring to a disease, usually malignant, for which surgical treatment is not an option, because of the extent of the disease or the condition of the patient.

masterly inactivity: same as benign neglect; a phrase first used, in a nonmedical context, by the British political writer Sir James Mackintosh (1765-1832).

medical: any form of treatment not involving surgery or physical manipulation.

monodrug therapy: treatment of a condition such as hypertension or malignancy with a single drug, rather than a combination of drugs.

palliative: referring to treatment of a severe or malignant disease that is intended to relieve pain or conserve function without removing the cause or effecting a cure.

physical therapy: treatment involving application of physical modalities (massage, exercise, heat, cold, ultrasound).

protocol: a therapeutic regimen, usually prescribed for malignant disease, consisting of fixed or proportionate doses of three or more drugs administered concurrently.

radical: a drastic program of treatment, medical or surgical, with a high risk of adverse effects, justified only by the severity of the patient's condition or the unfavorable prognosis.

regimen: a program or course of treatment, including diet, exercise, and drug therapy.

surgical: a mode of treatment involving physical or mechanical manipulation, usually by cutting into the body to repair or remove diseased or injured organs or tissues.

supportive: referring to a treatment regimen designed to preserve the patient's comfort, hydration, and nutritional status without affecting the underlying disease.

symptomatic: referring to treatment that is intended to relieve symptoms rather than abolish their cause.

synergism: a positive interaction between two or more drugs in which each boosts the effect of the others.

therapeutic trial: experimental administration of a drug in an effort not only to relieve symptoms but also to confirm the working diagnosis.

Space will not permit a full discussion of drug treatment. The student is advised to supplement material given here and in the following chapters by reading or referring to *Understanding Pharmacology* by Susan M. Turley, MA, CMT (Englewood Cliffs, NY: Regents/Prentice Hall, 1991).

The Diagnostic Process

The training of a physician includes an intensive study of diseases and their symptoms from two distinct points of view: learning the symptoms and signs of each disease, such as pneumonia and pericarditis; and learning all of the diseases that can produce any given symptom or sign, such as dyspnea or chest pain.

Training in diagnostics also includes learning to apply and interpret the four basic maneuvers of physical diagnosis as well as the full range of supplementary diagnostic tests available. Equipped with this battery of information and technical skills, the physician takes a history, performs a physical examination, orders diagnostic tests, and coordinates the resulting data to formulate a tentative or working diagnosis.

The **medical history and physical examination** are the cornerstone of all medical practice. For every patient admitted to a hospital, the physician must dictate or write a history and physical examination. Similar documentation of diagnostic findings, though often less extensive, is a part of most other medical office records and consultations. The history and physical shows the extent of the physician's evaluation of the patient and provides support for the diagnosis made. Conspicuous among the data reported in a history and physical examination are pertinent negatives—listing of symptoms and signs that are not present. Inclusion of these negatives is essential to providing a complete clinical picture and a complete account of the diagnostic procedures performed by the physician.

Sometimes the diagnosis is evident at once: a cut on the hand from a sharp tool; a foreign body in the eye. In other instances, diagnostic procedures may yield negative, normal, ambiguous, or contradictory results, and the tentative diagnosis must be based on a balancing of such probabilities as are suggested by the history. **Differential diagnosis** refers to this consideration and ranking of several alternative explanations of a patient's symptoms and physical findings. For example, the differential diagnosis (often shortened to just "the differential") of chest pain and shortness of breath includes myocardial infarction, spontaneous pneumothorax, rib fracture, pneumonia, and a number of other possibilities.

The diagnostician must always reckon with the possibility that the patient has two or more unrelated diseases, each of which is contributing to the total clinical picture. The likelihood that a patient has more than one disease at the same time increases with age.

comorbidity: the presence of two or more unrelated diseases in the same patient at the same time.

negative: said of a diagnostic test that reveals no abnormality ("The Romberg [test] is negative").

normal: within the range of expected or healthy sensations or diagnostic findings ("Alertness and mood have remained normal," "Cranial nerves II through XII are normal on examination"); often used synonymously with the preceding.

red herring (slang): a misleading diagnostic clue; for example, a history of having fallen and struck his head a few days ago, in a man who presents with headache and dizziness due to a brain tumor; the assumption that symptoms are due to the injury may delay or even prevent an evaluation that would reveal the true diagnosis.

tentative diagnosis: a diagnosis that seems most probable on the basis of available data, but which has yet to be confirmed.

working diagnosis: a preliminary diagnosis, often very general (fever of unknown origin, seizure disorder) on the basis of which therapy can be started and more specific diagnostic tests chosen.

Topics for Study or Discussion

1. Define: acute, chronic, etiology, sign, symptom, syndrome.

2. Give two examples of invasive and two examples of noninvasive diagnostic procedures.

3. What factors must a physician take into account in choosing what diagnostic tests to perform on a patient, and when to perform them?

4. It is often said that the patient's history provides more useful clues to the diagnosis than the physician's examination, and that the examination is more valuable than laboratory tests. Look through the discussions of genetic diseases in the next chapter and find examples of disorders that can be diagnosed by history alone; those in which physical examination is diagnostic; and those in which only laboratory testing can confirm the presence of genetic disease.

5. If you or a friend or family member has had an illness wrongly diagnosed by a physician, what factors do you think might have played a part in the error? (Suggestions: Misleading or incomplete information supplied by patient; absence of detectable abnormality on physical examination; conflicting laboratory data; examination or testing before the disease was fully manifest; failure to return to physician for followup.)sea, vomiting, and general malaise.

Chapter 2

Genetic Disorders

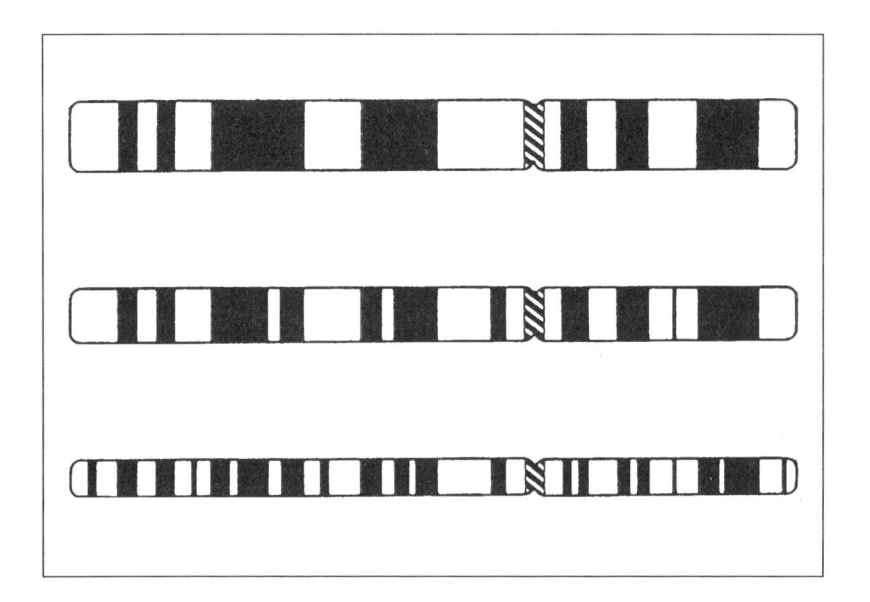

Learning Objectives

On completion of this chapter, the student should

- understand the biochemical basis of heredity;

- know basic information about the diagnosis of hereditary diseases and chromosomal abnormalities;

- know about some common inherited diseases;

- know about some common chromosomal abnormalities;

- know about oncogenes.

Congenital vs. Hereditary

This would be a good place to elaborate on two definitions that were given in the preceding chapter:
Congenital: beginning, occurring, or first being evident at birth.
Hereditary: inherited from one or both parents.

The distinction is often poorly understood. A **congenital disorder** is present at birth, but it is not necessarily transmitted genetically. For example, many congenital disorders result from environmental factors (maternal infections; maternal ingestion of certain medicines, drugs of abuse, or toxins such as dioxin or lead during pregnancy) or from faulty intrauterine development (umbilical cord tightly wrapped around an extremity and shutting off its blood supply). The birth process itself can lead to congenital disease or abnormality, as in the case of infections such as herpes simplex and chlamydia transmitted to the newborn from the birth canal, and cerebral palsy from difficult labor with compromise of blood flow to the baby's brain.

A **hereditary disorder** is genetically acquired; that is, it is transmitted to the affected individual by the genes of one or both parents. All of the diseases presented in this chapter are hereditary.

The Biochemical Basis of Heredity

The inheritance of physical traits (eye color, hair color, body build) as well as of some diseases and abnormal conditions depends on the transmission of genes from parents to offspring. A **gene** is a functional unit of heredity; each gene transmits a single trait or function. Every human cell nucleus contains more than 50,000 genes, arranged in bands along coils of protein and deoxyribonucleic acid (DNA) called **chromosomes**.

There are 46 chromosomes in the nucleus of a human cell, arranged in 23 pairs. One of these pairs, the **sex chromosomes**, determines the sex of an individual. Women have two X chromosomes (XX), and men have an X and a Y chromosome (XY). In women, one of the X chromosomes is genetically inactive. Hence all persons have one active X chromosome, and in addition men have an active Y chromosome.

The remaining 22 pairs of chromosomes are called **autosomes**; they are concerned with the transmission of traits having nothing to do with biological gender, and the members of each pair are basically identical to one another. Each gene has a fixed normal position, or **locus**, on a specific chromosome. The genes that occupy the corresponding loci on any given pair of chromosomes (and that transmit the same trait) are said to be **homologous**.

The autosomes are numbered from 1 to 22 in the order of decreasing length. Each is divided into a long arm (q) and a short arm (p), which are further divided into regions, bands, and subbands for the purpose of designating gene loci.

In the formation of human sex cells (female ovum, male sperm), *but in no other cells*, the chromosome pairs divide by a process called **meiosis**, which results in cells having only 23 chromosomes instead of 23 *pairs* of chromosomes. When sperm and egg unite, the full complement of 23 pairs of chromosomes is restored, one of each pair having come from each parent.

Body cells other than sex cells multiply by splitting into two identical daughter cells. Before this division takes place, the chromosomes replicate; each chromosome forms a copy of itself in a process called **mitosis**. This process, which occurs in several stages, results in the formation of two nuclei having identical sets of chromosomes, one for each daughter cell.

When **homologous genes** are identical (for example, when both genes for eye color are coded for blue eyes), the individual is said to be **homozygous** for the trait coded by that gene. When homologous genes are not identical (for example, one coding for blue eyes and the other for brown eyes), the individual is said to be **heterozygous** for eye color.

Some genes exert their effects only in homozygous individuals. That is, both genes at a given locus must be identical. Such a gene is said to be **recessive**, because if it appears on only one chromosome of a pair, the trait for which it codes is not expressed. An individual having only one recessive gene is called a carrier of that gene, because it can be transmitted to some or all offspring. A gene that has its effect even in a heterozygous individual, that is, when paired with a gene that is not identical to it, is said to be **dominant**. The basic pattern of normal inheritance is called **mendelian**, after Gregor Mendel (see box).

Geneticists distinguish between an individual's **phenotype**, which is the complex of traits as observed by inspection, measurement, biochemical testing, or other means; and the **genotype**, which is the actual

22 • Human Diseases

genetic composition of the individual's chromosomes, as determined by chromosomal analysis.

The fundamental concepts of the genetic transmission of traits from parents to offspring was evolved by a Bohemian amateur scientist, **Johann Gregor Mendel** (1822-1884). Mendel came of peasant stock and was unable to finish his college education for lack of funds. After becoming an Augustinian monk, he studied to be a teacher, but failed twice to obtain certification because his mind always went blank at examination time.

His leisure studies of the transmission of characteristics from one generation of peas to later generations provided the basis for his theories of the statistical distribution of parental characteristics among offspring and the notions of dominant and recessive genes and hybridization. He published his theories in 1865, but was rebuffed or ignored by professional biologists. Three years later he became the abbot of his monastery, and abandoned further research.

His work was rediscovered after his death and brilliantly vindicated by the studies of later scientists.

Genetic Abnormalities

Many things can go wrong in the process whereby a new individual is formed through the transmission of more than 50,000 genes. A **mutation** is a permanent, transmissible change affecting (usually) a single gene. Through mutation, an individual with normal parents can acquire an abnormal trait at conception and pass it on to some offspring, not necessarily in the first generation. Genetic defects in autosomes are called **autosomal** (dominant or recessive). Defects in sex chromosomes are called **sex-linked** or (since they all affect the X chromosome) **X-linked**. Not all genetic mutations cause evident abnormality. Fetuses with severe disorders are usually lost through spontaneous abortion.

Some mutations occur with sufficient frequency that their presence in a subject's genotype (chromosomal makeup) can be inferred from the resulting abnormal phenotype (physical appearance and biochemical composition and function). It is estimated that human beings are subject to at least 4,000 inheritable diseases.

Chromosomal aberrations are variations from the expected number and composition of chromosomes. These occur sporadically and result in a wide variety of abnormalities.

Nondisjunction means failure of chromosomes to divide and then pair up correctly during mitosis or meiosis. It results in an abnormal *number* of chromosomes (either more or less than the expected 46), a condition called **aneuploidy**. When the number is 47 (meaning that, for one kind of chromosome, 3 copies occur rather than 2) the condition is termed **trisomy**. A common example is **Down syndrome**, also called trisomy 21 because individuals so affected have 3 copies of chromosome 21. Down syndrome is discussed later in this chapter.

When the number of chromosomes is 45, the condition is called **monosomy**. A common example is **Turner syndrome** (monosomy X), in which the individual has only one X chromosome and no Y chromosome. This disorder is also discussed later in the chapter.

Mosaicism denotes a form of nondisjunction in which some of the cells of an individual have one genetic constitution (**karyotype**) while other cells have a different genetic constitution.

Breaks along the course of one or more chromosomes result in aberrations in their structure. **Deletion** is the complete loss of part of a chromosome that has broken away. In **inversion**, a separated fragment rotates end-for-end before reattaching. **Translocation** is an exchange of fragments between two chromosomes.

A few inherited disorders are called **multifactorial**, **nonmendelian**, or both, because they apparently result from abnormalities in more than one gene, involve an interaction between genetic material and environmental factors, and are transmitted in patterns other than the classical mendelian one. Examples include cleft lip and palate (discussed later in this chapter) and spina bifida (discussed in Chapter 18).

Diagnostic Procedures in Hereditary and Chromosomal Disorders

A number of diagnostic methods are available to establish or confirm a diagnosis of inherited disease or chromosomal aberration. Physical examination, measurements, or simple chemical tests may be sufficient to determine the presence of a specific genetic defect with reasonable certainty. The family history or pedigree of an individual, even an unborn one, can supply valuable clues about heritable disorders and patterns of transmission.

Cytogenetics (also called **chromosomal analysis** and **karyotyping**) is the examination of chromosomes by light microscopy. Cells for chromosomal analysis can be obtained in various ways: blood specimen, skin biopsy, and (from the fetus) amniotic fluid by amniocentesis and placental tissue by chorionic villus sampling.

Cells are first **cultured** (made to grow and divide in an artificial laboratory medium). Mitosis is induced by application of one chemical agent and then abruptly arrested by another. Cells are transferred to a microscope slide and stained by various methods that allow bands of genes on chromosomes to be distinguished. The slide is examined microscopically, and if chromosomes are clearly visible in several cells undergoing mitosis, these are photographed. Individual chromosomes appearing in the photograph are cut out and pasted on a form in standard order, autosomes 1 to 22 followed by sex chromosomes (X and, if one is present, Y).

The resulting karyotype shows the number of chromosomes and readily identifies gross structural aberrations such as deletion and inversion.

Another diagnostic modality is **biochemical genetics**. Most if not all single-gene heritable disorders involve the absence or insufficiency (occasionally, overabundance or overactivity) of one single substance, usually an enzyme or other protein, in body cells or tissues. Early in the twentieth century, the term *inborn errors of metabolism* was applied to genetic diseases that were known to involve such biochemical flaws. The term is now falling into disuse as it becomes increasingly apparent that a majority of genetic disorders can be so characterized.

Biochemical genetics refers to the detection of abnormally high or low levels, or the absence, of proteins and other substances in body fluids or tissues. Seeking and finding these biochemical markers is a more precise measure than karyotyping. For example, the discovery that the subject's plasma contains a very low level of coagulation factor VIII solidly confirms the presence of hemophilia A (discussed in Chapter 15).

A still more sophisticated diagnostic method is **DNA analysis** of chromosomes, sometimes called **molecular genetics**. In this procedure, abnormal DNA sequences are identified in individual genes by chemical analysis. This is the most specific and also the most expensive method of genetic diagnosis now in use. Very small quantities of specimen material can be amplified through **polymerase chain reaction** (**PCR**) technology, and specific sequences of DNA identified by **DNA probe**, an artificially fabricated strand of DNA that finds and fuses with the sequence being sought.

Some or all of these diagnostic methods may be used to reveal a suspected hereditary disorder in children with evident congenital deformity, mental or physical retardation, or delayed puberty. Indications for prenatal genetic studies include advanced maternal age (which increases the risk of Down syndrome), genetic disease in either parent or in other offspring, and abnormal findings on prenatal ultrasound examination.

Inherited Diseases

In this section a few of the more common inherited disorders are discussed. This is not an exhaustive catalog of such disorders. Several diseases described in other chapters (diabetes mellitus, muscular dystrophy, sickle cell anemia) are also hereditary. The reason for surveying some genetic diseases here is to provide a notion of the broad variety of their signs, symptoms, and severity.

This section will also serve as an introduction to the format used for discussing individual diseases throughout the book. Brief definitions of some terms are given on the page where they occur in the text. When you encounter other terms with which you are unfamiliar, always look them up in the index and find definitions or explanations of them where they appear in other chapters of the book.

Cystic Fibrosis

A disorder in which **exocrine glands** (bronchial mucous glands, pancreas, others) secrete abnormally thick mucus, which results in duct obstruction, damage to glandular tissue, and other adverse consequences. The most common lethal genetic disease in the United States, with an average incidence of one case for every 2000 Caucasian births.

Cause: Absence of a substance called cystic fibrosis transmembrane conductance regulator from mucous gland cells throughout the body. Autosomal recessive inheritance. Most patients have a family history of the disease.

History: In infancy, bowel obstruction due to abnormally thick meconium (**meconium ileus**). In childhood, failure to thrive, cough, dyspnea on exertion, recurrent respiratory infections (bronchitis,

bronchiectasis, pneumonia), atelectasis, pneumothorax, cor pulmonale. Malabsorptive nutritional deficiency, flatulence, steatorrhea (from failure to digest fats because of biliary and pancreatic obstruction). Infertility in males (due to spermatic duct malfunction and obstruction).

Physical Examination: Pallor, nutritional deficiencies, abdominal distention, basilar rales, hyperexpansion and hyperresonance of the thorax, digital clubbing, nasal polyps.

Diagnostic Tests: Anemia, hypoalbuminemia, low levels of fat-soluble vitamins (A, D, E, K) in serum. Arterial oxygen tension is reduced, and pulmonary function tests show reduction in forced vital capacity and in flow rate. Plasma levels of immunoreactive trypsinogen may be elevated. Chest x-ray may show peribronchial cuffing, emphysema, bronchiectasis, atelectasis, or pulmonary infiltrates. The sweat chloride level is elevated.

Course: Recurrent respiratory infections, nutritional deficiencies. Only one-half of patients survive beyond the age of 20. Complications and sequelae: cor pulmonale, hepatic cirrhosis, asthma, nutritional deficiency.

Treatment: Vigorous attention to general health and avoidance of respiratory irritants and infections. Physical therapy, postural drainage, aerosols, bronchodilators, prophylactic use of influenza and pneumococcal vaccines; corticosteroids for exacerbations of pulmonary symptoms. Nutritional supplements, pancreatic enzyme supplements.

Glossary

anemia: deficiency of red blood cells.

atelectasis: collapse of part of a lung.

basilar: pertaining to the bases (lowermost parts) of the lungs.

bronchiectasis: abnormal, irreversible dilatation of bronchi, related to chronic infection.

clubbing: club-shaped deformity of fingertips, seen in chronic pulmonary disease (see box).

cor pulmonale: dilatation, hypertrophy, or failure of the right ventricle due to acute or chronic pulmonary disease.

corticosteroid: cortisol or aldosterone (hormones of the adrenal cortex), or any synthetic drug having similar effects.

cuffing, peribronchial: thickening of bronchial walls as seen on chest x-ray.

Clubbing of the digits refers to a deformity of the tips of all ten fingers in which the distal phalanges are swollen, spongy, and warm to the touch, and the angles between the distal phalanges and the nails are flattened out.

Clubbing is a hereditary trait in certain families, but it usually points to some systemic disease, particularly in the pulmonary or cardiovascular system, such as congenital heart disease with inadequate oxygenation of the blood, infection of heart valves (bacterial endocarditis), chronic hepatic or intestinal disease, and malignancy or infection (particularly bronchiectasis or lung abscess) within the thorax.

When clubbing results from pulmonary disease it is sometimes called **hypertrophic pulmonary osteoarthropathy**.

An alternative term is **hippocratic clubbing**, referring to the Greek physician and medical writer **Hippocrates** (460-377 BC). The oldest known description of digital clubbing, in a case of empyema (local pus-forming infection in the pleural cavity), appears in Hippocrates's work *Prognostic*.

"Patients with empyema invariably present with the following symptoms and signs: unremitting fever, which is worse at night; drenching sweats; racking nonproductive cough; sunken eyes; flushed cheeks; abnormal curvature of the nails and warmth of the fingers, especially at the tips. . . ."

---

dyspnea: shortness of breath.

exocrine: referring to glands that discharge their secretions through ducts instead of into the bloodstream.

flatulence: excessive intestinal gas.

hypoalbuminemia: deficiency of albumin in the blood.

ileus: intestinal obstruction.

infiltrate: diffusion of inflammatory fluid or exudate into air cavities of the lung, or their walls, producing cloudiness of lung tissue on chest x-ray.

meconium: stool formed in the fetal intestine before birth.

prophylactic: preventive.

rale: a crackling or bubbling sound heard on auscultation of the lungs, due to accumulation of fluid in air passages or swelling of their walls.

steatorrhea: passage of excessive fat in stools.

Phenylketonuria (PKU)

An inborn error of metabolism causing mental retardation unless diagnosed and treated in early life.

Cause: Decreased activity of phenylalanine hydroxylase, an enzyme that normally converts phenylalanine to tyrosine. Phenylalanine is an essential amino acid whose principal dietary source is milk. In phenylketonuria, abnormally high levels of phenylalanine accumulate and cause irreversible damage to the central nervous system. Transmitted as an autosomal recessive trait, it occurs in one of 10,000 Caucasian births. Several clinical patterns are recognized.

History: The child appears normal at birth, but within a few months may display psychomotor retardation, hyperactivity, seizures, movement disorders, paralysis, and abnormally fair skin with a tendency to eczema.

Physical Examination: Fair skin, mental retardation, muscle weakness or paralysis, myoclonus, eczema. The urine has a mousy odor.

Diagnostic Tests: The serum level of phenylalanine is abnormally elevated, the level of tyrosine reduced. The urine contains phenylketones (phenylpyruvic acid and 2-hydroxyphenylacetic acid), hence the mousy odor and the name of the disease. Early detection of phenylketonuria is mandatory if treatment is to be successful.

Note: Testing of newborn blood for phenylalanine is standard pediatric practice. Testing is required by law in many states before hospital discharge of the newborn. With hospital stays for uncomplicated delivery restricted to 24 hours, many infants are tested before phenylalanine levels have begun to rise. Repeat testing must therefore be done a few days later in an outpatient setting.

Course: With dietary restriction of phenylalanine begun early, most patients lead normal lives. Sensitivity to phenylalanine may be outgrown in some cases.

Treatment: Restriction of dietary phenylalanine by feeding low-phenylalanine substitutes for milk. Avoidance of the artificial sweetener **aspartame**. Treatment should be begun before one month of age and continued as long as blood tests show a rise in phenylalanine after consumption of milk.

Glossary

eczema: an acute or chronic inflammation of the skin with itching, redness, blistering, weeping, crusting, and scaling, due to numerous causes.

hyperactivity: excessive physical activity, restlessness.
myoclonus: jerking or twitching of certain muscles or muscle groups.
paralysis: complete loss of motor function in muscles.
psychomotor retardation: delayed development in both motor skills (muscle strength and coordination) and mental function (ability to understand and learn).

Acute Intermittent Porphyria
An inborn error of metabolism causing crises of abdominal pain after ingestion of certain drugs.

Cause: Deficiency of the enzyme porphobilinogen deaminase, which normally breaks down porphyrins (products of red blood cell metabolism), leads to a rise of porphyrins in blood, with resulting neurologic symptoms, most often attacks of severe abdominal pain. Such attacks are triggered by ingestion of alcohol, various medicines (barbiturates, sulfonamides, and many others), or a low-carbohydrate diet. Autosomal dominant inheritance. Many if not most persons carrying the gene for acute intermittent porphyria have no symptoms. Most patients with symptoms are women, and symptoms often begin before age 25.

Note: The term *porphyria* (from Greek *porphyra* 'purple') refers to the color of the urine after standing. Several other diseases, not all hereditary, are also called porphyrias because they cause a rise in the level of porphyrins in the blood and of their products in the urine. The symptoms of the porphyrias vary widely.

History: Attacks of severe abdominal cramps, often with vomiting and constipation; the pain arises in the middle of the abdomen but may radiate widely; less commonly, paralysis, seizures, or psychosis. Occasionally seizures or hallucinations. Urine turns deep pink, brick red, or brown on standing. Between attacks, no symptoms.

Physical Examination: During abdominal crises, evidence of severe distress, usually without abdominal tenderness, spasm, distention, or fever. Rarely, jaundice. Weakness or paralysis of muscles, including respiratory muscles. Between attacks there are no abnormal signs.

Diagnostic Tests: The white blood count and differential are normal. Porphyrin levels are elevated in blood, urine, and stool. Urinary excretion of porphobilinogen and delta-aminolevulinic acid is increased. The blood level of sodium may be far below normal.

Course: With avoidance of low carbohydrate intake (starvation diets), alcohol, and drugs known to precipitate crises, patients should be able to lead normal lives.

Treatment: Strict avoidance of alcohol, precipitating medicines, and low carbohydrate intake. For crises, supportive treatment as needed; intravenous glucose (to raise blood sugar) and hematin (to inhibit the synthesis of porphyrins).

Marfan Syndrome

An inherited disorder of connective tissue affecting primarily bones, the cardiovascular system, and the eye.

Cause: Abnormal synthesis of the protein fibrillin (a major component of connective tissue) due to an abnormal gene on chromosome 15. Autosomal dominant inheritance.

History: Lax joints, subject to dislocation; unusually tall stature. Dislocation of ocular lens, severe myopia, retinal detachment. Symptoms of cardiac failure.

Physical Examination: Characteristic habitus: long, spindly extremities and digits, often with pectus excavatum and scoliosis. Lax joints. Evidence of ectopia or dislocation of ocular lens(es); mitral regurgitation, evidence of aortic dilatation, aortic regurgitation.

Diagnostic Tests: There are no known biochemical markers. Echocardiography reveals mitral valve prolapse in most patients. Chest x-ray may show dilatation of the aorta.

Course: Progressive dilatation of the aorta often leads to aortic rupture in middle life. Recurrent dislocation may damage joints. Scoliosis may become severe and is irreversible after adolescence. Ocular abnormalities often lead to severe visual impairment.

Treatment: Avoidance of strenuous physical exertion and prophylactic use of beta-blockers to delay aortic dilatation. Close observation of vision and correction of myopia with glasses. Monitoring of aortic diameter and cardiac valvular function. Prophylactic grafting of the aorta when dilatation is severe. Endocarditis prophylaxis before surgery or dental work.

Glossary
ectopia: abnormal location or position.
habitus: body build, physique; overall appearance.

myopia: nearsightedness.

pectus excavatum: funnel chest, hollow chest; a deformity of the thorax in which the breastbone appears sunken.

prolapse, mitral valve: abnormal movement of the valve between the left atrium and the left ventricle of the heart, allowing regurgitation of blood during systole (ventricular contraction).

regurgitation: when referring to a cardiac valve, an abnormal backflow of blood through the valve.

scoliosis: lateral curvature of the spine.

Cleft Lip and Palate

A group of congenital deformities of the face and the roof of the mouth.

Cleft lip is a gap in the upper lip near the midline, and cleft palate is a similarly located fissure dividing part or all of the roof of the mouth. Either may occur without the other. Deformity is evident at birth and may cause severe feeding difficulties. Some cases are due to chromosomal abnormalities, and may occur in conjunction with other congenital disorders of the lower jaw, eyes, or ears. Other cases may be related to maternal ingestion of alcohol or certain drugs (for example, phenytoin). Treatment is surgical repair of cleft lip before the age of 3 months and of cleft palate by the age of one year. Patients with cleft palate usually require speech therapy and orthodontic treatment.

Chromosomal Aberrations

Down Syndrome (Trisomy 21, Mongolism)

A genetic aberration producing characteristic physical stigmata and mental retardation.

Cause: The presence of an extra chromosome 21. In most instances the mother is over 40.

Physical Examination: Small head, characteristic facial features (slanted eyes, flattened bridge of nose, small ears, large tongue with gaping mouth), short flat hands with single transverse "simian" crease, hypotonia, retarded physical and mental development (IQ around 50). Brushfield spots in iris during first year of life.

Course: Life expectancy is reduced (under 50). Heart disease, acute leukemia, and an Alzheimer-like dementia often develop before age 30.

Glossary
hypotonia: diminished muscle tone.
spots, Brushfield: small white spots in the irises of the eyes.
stigma (plural, **stigmata**): a peculiarity or abnormality characteristic of a specific disease.

Turner Syndrome

A chromosomal aberration consisting of loss of an X chromosome (XO pattern). All patients are female. Several variants occur, some due to **mosaicism**. Signs and symptoms include short stature, facial abnormalities, webbed neck, failure of ovarian development with amenorrhea and sterility, structural abnormalities of the skeleton, the cardiovascular system, and the kidneys. Treatment with growth hormone and estrogen leads to correction of some deformities but does not restore fertility.

Glossary
amenorrhea: absence of menstrual periods.
sterility: inability to become a parent because of physical abnormality of the reproductive system.

Klinefelter Syndrome

A chromosomal aberration consisting of an extra X chromosome (XXY pattern). All patients are males. At puberty, the arms and legs grow disproportionally long, the testicles fail to develop, and gynecomastia occurs. All patients are sterile; many have subnormal intelligence or learning disorders. There is a higher risk of breast cancer and diabetes mellitus than in the general population. Diagnosis is confirmed by karyotyping. Treatment with testosterone may correct abnormalities of habitus but will not reverse sterility.

Glossary
gynecomastia: abnormal breast development in a male.

Oncogenes and Tumor Suppressor Genes

Some individuals inherit a predisposition to certain malignancies. **Oncogenes** are abnormal autosomal genes that arise by mutation from pre-existing normal genes (proto-oncogenes) and, under certain conditions, can induce neoplastic transformation of cells. Oncogenes cause certain body cells to secrete abnormal proteins (or normal proteins, such as cellular growth factors and regulators, in abnormal amounts), with resultant uncontrolled growth and development.

Various factors can lead to the formation of an oncogene. Some viruses (such as the **human papillomavirus**) contain oncogenic strands of DNA in their chromosomal makeup. Infection with one of these viruses can cause incorporation of such abnormal genetic material into body cells. Some oncogenic mutations are triggered by exposure to ionizing radiation or to toxic chemicals (**carcinogens**), such as benzpyrene in cigarette smoke, benzene, and asbestos. **Genetic instability** (a heightened risk of chromosomal aberrations) occurs in some inherited diseases, such as Down syndrome, in which the risk of leukemia is 20 times that in the general population.

Tumor suppressor genes (**anti-oncogenes**) are normal genes whose function is to suppress malignant transformation in cells. Their inactivation through deletion or mutation results in increased risk of such malignant transformation.

It is now possible to identify a number of oncogenes, and to detect inactivation of anti-oncogenes, by DNA analysis.

Topics for Study or Discussion

1. Distinguish congenital (but not inherited) disorders from hereditary disorders, and give examples of each type.

2. Define: chromosome, gene, autosomal dominant, nondisjunction, trisomy.

3. What are the three basic laboratory methods of genetic diagnosis?

4. Give two examples of genetic diseases that cause obvious physical deformity, and two examples of genetic diseases that cause problems only intermittently.

5. What are some advantages and disadvantages of the medical progress that has enabled many persons with cystic fibrosis to survive past puberty?

Chapter 3

Infectious Diseases

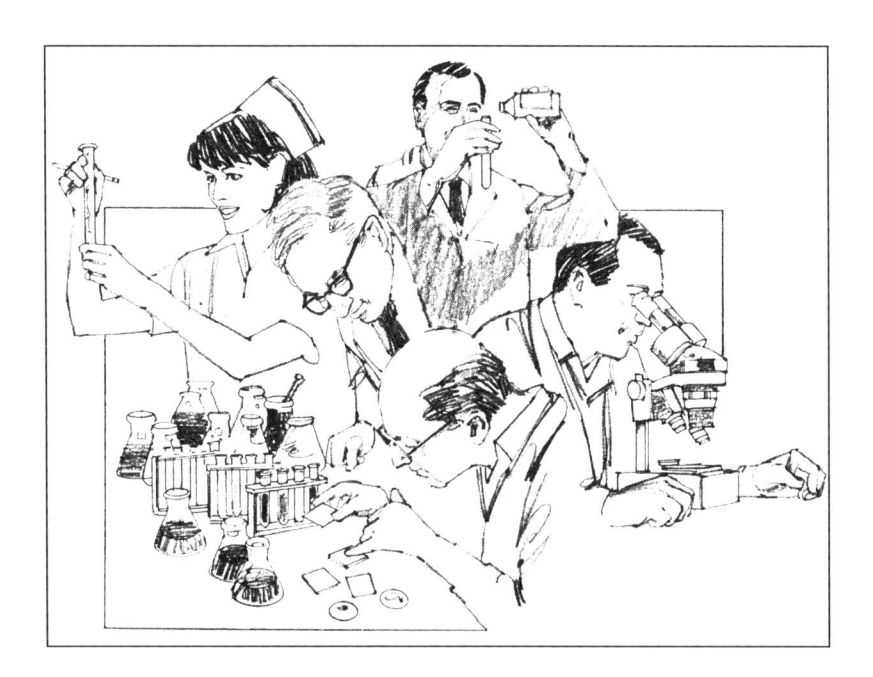

Learning Objectives

On completion of this chapter, the student should

- understand the general concepts of infection, transmission of infectious diseases, and immunity;

- have a general knowledge of the types of infecting organisms, the ways in which they cause disease, and patterns of transmission;

- know how infectious diseases are diagnosed;

- know general principles of treatment of infectious diseases.

An Overview of Infectious Diseases

An **infection** is a disease or process resulting from the growth of certain microorganisms (sometimes, larger organisms) in the living body. Infections may be **local** (an abscess of the elbow), **generalized** (septicemia, defined later in this chapter), or **local with systemic effects** (pulmonary tuberculosis). They may be **trivial** and **self-limiting** (the common cold), **life-threatening** (acute bacterial meningitis), or uniformly **lethal** (AIDS). They may be readily **responsive** to treatment (strep throat) or essentially **untreatable** (rabies).

The subject of infectious disease is far too broad to be fully explored within the scope of a single chapter. The following pages provide a survey of basic concepts. The chapter concludes with discussions of selected infectious diseases, to provide some notion of their variety. Most of the remaining chapters in this book also contain discussions of infectious diseases. If you encounter an unfamiliar term that is not immediately defined in the text, look in the glossary at the end of the chapter.

The term **pathogen** denotes any organism that is capable of inducing disease through infection. The following types of pathogens cause infections in human beings:

bacteria (singular, **bacterium**): one-celled organisms on the borderline between animals and plants, varying enormously in structure, physical and chemical properties, and disease-causing capabilities. Examples: staphylococci (staph), streptococci (strep), chlamydia.

fungi: simple microscopic mold- or yeast-like organisms. Examples: ringworm fungus, yeast-causing thrush and vaginitis.

parasites: members of the animal kingdom, including one-celled organisms, worms, and arthropods (insects and related animals), that live on or in the human body, deriving their nourishment from it and often causing severe or chronic disease in the process; the term *infestation* is usually preferred to *infection* with respect to parasites. Examples: Trichomonas, pinworm, pubic lice.

viruses: fragments of genetic material incapable of independent existence; they cause disease by entering living cells, taking over their operation at the molecular level, and using them as breeding grounds for hundreds of thousands of new viral particles, ultimately destroying them. Examples: herpes simplex virus, chickenpox virus.

Pathogenic microorganisms induce disease by a wide variety of mechanisms. They may cause local erosion or destruction of tissue; interfere with the functions of cells, tissues, or organs; or elicit an inflammatory reaction in the host that becomes the dominant clinical problem.

Inflammation is a complex but stereotyped pattern of reaction whereby living tissue responds to injury in the broad sense (direct physical injury, burning or freezing, chemical or biological irritants, or poisons). In local inflammation there is generally an increase in blood flow through the affected part, causing redness, warmth, and (because fluid is released from the circulation into tissue spaces) swelling.

The nature of the tissue in which an inflammatory reaction occurs determines in some measure the resulting symptoms: in the respiratory tract, congestion and increased secretions; in the digestive system, abdominal pain, vomiting, and diarrhea; in the skin, itching, blistering, and crusting. An inflammatory reaction also includes production by the patient's tissues of chemical substances that attract white blood cells to the area to repel, engulf, or destroy invading or proliferating microorganisms.

Suppuration refers to the process of pus formation. **Pus** is a mixture of white blood cells, dead tissue, and killed or inactivated pathogens. A local accumulation of pus, surrounded by a wall of inflamed tissue, is called an **abscess**.

Many pathogens have "inborn errors of metabolism"—that is, they are biologically defective in some way, so that they depend on their host for sustenance, or produce waste products that are harmful to the host, or both. Such waste products, considered from the point of view of the host, are called toxins. A **toxin** (as the term is used here) is a chemical substance produced by pathogenic organisms and causing harmful effects to the host. These effects vary widely from one pathogen to another, and include local inflammation, rash, and muscular paralysis. Some microorganisms (for example, some streptococci) produce toxins that break down body proteins and permit spread of the pathogens through tissue spaces. An infection characterized by such wide infiltration of tissues by pathogens is called **cellulitis**. Toxin formation is an important mechanism of disease production by many pathogens.

Any severe or systemic infection may produce nonspecific symptoms such as fever, chills, headache and muscle aches, loss of appetite, nausea, vomiting, and general malaise.

Transmission of Infection

Some infections (chickenpox, genital warts) can be spread from one person to another by various routes; others (sinusitis; pyelonephritis, an infection of the kidney and ureter) cannot. The following terms relate to the transmission of infectious diseases.

airborne: infections that can be spread through the air, usually by droplets of respiratory secretions but sometimes on particles of moisture or dust, or free-floating.

bloodborne: referring to infections transmitted by blood transfusion, surgical or dental instruments contaminated with the blood of an infected person, needles shared by intravenous drug abusers, and occasionally through sexual or other intimate contact, with transfer of blood from one person to another.

carrier: a person who has recovered from a communicable disease (hepatitis B, typhoid fever) but still harbors living and virulent organisms and can transmit them to others.

communicable disease: an infection that is capable of being transmitted in any way from one person to another.

congenital: referring to infections acquired before or at birth.

contagious: transmitted by close exposure (direct touch, sexual contact, exposure to respiratory, digestive tract, or other secretions).

droplet spread: transmission of respiratory and other infections by fine mists of respiratory secretions expelled into the air by coughing or sneezing.

epidemiology: the branch of medicine and public health that deals with patterns of disease causation and spread (not necessarily infectious diseases).

fecal-oral route: the route by which some intestinal and other pathogens are transferred from person to person; contamination of food or water, or direct physical contact, with the infected person's feces leads to ingestion of the pathogen.

fomite: any inanimate object, such as a washcloth, drinking glass, or doorknob, that can be the means whereby pathogenic microorganisms are transmitted from an infected person to others.

host: a living organism on or in which another organism, usually a parasite, lives.

infectious disease: any disease caused by infection; sometimes used in the narrower sense of transmissible disease.

period of communicability: the length of time, often beginning before the appearance of symptoms, during which a person with an infectious disease can spread it to others in some way.

sexually transmitted disease (STD): any infection that is transmitted from person to person through sexual activity.

transmissible: able to be spread from person to person.

tropical disease: an infection or infestation that occurs predominantly or exclusively in tropical latitudes.

vector: a living organism that transmits pathogens from an infected person to a healthy person (such as mosquitoes that transmit the causative organisms of yellow fever or malaria).

venereal disease (VD): sexually transmitted disease.

Clinical Features of Infectious Diseases

Numerous factors influence the signs and symptoms of infectious diseases, their course and severity, the diagnostic procedures whereby they can be identified, and their response to treatment. By and large, the most important of these factors is the identity of the infecting organism. That is, any given pathogen (chlamydia, hepatitis A virus, ringworm fungus) tends to produce the same basic disease or group of diseases in all infected persons.

But the extent and severity of the basic disease process can be modified by a number of variables. The **virulence** of a pathogen is its innate capacity to do harm. Some strains of an infecting organism may be more virulent than others, and may thus be better able to overcome the resistance of the host and to escape destruction by medicines. The **mode of exposure** (inhalation, ingestion, introduction into the bloodstream) and the **dose** (100 organisms or 100 billion) have a bearing on the extent and severity of illness produced, if any.

Host resistance refers to the whole gamut of defenses by which a living body is able to repel, inactivate, or destroy pathogens that threaten to invade it. General state of health, nutritional status, the integrity of skin and mucous membranes, and most importantly the effectiveness of the immune system, all influence host resistance.

Immunity (discussed more fully below and in the next chapter) is a biological response of the living body to invading microorganisms or other noxious materials. Upon recovery from many diseases, one acquires a lasting, perhaps lifelong, ability to resist infection by the same organism. More immediate immune responses reduce the capacity of organisms to invade in the first place. When the immune system is impaired by congenital or acquired disease, infections may prove much more severe, even lethal. In addition, organisms that are ordinarily unable to infect human beings may produce opportunistic infections in persons with deficient immunity.

The interval between invasion by microorganisms and the first appearance of symptoms is called the **incubation period** of an infection. For some infections (the common cold, viral gastroenteritis) this may be less than one day; for others (malaria, hepatitis B, leprosy) it may be more than six months.

Once a pathogenic organism has gained entrance to the body, it can spread by various routes, depending chiefly on the nature and virulence of the organism but also on host defenses. Some pathogens are spread by the **hematogenous route** (through the bloodstream). Others move through **lymphatic channels**. **Bacteremia** denotes the presence of bacteria in the blood, as detected by laboratory tests. **Toxemia** means the presence of toxic products of an infecting organism in the blood. When large numbers of virulent organisms and their toxic products are circulating in the blood, the condition is called **septicemia**. Microorganisms can also spread along the surface of skin or mucous membranes.

Immunity to Infection

The topic of immunity will be more fully discussed in the next chapter. Here it will suffice to state a few general principles.

Immunity is the capacity of a living body to repel or destroy invading microorganisms or other noxious substances, and in particular to resist a second attack by a pathogen that has already invaded and caused disease. Immunity involves a large number of processes depending primarily on white blood cells (**cellular immunity**) and antibodies (**humoral immunity**). An **antibody** is a complex protein, formed by cells of the immune system, that can recognize a specific target organism, combine with it, and bring about its inactivation or destruction.

Immunity plays three important roles with respect to infectious disease:
1. It can strongly influence and alter the course and prognosis of an infectious disease.
2. An antibody produced by the immune system in response to a specific pathogenic organism, and circulating in the patient's blood, can be used diagnostically to identify the organism.
3. Vaccines consisting of killed or inactivated pathogens can cause the immune system to produce antibody conferring resistance to those pathogens, just as if the subject had already had the disease and developed natural antibody.

The Diagnosis of Infectious Disease

Besides the basic diagnostic procedures described in Chapter 1, the physician uses numerous other measures to diagnose infections. These can only be sketched here; specific examples and elaborations will be given throughout the remaining chapters of the book.

The findings of the basic physical examination can be supplemented by various diagnostic tests. **X-rays**, **scans**, and **endoscopy** can provide more specific information about the location and character of an infection. **Blood tests** such as the white blood count, the differential white blood count, and the erythrocyte sedimentation rate can provide nonspecific clues to the presence of infection.

But generally the principal goal of diagnostic maneuvers in infectious disease is to identify the pathogen. For many if not most infections, knowing the exact identity of the causative organism leads to the most accurate prediction of the course of the disease and the most precise selection of effective therapy. The causative organism can be identified in one of two ways: by removing a specimen from the body and visually observing the pathogen in the specimen, or by detecting antibodies to the pathogen in the patient's blood.

Methods leading to direct visual identification of pathogens pertain to the field of microbiology. Technologists in this field process and examine specimens of blood, urine, stool, or tissue obtained at surgery or by biopsy; and secretions, pus, or any other material that is likely to contain visible organisms. A **smear** may be made from the specimen on a microscope slide and inspected by light microscopy. Ordinarily a **microbiologic smear** is prepared for examination by the application of one or more stains. These are variously colored dyes that render microorganisms more readily visible or that bring out distinctive structural or biochemical features.

The **Gram stain** is a standard bacteriologic procedure that highlights structural features of bacteria and permits them to be separated into two large categories. **Gram-positive** organisms take up crystal violet stain in the presence of iodide, and hence appear blue or purple in a smear. **Gram-negative** organisms do not take up crystal violet in the presence of iodide, and so would appear colorless in a smear if a second stain (**counterstain**) in a contrasting color (red or pink) were not applied after the first.

The **acid-fast stain** is used to identify **mycobacteria**, which cause tuberculosis and leprosy. These organisms take up fuchsin and certain other organic dyes so avidly that they cannot be washed away with acid-alcohol. (Mycobacteria, and often the infections they cause, are thus loosely termed "acid-fast.") Many other specialized staining procedures are available for the identification of certain organisms, including fungi and parasites.

Viruses cannot be seen by **light microscopy**. Some viruses, however, induce changes in cells (inclusion bodies, vacuolization) that can be seen in preparations of tissue or certain fluids, and can strongly support the diagnosis of a specific viral infection. Viruses can be seen by **electron microscopy**, but the principal method used to identify viral infection is testing for antibody in the patient's blood.

When a specimen is thought to contain too few pathogenic microorganisms for them to be observed in a smear, their number can be amplified by allowing them to multiply under controlled laboratory conditions. A **culture** is a colony of microorganisms grown in a laboratory. A culture grows on or in a **medium** (plural, media): a mixture of nutrients and other substances (minerals, antibiotics, agents to modify the texture of the medium) that is designed to favor the growth of certain organisms of interest and often to inhibit the growth of others.

Cultures are grown in specially designed dishes, bottles, or tubes. Media may be solid, semisolid, or liquid. Media for growing viruses and chlamydias contain living cells. A culture medium into which microorganisms are introduced is said to be **inoculated** with them. Growth of organisms in a culture medium is called **incubation**, especially when the culture is placed in an incubator that maintains a specific temperature (usually around human body temperature, 37°C). Examining blood serum or other specimens for evidence of antibody to specific infectious organisms pertains to the field of **immunology** or **serology**. A number of highly precise techniques are currently available to find and measure antibodies to a large number of pathogenic organisms. Space does not permit elaborate discussion of this complex subject.

Treatment of Infectious Disease

Physicians use numerous medicines to control or mitigate symptoms of infectious disease such as fever, pain, inflammation, cough, respiratory congestion, intestinal spasm or irritability, itching, and so forth. But for most of the most common infectious diseases, modern medicine has antimicrobial agents: specific drugs intended to destroy or inactivate pathogenic microorganisms in or on the body.

All antimicrobial agents are poisons. The basic principle underlying their use is **selective toxicity**: the drug must be able to combat the infecting organism without harming the host. Some antimicrobial agents, such as alcohol, hexachlorophene, and povidone-iodine, are effective against a wide variety of pathogens but are used only on skin or mucous membranes (for example, as a preoperative scrub) because they are too toxic to the host for systemic use. These are called **disinfectants**.

Most of the antimicrobial drugs in current use are effective against a narrower range of organisms but have low enough toxicity for the host that they can be administered **systemically** (by mouth or by injection). These are the **antibiotics**, the **sulfonamides**, and certain **chemotherapeutic agents**.

All natural **antibiotics** are produced by molds and are toxic to certain classes of microorganisms, sometimes including other molds. Modern technology can greatly amplify the yield of antibiotic from a culture of mold, and chemical alteration of the antibiotic molecule can produce a drug that is less toxic to the host than the parent molecule, more potent and specific in attacking pathogens, or both.

Sulfonamides (see box) are chemicals produced in the laboratory that work much like certain antibiotics. Some drugs used to treat malaria and other parasitic diseases are also laboratory fabrications.

> During the years immediately following the discovery of penicillin by Alexander Fleming in 1928, researchers around the world were testing thousands of substances, natural and synthetic, for activity against pathogenic microorganisms.
>
> In 1932 **Gerhard Domagk** (1895-1964), a physician and biochemist at one of Bayer's chemical plants in Germany, found that a red dye for leather, marketed as Prontosil, had such activity.
>
> Domagk conducted exacting experiments in mice and showed that Prontosil and its derivatives were both effective and safe in controlling infections, including those due to streptococci (discussed later in this chapter).
>
> The usefulness of the new drug in human patients was put to a dramatic test when Domagk's own daughter Hildegarde injured her finger on a knitting needle and developed severe septicemia. She was dying when Domagk injected her with Prontosil. The experiment was brilliantly successful. The child recovered rapidly and completely.
>
> Further research on Prontosil showed that in the body it split into two compounds, and that one of these, sulfanilamide, was responsible for its antimicrobial activity. This was the beginning of the sulfonamide era, which continues to this day.
>
> Numerous other sulfa compounds with greater effectiveness and fewer side effects have been synthesized. Drugs in this class are widely used nowadays in the treatment of respiratory and urinary tract infections and other conditions. However, the sulfonamides are no longer considered appropriate treatment for streptococcal infections.
>
> Gerhard Domagk received the Nobel Prize for Medicine or Physiology in 1939, but was forbidden to accept it by Adolf Hitler.

Along with the sulfonamides, these are sometimes called chemotherapeutic agents in contradistinction to antibiotics, all of which originally came from molds. (Some antibiotics, such as chloramphenicol, were originally natural mold products but are now synthesized "from scratch" in the laboratory.)

Antibiotics and chemotherapeutic agents destroy pathogens or inhibit their growth by various mechanisms: by preventing them from forming cell walls (penicillins, cephalosporins), by affecting cell wall permeability (amphotericin B, polymyxin B), by inhibiting protein synthesis (erythromycin, tetracycline), or by inhibiting nucleic acid synthesis (sulfonamides, nalidixic acid). No antibiotic is effective against all pathogens. Virtually no antibiotic or sulfonamide is effective against any virus.

The range of organisms against which an antibiotic can be used is called its **spectrum**. The sensitivity of infecting organisms to antibiotics can be tested in the laboratory by applying small paper discs impregnated with various antibiotics to the surface of a culture medium inoculated with the organism in question, and observing which ones inhibit bacterial growth.

The dose, route of administration, and duration of treatment with an antibiotic depend on many considerations: the identity of the pathogen, the severity of the infection, the patient's general condition, other drugs the patient is already receiving, the antimicrobial spectrum of the drug, its physical and biochemical properties, its expected side effects, and even its cost. Some antibiotics are not adequately absorbed from the digestive system and so must be given by injection.

Prophylactic administration of antibiotics refers to their use in preventing rather than in treating infection. Antibiotic prophylaxis is generally considered inappropriate except in a limited number of circumstances: before or after certain types of surgery (particularly if the patient has a chronic condition such as valvular heart disease) and in certain disorders in which recurring infection is likely (emphysema, chronic bronchitis, certain urinary tract problems).

Two factors limit the usefulness of antibiotics in combating human infections: **drug resistance** and **side effects**. Many pathogens resist the toxic effects of some or all antimicrobial agents simply because of their innate biochemical makeup. But most cases of drug resistance in pathogens are due to genetic mutation. That is, one or more organisms undergo a change in their genetic composition that confers on them and their offspring the ability to escape the toxic effects of certain antimicrobials.

If microorganisms that are resistant to a certain antibiotic emerge in a patient who is taking that antibiotic, then the organisms that have not undergone mutation will die, while those that have developed resistance will quickly multiply and form a whole colony of resistant organisms. From then on, the antibiotic in question will be of no use in treating that patient's infection. Drugs chemically related to the first antibiotic may also prove ineffective, by a phenomenon called **cross-**

resistance. Moreover, if resistant organisms are transmitted to other persons and cause infection, antibiotics to which they are resistant will be ineffective from the first.

Adverse effects of antimicrobial drugs on the host are of various types. They may cause chemical **toxicity**, as when streptomycin and related drugs damage the eighth pair of cranial nerves, with resulting impairment of hearing or loss of balance sense. Peak and trough (maximum and minimum) blood levels of certain antibiotics may be monitored chemically to ensure that the dose is adequate (high enough to control the infection) but not excessive (likely to cause serious adverse effects).

Many adverse effects of antibiotics and sulfonamides are due to **allergy**, an acquired hypersensitivity to a drug, leading to rash, respiratory distress, or other problems, some of which can be fatal, when that drug is administered. Finally, an antimicrobial agent may so **alter the patient's normal microbial flora** that organisms not affected by the drug overgrow and produce symptoms. For example, antibiotic treatment often suppresses normal intestinal or vaginal germ populations so that virulent and toxigenic strains of resistant bacteria, or Candida and other yeasts, can become the predominant organisms present and produce disease.

As mentioned earlier, antibiotics and sulfonamides are ineffective against viruses. Physicians have a limited but growing arsenal of antiviral agents, most of them chemical substances synthesized in the laboratory:
    acyclovir, used in chickenpox and herpes simplex
    amantadine and rimantadine, in influenza
    famciclovir and valacyclovir, in zoster
    foscarnet and ganciclovir, in cytomegalovirus retinitis
    idoxuridine, in herpetic infections of the cornea
    didanosine, zalcitobine, and zidovudine, in AIDS

Interferons are natural substances, induced in human beings by viral and other types of infection, that boost and regulate host defense. Synthetic interferons are now used in various viral infections, including hepatitis B and C and genital warts.

Antibodies, usually in the form of immune globulin, may be administered to some persons after exposure to certain diseases (hepatitis A, hepatitis B, rabies) to prevent or modify infection. **Antitoxins** are antibodies directed against toxins rather than against the organisms that produce them. They are useful in modifying certain uncommon diseases, such as botulism and diphtheria.

Examples of Some Infectious Diseases

The chapter concludes with discussions of selected examples of infectious diseases. Many infectious diseases are discussed in following chapters.

Infectious Mononucleosis (IM)

A contagious viral infection involving primarily the lymphatic system (spleen, lymph nodes, and liver).

Cause: The **Epstein-Barr virus** (**EBV**), a member of the herpesvirus family. The virus is transmitted from person to person chiefly in saliva, hence most often through kissing or sharing of food, or of eating or drinking utensils.

History: After an incubation period of about 6 weeks, fever, headache, sore throat (often severe), glandular swelling, malaise, and a sense of fatigue. Less often, rash, jaundice, palpitations, chest or abdominal pain.

Physical Examination: Fever; inflammation of the pharynx with redness, swelling, and exudate; swelling of lymph glands, particularly on the back of the neck, but sometimes also in the groins and armpits; enlargement and tenderness of the spleen and, less often, the liver; occasionally jaundice (due to liver involvement), rash, or both; sometimes rapid or irregular pulse (due to cardiac involvement).

Diagnostic Tests: The lymphocyte count is elevated, with many **atypical lymphocytes** (also called reactive lymphocytes or virocytes). A few patients develop transitory hemolytic anemia. Liver function tests show slight or marked elevation of bilirubin and of hepatic enzymes, particularly alkaline phosphatase. **Heterophile antibodies** (nonspecific and nonprotective against further attacks of illness) appear in the blood by the second week of illness. More specific antibodies directed against components of EBV (viral capsid antigen, viral nuclear antigen) appear eventually, some persisting throughout life and conferring immunity to further attack. Chest x-ray may show enlargement of hilar lymph nodes. The electrocardiogram may demonstrate abnormalities if there is involvement of heart muscle (myocarditis) or of the conduction system of the heart.

Course: Despite the severity of symptoms in the acute phase, most cases resolve completely in 2-3 weeks. Complications such as severe hemolytic anemia, airway obstruction, rupture of the spleen, and severe liver involvement occur rarely.

Treatment: Largely supportive: symptomatic medicines for relief of pain and fever; rest, fluids, and diet as tolerated during the acute phase (7-10 days). With severe swelling of the neck and throat and high fever, nonsteroidal anti-inflammatory drugs are often supplemented with corticosteroids.

Lyme Disease (Lyme Borreliosis)

An acute and chronic infectious disease affecting successively the skin, the nervous system, and the joints.

Cause: *Borrelia burgdorferi*, a spirochete, which is transmitted by ticks of the genus *Ixodes*. Nymphs and larvae of the tick vector feed on the white-footed mouse, adults on the white-tailed deer. Infected ticks in any of these stages of development can transmit spirochetes to human beings, but usually only after feeding on the human host for at least 24 hours.

History: During the initial stage (starting about one week after infection), most patients develop either a characteristic expanding rash called **erythema chronicum migrans**, or a flu-like illness with fever and muscle aches, or both. In some infected persons, this stage passes without any symptoms. In the second stage, days or weeks after infection, spread of spirochetes to certain organs and tissues causes a highly variable clinical picture. Fever, headache, muscle and joint pains, secondary skin lesions not related to tick bites, irregular heartbeat, and involvement of the central and peripheral nervous systems (encephalitis, Bell palsy) all may occur during this stage. The third stage, which occurs months or years after infection, causes painful chronic inflammation in joints, tendons, and muscles.

Physical Examination: Expanding red or purple rash at site of tick bite, often with a bull's-eye appearance. Fever, other nonspecific rashes, evidence of muscle weakness or abnormal reflexes, cardiac irregularities. Signs of local inflammation in joints.

Diagnostic Tests: Blood cell studies are nonspecific. The electrocardiogram or electromyogram may detect abnormalities in conduction. Antibody to the causative spirochete appears early in the disease, but currently available methods of detecting it often fail to meet acceptable standards of sensitivity, specificity, or reproducibility. The diagnosis should be based on clinical findings, not laboratory studies; otherwise the disease will continue to be both underdiagnosed and overdiagnosed—that is, some cases will be missed, and other diseases will be misdiagnosed as Lyme disease.

Course: This has already been described under History. Some patients, particularly those in whom diagnosis and appropriate treatment are delayed, have residual musculoskeletal, neurologic, or mental impairment.

Treatment: Tetracyclines, azithromycin, ampicillin, and other antibiotics generally produce a cure within 2-3 weeks if administered during the first stage. Chronic symptoms may be less amenable to antibiotic therapy. A variety of treatments may be prescribed for symptoms, including physical therapy.

Streptococcal Disease

A group of infections caused by bacteria of the genus *Streptococcus*.

Streptococci are gram-positive bacteria with a broad range of potential effects on human hosts. Many species are highly virulent and aggressive. Streptococci are involved in infections of the skin (impetigo, cellulitis, erysipelas), the respiratory tract (streptococcal pharyngitis or "strep" throat, pneumococcal pneumonia), the ears and sinuses, heart valves (endocarditis), joints (infectious arthritis), and many other tissues.

Group A beta-hemolytic streptococci (GABHS) are both widespread and highly virulent. One strain produces a toxin that induces a generalized red rash (**scarlet fever**). Pharyngeal or other infections with GABHS, unless adequately treated, can stimulate the host's immune system to produce antibodies that attack the heart and the joints (acute rheumatic fever) or the kidney (acute glomerulonephritis).

The diagnosis of streptococcal infection is based on clinical findings and laboratory studies, particularly identification of the organism by smear, culture, or antibody tests. The **strep screen**, a rapid slide test for streptococci in pharyngeal secretions, permits prompt and reliable identification of streptococcal pharyngitis, a highly prevalent disease, particularly in children.

Several antibiotics are effective in controlling streptococcal infections, but not all of these are approved for prevention of rheumatic fever. Penicillin (intramuscularly in long-acting form, or orally), erythromycin, and some cephalosporins reliably prevent rheumatic fever. When given orally these drugs must be administered for ten days.

Varicella-Zoster
Two infections caused by the same virus, but with different manifestations: varicella and zoster.

Varicella (Chickenpox)
A febrile exanthem usually contracted in childhood.

Cause: The varicella-zoster virus, which can be spread from persons with chickenpox by direct contact or by respiratory droplets. It can also be acquired by direct contact with the lesions of zoster.

History: After an incubation period of about two weeks, fever for a day or two before and after the appearance of a rash consisting of small vesicles that rapidly evolve into pustules and then slough to form crusted ulcers. Three or four crops of lesions may appear over the next 3-5 days. The face, scalp, and trunk are most prominently involved; lesions may also appear in the mouth and throat. Itching can be severe, and scratching can result in secondary bacterial infection. Fever, headache, malaise, and cough are variable.

Physical Examination: Characteristic lesions involving the face and trunk more than the extremities. An early (vesicular) lesion resembles "a drop of honey on a rose petal." Crops appear on 3-5 successive days.

Diagnostic Tests: The white blood count may be low. A Tzanck smear of material from skin lesions shows multinucleated giant cells. Virus can be cultured from vesicle fluid, but identification of viral antigen by immunofluorescence is simpler.

Course: Fever generally disappears within 1 week of onset, and the skin lesions heal completely in 2-3 weeks. Secondary bacterial infection of lesions can lead to scarring or septicemia. Other possible complications are pneumonitis, meningitis, and (after treatment with aspirin) Reye syndrome. Maternal varicella during early pregnancy can lead to death or deformity of the fetus.

Infectious Diseases • 51

Treatment: Largely symptomatic and supportive. Aspirin is withheld because of the risk of Reye syndrome. The antiviral drug acyclovir mitigates symptoms and shortens the period of illness. Patients are isolated from susceptible persons. Varicella is reliably prevented by a live vaccine now recommended for all children at age one year and for susceptible household contacts of patients. Varicella-zoster immune globulin (VZIG) is given to exposed persons with immune deficiency.

Zoster (Herpes Zoster, Shingles)

A reactivation of varicella-zoster infection, with local involvement of nerves and skin.

Cause: After recovery from chickenpox, the varicella-zoster virus remains in the body for life, lying dormant in cells of the dorsal spinal nerve roots or in ganglions of cranial nerves. Reactivation of the virus leads to the clinical syndrome known as zoster.

History: Stinging or burning pain, almost always in the distribution of a single dorsal nerve root; usually on the trunk but occasionally on the face or in the ear. Before or after the onset of pain, a rash appears within the dermatome of a single nerve root. On the trunk, this is a band about 7.5 cm in width, running around half of the body from back to front (see box). Pain and rash are both in the same dermatome, but not necessarily in exactly the same places within that dermatome.

When the rash of **zoster** appears on the trunk of the body, it is so distinctive that the diagnosis can hardly be missed. Even many laypersons can accurately recognize it. When fully developed, the cutaneous eruption looks like a belt or sash running around half of the body.	*Zoster* is a Greek word for 'belt'. Another is *zone*, which in its latinized form *zona* was formerly used as a name for this condition. The lay English term *shingles* is a corruption of Latin *cingulum*, which also means 'belt, girdle'.

Physical Examination: Fever is generally absent. Skin lesions are highly typical, consisting of one or more clusters of vesicles, each cluster surrounded by a zone of erythema. Involvement of the geniculate ganglion of the facial (seventh cranial) nerve can lead to facial paralysis and lesions of the outer ear.

Diagnostic Tests: Diagnosis is clinically evident. Fluid from vesicles gives a positive Tzanck test (see under *Varicella*).

Course: Symptoms are more severe in persons over 40. Pain and skin lesions usually resolve within 2-6 weeks. However, one-half of patients over 60 will develop postherpetic neuralgia, a chronic neuritic pain that can persist for months or years.

Treatment: Mild cases in younger persons are treated symptomatically. In severe disease, in older or immunodeficient persons, or when there is involvement of the eye or ear, antiviral agents (famciclovir, valacyclovir) shorten the duration of symptoms and reduce the risk of postherpetic neuralgia.

Glossary

dermatome: a segment of the body surface supplied by a single spinal nerve root.

encephalitis: inflammation of the brain, generally due to infection.

erythrocyte sedimentation rate (ESR): the rate at which erythrocytes (red blood cells) settle in a glass column under standardized laboratory conditions; the rate is often elevated in cases of infection, inflammation, or malignant disease.

exanthem: an eruption on the skin resulting from some internal or systemic disease, usually an infection.

febrile: pertaining to or accompanied by fever.

flora: the total bacterial population of the human body, or of a specific area (mouth, colon, skin).

gastroenteritis: inflammation of the stomach and intestine, usually due to infection, causing nausea, vomiting, abdominal cramping, and diarrhea.

humoral: a general term referring to chemical substances produced in the body and having an effect at a site remote from the place of production; for example, hormones, antibodies.

impetigo: a superficial skin infection due to staphylococci, streptococci, or both, and characterized by spreading red, weeping, crusting lesions.

inclusion body: an abnormal structure found inside certain cells that are infected with certain viruses.

lesion: any local injury or other abnormality that causes disease or impairment of function.

lymphocyte: one of the principal types of white blood cell, concerned with immunity.

microorganism: any living thing that is too small to be seen without a microscope.

multinucleated giant cells: abnormal cells formed by the amalgamation of many cells in certain infections and in foreign body reactions.

neuritic: referring to neuritis, inflammation of a nerve; neuritic pain is described as stinging, burning, or shock-like.

Reye syndrome: a severe metabolic disorder occurring in children or adolescents with influenza, varicella, and other infections who are treated with aspirin, resulting in vomiting, brain swelling, seizures, and often death.

synthesis: the formation of a complex chemical substance, by combination or alteration of other substances.

thrush: an infection of the mouth and throat by Candida (yeast).

Tzanck smear: a stained smear of fluid from skin scrapings or vesicular fluid, which may show characteristic changes (multinucleated giant cells, inclusion bodies, vacuolization) in viral diseases such as herpes simplex and varicella-zoster.

vacuolization: formation of vacuoles (bubbles of air or gas) inside cells.

vesicle: a small blister on the skin.

54 • Human Diseases

Topics for Study or Discussion

1. Name four general classes of pathogen, four routes by which infecting organisms can be transmitted from person to person, and four classes of drug used in infectious disease.

2. What are some nonspecific symptoms or signs that occur in many different infections? Do these always indicate the presence of infection?

3. What is the most important single piece of information that the physician needs in order to make a rational forecast of the course of most infectious diseases, and an informed choice of therapeutic agents? How can this information be obtained?

4. Name several infectious diseases that readily respond to treatment with antimicrobial agents, and several others that do not respond to such treatment at all.

5. What factors have been responsible for the emergence of many drug-resistant strains of pathogenic microorganisms? What can be done to combat this problem or prevent it from getting worse?

Chapter 4

The Immune System

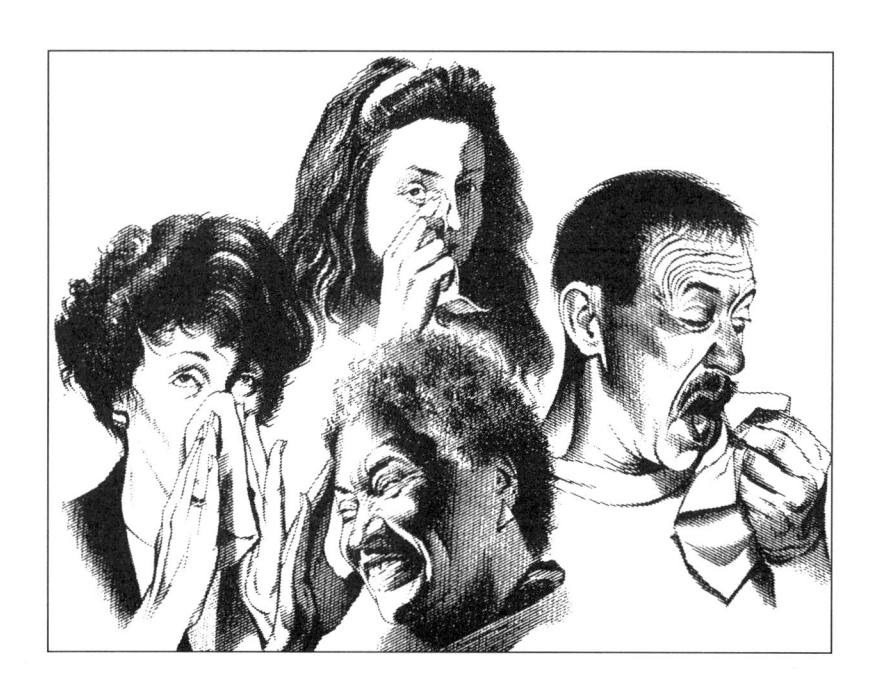

Learning Objectives

On completion of this chapter, the student should

- understand the basic structure and function of the immune system;
- know something about immunodeficiency;
- be aware of the nature and various manifestations of allergy;
- have basic knowledge of autoimmunity.

After a brief survey of normal immunity, this chapter discusses immunodeficiency (especially AIDS), allergy, and autoimmune disorders. If you encounter unfamiliar terms, look them up in the glossary at the end of the chapter.

Description of the Immune System

Immunity was briefly described in the previous chapter. Here a more elaborate discussion is in order.

Immunity refers to a set of protective responses in the living body by which infections and other threats from outside can be repelled or inactivated. Human immunity has three cardinal features: it is stimulus-activated, directed against a specific target, and persisting. Immunity is a *response*: it does not come into play until some assault has been launched on the integrity of the body from without. Moreover, the response is *specific*: the immune system not only recognizes invading microorganisms as being foreign to self, but reacts to them in ways that are closely linked to their biochemical structure. Finally, the immune system has a *memory*: it retains the ability to recognize and repel previous invaders long after the first assault is over.

The immune system consists of the spleen, lymph nodes, and smaller aggregations of lymphoid tissue throughout the body; **lymphocytes**, which are white blood cells formed in lymphoid tissue; and other white blood cells formed in bone marrow. Lymphocytes are of two basic types: **B lymphocytes**, which (after being converted into plasma cells) produce antibodies; and **T lymphocytes**, which have a variety of subtypes with various functions.

The most important protective responses of the immune system are classified as either humoral or cell-mediated. **Humoral immunity** depends on the formation of antibodies by B lymphocytes. (Subtypes of **T lymphocytes**, called helper T cells and suppressor T cells, help to regulate antibody formation.) An **antibody** is a complex protein that reacts with a specific foreign material or organism by meshing chemically with it. Any substance that elicits the formation of an antibody is called an **antigen**.

Antibodies are part of the **globulin** fraction of plasma. The **immune globulins** are subdivided on the basis of chemical structure and immune function into five classes. **IgG**, the largest group, includes antibodies and antitoxins that are important in providing lasting protection against infection. **IgA** antibodies protect surfaces and membranes. **IgM** antibodies are formed early in the immune response and often fade soon after recovery from infection. **IgD** is chemically bound to lymphocytes and serves as their link or attachment to antigens. **IgE** is concerned in allergic and hypersensitivity reactions and in protection against parasites.

Cell-mediated immunity depends on a direct attack by cytotoxic or killer T lymphocytes on foreign cells. **Killer T lymphocytes** recognize these cells as foreign and react specifically to them, but without the involvement of antibodies. Other white blood cells (neutrophils, eosinophils, basophils, monocytes) and certain tissue cells (macrophages, mast cells) serve specialized functions. These cells function either by **phagocytizing** (engulfing and destroying) foreign cells and materials or by releasing into the blood or the tissues **chemical mediators** (histamine, prostaglandins, leukotrienes, cytokines) that trigger or modulate various features of the immune response.

Not all infections lead to the formation of protective antibodies. A mild infection may elicit only feeble or transitory immune response, so that some time after recovery the subject becomes vulnerable to the same pathogens. Other infections (the common cold, staphylococcal infections) generate no protective immunity at all.

A **vaccine** is a material administered to stimulate immunity (see box). A **live vaccine** contains living pathogenic organisms that have been attenuated (weakened chemically or otherwise, so as to be unable to cause disease). A **killed vaccine** contains only nonliving pathogens, and sometimes only part of their protein structure. Some vaccines currently in use are chemical fabrications, made by recombinant DNA technology. They duplicate part of the protein structure of a pathogen, but are not derived from pathogens and are therefore incapable of inducing infection. A **toxoid** is a preparation of a weakened toxin (for example, the paralytic toxin produced by tetanus organisms) that causes the immune system to form antibody to the toxin (**antitoxin**) rather than to the pathogen. Use of these materials is called **active immunization**, since they all elicit an active response from the host's immune system.

In contrast, **passive immunization** is the administration of antibodies, including antitoxins, that have been formed by an immune system other than that of the recipient—that is, by human subjects or animals

> The term **vaccine** comes to us from *vaccinia*, the Latin name for cowpox. Late in the 18th century, the English physician Edward Jenner (1749-1823) made experiments to test the folk belief that infection with cowpox (a skin eruption of cattle sometimes contracted by herdsmen and milkmaids) could confer protection against smallpox.
>
> At that time smallpox was one of the most dreaded diseases in the world. Caused (as we now know) by a virus, it had a mortality rate as high as 30% and usually left survivors marked with pits or scars for life. Down through history, epidemics of smallpox wiped out entire royal families, entire armies, and entire nations.
>
> Inoculation of healthy persons with material from smallpox lesions had been imported into England from Turkey several decades before Jenner made his experiments. Although inoculation did elicit immunity, it might also bring on a disfiguring or fatal case of the disease.
>
> Jenner's experiments were brilliantly successful. In 1806, the American President Thomas Jefferson wrote to Jenner, "You have erased from the calendar of human afflictions one of its greatest . . . Future nations will know by history only that the loathsome smallpox existed."
>
> But resistance to "vaccination" (for which no scientific rationale then existed) was violent among both the medical profession and the lay public. Not until 1979 did an official declaration that smallpox is extinct fulfill Jefferson's prophecy of 173 years earlier.

(rabbits, horses). Passive immunization is used when the patient's immune system is impaired, when protection against a specific infection is needed immediately and cannot wait for the formation of antibody after active immunization, or when no active vaccine is available.

It is currently recommended that all children receive active immunization against ten diseases (diphtheria, hepatitis B, measles, mumps, poliomyelitis, *Haemophilus influenzae* type b infection, pertussis (whooping cough), rubella, tetanus, and varicella-zoster) by the age of 15 months, with booster doses for some of these at prescribed intervals throughout life.

Immunodeficiency

Immunodeficiency is a general term for impairment of any part or function of the immune system that leaves the body vulnerable to infectious diseases. Persons with immunodeficiency are more susceptible than normal persons to certain bacterial, viral, and fungal infections. In addition, they may be subject to **opportunistic infections** (infections due to pathogens to which persons with intact immune systems are virtually invulnerable).

Immune deficiencies are divided into two large classes: **congenital** and **acquired**. Congenital disorders of immunity are virtually all due to inherited defects in the functioning of some component of the immune system. Some run in families; many are lethal in early childhood. The following are some of the more common congenital immunodeficiency syndromes.

agammaglobulinemia: inability to form antibodies, due to inherited B lymphocyte dysfunction. Serum levels of immunoglobulin are low, and patients are subject to recurrent bacterial infections, including abscesses and purulent infections of the ears, sinuses, and lower respiratory tract.

Chédiak-Higashi disease: reduction in the number of circulating neutrophils, with impairment of their ability to destroy bacteria due to enzyme deficiencies and failure to respond to chemical signals. Children with this disorder also have congenital abnormalities of the skin and central nervous system.

DiGeorge syndrome (thymic hypoplasia): inherited T lymphocyte dysfunction, leading to susceptibility to local or systemic infection with fungi, viruses, mycobacteria, and protozoan parasites.

Job syndrome: a disorder of neutrophil function, with eosinophilia and increased IgE antibodies. Children with this disorder are vulnerable to recurrent staphylococcal infections of the skin and respiratory tract.

severe combined immunodeficiency disease (SCID): failure of both B and T lymphocyte function, with heightened risk of certain infections (bacterial diarrhea, *Pneumocystis carinii* pneumonia). Even a seemingly trivial infection can prove lethal, and few patients survive beyond childhood.

Wiskott-Aldrich syndrome: combined B and T lymphocyte dysfunction complicated by thrombocytopenia and eczema.

60 • Human Diseases

Treatment of these disorders is limited to supportive care, avoidance of exposure to infectious organisms (sometimes by lifelong isolation), and vigorous treatment of infections when they occur.

Acquired immunodeficiency can result from malignancies affecting the immune system, radiation therapy, prolonged administration of corticosteroids, and deliberate suppression of immune function with cytotoxic drugs and antimetabolites in the treatment of autoimmune disorders and malignant tumors. The best-known and most significant form of acquired immunodeficiency is that caused by the **human immunodeficiency virus (HIV)**, and known as AIDS (acquired immunodeficiency syndrome).

The following discussion begins with general remarks on history, physical findings, results of diagnostic tests, and treatment, and concludes with more detailed information about several of the more common opportunistic infections that occur in AIDS.

Acquired Immunodeficiency Syndrome (AIDS)

A uniformly lethal impairment of T lymphocyte function caused by a virus.

Cause: The **human immunodeficiency virus (HIV)**, which is transmitted almost exclusively by sexual contact or sharing of needles by intravenous drug abusers. After a latent period of 10-12 years, the virus causes wholesale destruction of helper T cells, with resultant loss of immunity to many opportunistic pathogens.

History: Primary HIV infection sometimes causes a self-limited flu-like illness and later, dementia. Any of a number of opportunistic infections may induce symptoms of weakness, weight loss, diarrhea, pneumonia, or cutaneous lesions.

Physical Examination: Findings depend on the nature of the infection. Often there are fever, weight loss, and muscle wasting.

Diagnostic Tests: The absolute lymphocyte count is low, and in particular the **CD4+** (T_4, helper T) **lymphocyte count** is below 800/μL. The serum contains antibody to HIV. Other findings (anemia, abnormal chest x-ray, organisms in sputum or stool) depend on specific infections contracted.

Course: Recurrent and increasingly severe infections lead to death within three years after the diagnosis of AIDS in most patients.

Treatment: Zidovudine, an antiviral drug that limits damage to T4 lymphocytes by HIV, is administered when the T4 count falls below 500. Drugs to prevent *Pneumocystis carinii* pneumonia (PCP, the most common and most frequently fatal opportunistic infection in AIDS) are administered when the T4 count drops below 200, or when PCP infection is diagnosed; these include pentamidine, atovaquone, and trimethoprim-sulfamethoxazole.

Opportunistic Infections in AIDS

bacillary angiomatosis: formation of vascular tumors in the skin, bone, liver, and other tissues, due to infection with species of *Rochalimaea*, which are rickettsias. Erythromycin, doxycycline, and other antibiotics provide a measure of control.

candidosis: a superficial fungal infection due to *Candida albicans* and related species. This is a common pathogen in the general population, where it causes oropharyngeal lesions (thrush) and cutaneous and vaginal candidosis. In persons with AIDS, *Candida* often extends into the esophagus and the intestine. Superficial infections are treated with clotrimazole, miconazole, nystatin, and other topical antifungals. Amphotericin B and ketoconazole are used in systemic infection.

cytomegalovirus (CMV) infection (cytomegalic inclusion disease): a common mild or subclinical infection in the general population. In AIDS, the virus causes disease of the respiratory system (pneumonia), gastrointestinal tract (ulcerative enterocolitis with bloody diarrhea), the eye (retinitis leading to blindness), and the nervous system (ascending polyradiculopathy). Treatment with ganciclovir or foscarnet slows progression of disease, particularly retinitis.

herpes simplex: the familiar cold-sore and genital herpes are both caused by herpes simplex viruses. In AIDS, herpes simplex can present as an extensive and chronic ulceration of skin or mucous membrane (mouth or esophagus), bronchitis or pneumonia, or as systemic infection. Acyclovir and foscarnet provide some antiviral effect.

histoplasmosis: infection with *Histoplasma capsulatum*, a fungus that causes mild or subclinical respiratory infection in persons with intact immunity. In AIDS it is sometimes associated with severe pulmonary disease and respiratory failure. It may also become disseminated throughout the body. Treatment is with amphotericin B and itraconazole.

Kaposi sarcoma: a malignant tumor formed of cutaneous or mucosal blood vessels and appearing as one or several pink or purple plaques or nodules. The cause is probably a virus or other pathogen that is normally suppressed by the immune system. Kaposi sarcoma occurs in about one-third of all AIDS patients. The tumors may spread to the respiratory and digestive system and the abdominal viscera. Some control may be provided by treatment with interferon alfa.

oral hairy leukoplakia: a shaggy whitish plaque of abnormal oral mucosa, induced by infection with the Epstein-Barr virus (the cause of infectious mononucleosis) in AIDS. Antiviral drugs may suppress the lesion satisfactorily, but in about 5% of cases it progresses to oral cancer.

Pneumocystis carinii **pneumonia** (plasma cell pneumonia, PCP): an infection of the lungs due to a protozoan parasite, which eventually affects about three-fourths of all AIDS patients and is the cause of death in many. Symptoms include fever, cough, and progressive respiratory failure. There may be no specific findings on physical examination or x-ray. Silver stains demonstrate the causative organism in smears of respiratory secretions or bronchoalveolar washings. Treatment is with adrenocortical steroids, atovaquone, pentamidine, primaquine, and trimethoprim-sulfamethoxazole.

toxoplasmosis: infection with the intracellular parasite *Toxoplasma gondii*, which causes encephalitis (manifested as headaches, seizures, and personality change), pneumonitis, myocarditis, and disseminated infection. Treatment is with clindamycin, pyrimethamine, sulfadiazine, and other agents.

tuberculosis: pulmonary infection due to *Mycobacterium tuberculosis* and, more commonly, intestinal or disseminated infection due to *M. avium, M. intracellulare*, or other members of the *M. avium complex* (MAC). Multidrug regimens including isoniazid, rifampin, ethambutol, and other antibiotics or chemotherapeutic agents are commonly required to control tuberculosis in AIDS.

varicella-zoster infection: the virus that causes chickenpox (varicella) and **herpes zoster** can produce a severe and protracted form of zoster in persons with AIDS. Treatment is with acyclovir, famciclovir, foscarnet, or valacyclovir.

Allergy and Delayed Hypersensitivity

An immunologically mediated sensitivity to a foreign antigen (allergen), with resultant tissue inflammation and organ dysfunction.

Allergy includes a broad variety of local and systemic reactions to foreign materials, which may be inhaled (dusts, pollens, molds), ingested (foods, medicines), injected (medicines, insect venoms), or brought into contact with skin (household or industrial chemicals, plant toxins). In all true allergy, prior exposure and sensitization must have occurred before the allergen elicits a reaction. Two basic types are distinguished.

In IgE-mediated (immediate) hypersensitivity reactions, release of histamine and other substances from mast cells leads to local or systemic symptoms within minutes after exposure. Examples are allergic rhinitis (hay fever, nasal allergies to cats), atopic dermatitis (intensely itchy rashes), urticaria (hives), anaphylaxis (a life-threatening syndrome of urticaria, swelling of respiratory mucosa, and shock), and serum sickness (fever, urticaria, joint pains, swollen lymph nodes).

In T-cell-mediated (delayed) hypersensitivity, a latent period of 48-72 hours elapses between exposure and onset of symptoms. Examples are allergic contact dermatitis (poison ivy rash) and hypersensitivity pneumonitis.

History: Depending on the inciting cause and target organ, the range of symptoms includes watery rhinitis, sneezing, wheezing and cough, itching and rash, intestinal cramping and diarrhea, joint pain and swelling, dyspnea, hypotension and collapse.

Physical Examination: May show tachycardia, hypotension, edema, erythema, wheals, copious nasal secretion, nasal polyps, bronchial wheezing, fever, or other local or systemic signs of allergy.

Diagnostic Tests: The eosinophil count may be elevated, and eosinophils may be seen in smears of nasal scrapings or nasal or bronchial secretions. Provocative skin testing or challenge with certain foods may confirm specific causal agents. **Radioallergosorbent testing (RAST)** can identify specific antibody in serum.

Treatment: Avoidance of known causes is paramount in preventing allergic disorders. Antihistaminic drugs are used to control local and generalized symptoms due to histamine release. Cromolyn and related drugs stabilize mast cells and exert a protective effect if administered before exposure. Sympathomimetic drugs (epinephrine, albuterol) can block some of the local or general effects of histamine and other mediators of allergic symptoms. Adrenocortical steroids are used in severe allergy. Immunotherapy consisting of periodic injection of known allergens in increasing doses provides an apparent desensitization in some patients.

Autoimmunity

Autoimmunity results when the body's immune system forms antibodies against some component of itself. Autoimmune disorders are common and exceedingly diverse. The formation of antibodies against self can come about through various mechanisms: failure of suppressor T cells to regulate the immune process; failure of the immune system to recognize some component of the body as self; formation of antibody to an infecting organism that happens to have a similar protein composition to some body tissue, which is then attacked by the antibody; and disorders of lymphocytes causing them to form abnormal antibodies that happen to attack body tissues.

Susceptibility to autoimmune disease runs in families, and persons who have one autoimmune disorder tend to have others. The so-called collagen or connective-tissue diseases (rheumatoid arthritis, lupus erythematosus, and others) are all caused by autoimmune phenomena.

The following survey of autoimmune diseases is by no means exhaustive. Discussions of several autoimmune disorders (insulin-dependent diabetes mellitus, Graves disease, Hashimoto disease, pernicious anemia, chronic hepatitis B) appear in other chapters of this book.

Rheumatoid Arthritis

A chronic systemic disease causing inflammatory changes in many tissues, particularly joint membranes.

Cause: Formation of antibody to one's own tissues, particularly synovial membranes. About 1-2% of the population are affected, and the disease is three times more common in women. It tends to run in families. Onset is typically between 20 and 40. The onset may be triggered by emotional or physical stress, surgery, or childbirth.

History: Gradual onset of pain, stiffness, and warmth in joints, particularly smaller joints (proximal interphalangeal and metacarpophalangeal joints, wrists, knees, ankles, and toes). Stiffness is worse in the morning ("gelling"). Malaise, fever, and weight loss may accompany the onset of the disease.

Physical Examination: Tenderness, warmth, stiffness of affected joints. Enlargement and deformity of joints, including ulnar deviation of finger joints, may occur late. About 20% of patients have subcutaneous nodules over bony prominences on extremities.

Diagnostic Tests: The erythrocyte sedimentation rate is elevated. A mild anemia is common, and platelets may be increased. Testing for rheumatoid arthritis factor is positive in about 75% of patients, and for antinuclear antibody in about 20%. Serum protein studies may detect an increase in immune globulin. X-rays are normal early in the disease but eventually show osteoporosis of bone near affected joints, erosion of joint surfaces, and narrowing of joint spaces.

Course: In as many as one-half of all patients, symptoms remit largely or completely within two years. Patients in whom symptoms continue may have intermittent or persistent pain and stiffness, with increasing deformity and fusion of affected joints. Extra-articular manifestations include pericarditis, pleurisy with effusion, lymphadenopathy, splenomegaly, vasculitis, dry mouth and eyes (Sjögren syndrome, discussed below) and peripheral nerve entrapment problems such as carpal tunnel syndrome (see Chapter 18).

Treatment: The standard treatment is aspirin (ASA), but other nonsteroidal anti-inflammatory drugs (NSAIDs) may also be used. In refractory cases a number of other drugs may prove useful, including methotrexate, antimalarials, gold salts, and adrenal corticosteroids. All of these drugs have problematic side effects or toxicities. Physical therapy is important in maintaining mobility. Surgery to correct severe deformity.

Lupus Erythematosus

A chronic inflammatory disorder of connective tissue due to formation of antibody to nucleoprotein.

Cause: Unknown. Ninety percent of patients are young women. Antinuclear antibody and anti-DNA antibody are found in the serum.

History: Gradual or abrupt onset of widely varying symptoms: joint pain, butterfly rash over the cheeks, discoid lesions and other skin changes (purpura, alopecia), fever, chest pain, mood changes and other psychiatric symptoms.

Physical Examination: Fever, signs of swelling and inflammation in joints, malar "butterfly" eruption, lymphadenopathy, splenomegaly, pericardial or pleural friction rub heard on auscultation.

Diagnostic Tests: The erythrocyte sedimentation rate is elevated, white blood cells (particularly lymphocytes) and platelets are decreased. The LE-cell preparation, antinuclear antibody, and anti-DNA antibody tests are often positive. Serologic test for syphilis may be falsely positive. Urinalysis may show proteinuria, red blood cells, and casts in lupus nephritis.

Course: The disease is chronic and relapsing, with spontaneous remissions and exacerbations. With treatment the ten-year survival rate is about 95%. Death is usually due to renal failure.

Treatment: Nonsteroidal anti-inflammatory drugs (NDAIDs) and general supportive measures may suffice to control symptoms. Antimalarial drugs (hydroxychloroquine and others), adrenal corticosteroids, and immunosuppressive drugs (azathioprine, cyclophosphamide) are useful in more severe cases.

Discoid Lupus

A variant of systemic lupus erythematosus in which abnormalities are confined to the skin.

The disease occurs almost exclusively in young women. Round erythematous papules with plugging of oil gland ducts occur on the cheeks, nose, ears, and other cutaneous surfaces, particularly those exposed to sunlight. Involvement of mucous membranes and of the scalp (sometimes leading to alopecia) may also occur. About 10% of patients with these symptoms are found on evaluation to have systemic lupus erythematosus; in the rest, disease is limited to the skin eruption. Treatment is avoidance of sunlight, use of sunscreens, and, when necessary, topical steroids and oral antimalarials.

Sjögren Syndrome

An autoimmune disorder of certain exocrine glands, causing dryness of the mouth and eyes.

Nearly all patients are middle-aged women. Dysfunction of lacrimal glands causes dryness and burning of the eyes. Abnormality of salivary glands leads to swelling of the glands (particularly the parotids), dry mouth, dysphagia, and dental caries. Other gland tissue impairment may affect the skin, the pancreas, the lower respiratory tract, and the vagina. The disorder frequently occurs in association with other autoimmune diseases (rheumatoid arthritis, systemic lupus erythematosus, Hashimoto disease). Many patients eventually develop renal disease or lymphoma. Treatment is supportive, with artificial tears, strict oral hygiene, and attention to diagnosis and treatment of associated disorders.

Acute Rheumatic Fever

An autoimmune disorder affecting the heart, the joints, and the skin.

Cause: Antibody formed to group A beta-hemolytic streptococci (during streptococcal pharyngitis) attacks certain tissues of the patient's body. Rheumatic fever follows streptococcal infection after an interval of 2-4 weeks. It occurs almost exclusively in children and adolescents. The incidence is higher during cold, damp weather and in children from lower socioeconomic levels. Susceptibility to acute rheumatic fever seems to run in families.

History: Fever, joint pain, rash, nontender subcutaneous nodules, weakness, shortness of breath, chest pain, rapid pulse, cough, chorea (see box).

Physical Examination: Fever, tachycardia, a macular rash called erythema marginatum, swelling and tenderness in certain joints, irritability, muscle twitching, heart murmurs indicative of mitral or aortic valve disease or both, evidence of congestive heart failure. (Valvular disease and congestive failure are fully discussed in Chapter 8.)

Diagnostic Tests: Neutrophilia, mild anemia, elevated erythrocyte sedimentation rate. The serum contains C-reactive protein during the acute phase, and eventually the antistreptolysin O (ASO) titer rises. Chest x-ray may show cardiomegaly, pericardial effusion, or signs of cardiac failure. Electrocardiography, echocardiography, and cardiac catheterization provide more specific clues to the extent and severity of disease.

Course: Most of the manifestations of acute rheumatic fever resolve spontaneously. However, various forms of carditis (inflammation of the heart), which occur in about one-half of all patients, can lead to severe heart damage, with chronic, progressive, or even rapidly fatal malfunction

> **Chorea** (from Greek *choreia* 'dancing') denotes a clinical disorder manifested by recurring sudden, intricate, well-coordinated but involuntary muscle movements, which may affect gait, use of the arms and hands, and even speech. Several forms of chorea are recognized and distinguished.
>
> Huntington chorea, named after the American physician George S. Huntington (1850-1916) is inherited as an autosomal dominant trait. Onset usually occurs in the thirties or forties and death, due to progressive neuromuscular dysfunction and dementia, follows in about 15 years.
>
> Sydenham chorea, named after the English physician Thomas Sydenham (1624-1689), is the type that occurs in acute rheumatic fever. (Another name for this disorder is St. Vitus dance, after the Christian martyr whose intercession was believed helpful in various forms of movement disorder and "dancing mania" during the Middle Ages.) Patients display abrupt, jerky, complex, involuntary movements of the trunk and extremities, and often mild personality changes. This type of chorea is invariably self-limited, resolving without any neurologic, psychologic, or muscular sequelae.

of heart valves. About 20% of persons recovering from acute rheumatic fever will have a recurrence within five years.

Treatment: Streptococcal infection must be eradicated with penicillin, erythromycin, or another antibiotic known to be effective in preventing rheumatic fever. Bed rest is enforced until resting pulse, temperature, sedimentation rate, and electrocardiogram have returned to normal (often longer than one month). Most symptoms can be controlled with aspirin; corticosteroids are used as needed. Valvular heart disease and congestive heart failure may require vigorous treatment during the acute phase. Severe chronic involvement of the mitral or aortic valve may require long-term treatment, including surgery. Monthly injections of repository penicillin are continued for five years or until age 25, whichever comes first, to prevent recurrences of acute rheumatic fever.

Glossary

alopecia: local or widespread loss of scalp hair.
cardiomegaly: enlargement of the heart.
extra-articular: affecting or pertaining to structures other than joints.
dementia: deterioration of mental function.
discoid: consisting of small flat plaques.
effusion: an abnormal accumulation of fluid in a body cavity, such as the pleural space or pericardium.
enterocolitis: inflammatory disease of both the small and large intestines.
erythematous: having an abnormal red color.
hypotension: an abnormally low blood pressure.
lymphadenopathy: disease of lymph nodes, manifested by swelling, tenderness, or both.
macular: consisting of flat, abnormally colored spots (macules) on the skin.
malar: pertaining to or situated on the cheeks.
nephritis: inflammation of the kidney.
pericarditis: inflammation of the pericardium, the membranous sac surrounding the heart.
pleurisy (pleuritis): inflammation of the pleura.
purpura: an eruption of purple spots on the skin due to local hemorrhages.
purulent: pertaining to the formation of pus.
retinitis: inflammation of the retina, the light-sensitive membrane at the back of the eyeball.
rhinitis: inflammation of nasal mucous membranes, usually accompanied by nasal obstruction, excessive secretions, and sneezing.
splenomegaly: enlargement of the spleen.
vasculitis: inflammation of blood vessels.
wheal: a rapidly appearing and disappearing zone of circumscribed swelling in the skin, usually white with a red halo, due to various types of allergic reaction; the characteristic lesion of hives.

Topics for Study or Discussion

1. Give a brief definition of immunity, including its 3 cardinal features.

2. Name 3 kinds of congenital immunodeficiency and 3 opportunistic infections typical of the acquired immunodeficiency syndrome (AIDS).

3. Define or explain: allergy, anaphylaxis, antibody, antigen, autoimmunity, opportunistic infection.

4. Name and briefly describe 3 autoimmune disorders.

5. Discuss the pros and cons of having an immune system.

Chapter 5

Neoplasia

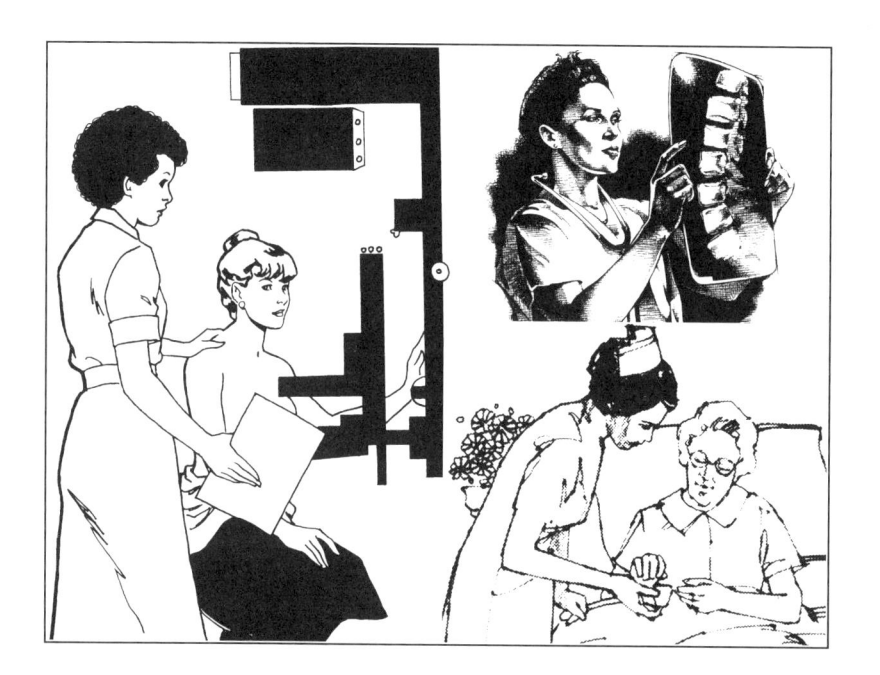

Learning Objectives

Upon completion of this chapter, the student should

- understand the meaning of neoplasia and be able to distinguish benign from malignant neoplasms;

- know something about the diagnosis, grading, staging, and treatment of malignant diseases;

- have basic information about the more common cancers.

The Nature of Neoplasia

Neoplasia refers to any growth of cells or tissues that is erratic, not in accord with normal bodily needs or patterns of growth and development, and not under the control of normal regulatory mechanisms. Neoplasia results in the formation of a **neoplasm** (growth, tumor).

The causes of neoplasia are not fully understood. The process begins with normal cells. Cellular mutation, induced by chemical toxins (**carcinogens**), radiation, chronic inflammation, or certain infections, can lead to formation of a clone or colony of cells whose internal structure and biochemical nature are aberrant or atypical and whose proliferation and behavior do not respond to normal controls. An inherited tendency to develop some kinds of neoplasm has been recognized for many years. Oncogenes were discussed at the end of Chapter 3. Many neoplasms result from cell stimulation by abnormal growth factors, or by normal hormones in abnormal amounts. A **tumor** is said to be hormone-dependent if it develops in a tissue that is stimulated by a hormone normally present, and can be suppressed by withdrawing this hormone (for example, prostate cancer is androgen-dependent).

Neoplasms are divided into two large classes: **benign** and **malignant**. A malignant tumor is one that, if unchecked, tends to cause death; a benign tumor has no such inherent tendency.

A more precise delineation of malignancy can be seen in the following four distinctions:

1. A malignant tumor is found on histologic examination to contain cells that are more primitive, undifferentiated, or anaplastic than those composing a benign tumor, or a higher proportion of such cells than in a benign tumor.

2. A malignant tumor enlarges by infiltrating and invading adjacent tissues, whereas a benign tumor simply gets bigger, without sending out neoplastic extensions into adjacent normal tissue.

3. A malignant tumor characteristically grows much faster than a benign one arising from the same cell type.

4. A malignant tumor can spread by **metastasis**—transmission of malignant cells or groups of cells by the bloodstream, the lymphatic channels, or other routes to establish new foci of malignancy at remote sites in the body.

These distinctions are not absolute. Although most cancers arise as malignant tumors, some develop by malignant degeneration of benign tumors. Skin cancers other than melanomas, though they are histologically malignant, seldom metastasize or cause death. A benign tumor can prove lethal if it compresses a vital structure or causes severe hemorrhage.

Malignant tumors, commonly called **cancers** (see box), can arise in virtually any cell, tissue, or organ of the body. A malignant tumor can cause death in a broad variety of ways: by outgrowing its blood supply and undergoing necrosis and hemorrhage, by producing toxic substances, by eroding into a major blood vessel, by invading or metastasizing to a vital organ such as the brain, or by impairing nutrition, immunity, or some other life-sustaining biochemical function.

The term *cancer*, the Latin word for 'crab', was used for malignant ulcerations by the Roman medical writer Celsus (lst century AD). Much earlier, Greek writers including Hippocrates used the Greek word *karkinos*, also meaning 'crab', and its derivative *karkinoma*, for malignant disease.

The association between malignancy and crabs has been variously explained. One theory is that malignant tumors were thought to gnaw or erode tissue like the pincers of a crab. According to another view, the dilated veins on the surface of a cancerous breast seemed to suggest the outline of a crab with outstretched pincers.

Cancer nomenclature is highly complex and constantly changing. Two main types of malignant tumor are distinguished on the basis of their tissues of origin. **Carcinoma** (by far the more common) develops from epithelium, either glandular (adenocarcinoma) or squamous (squamous carcinoma). **Sarcoma** (from a Greek word meaning 'to become fleshy') denotes a tumor arising from connective tissue (muscle, bone).

Because of their built-in lethal potential, the diagnosis and treatment of malignant tumors are more critical than those of benign tumors. Both benign and malignant tumors are discussed in other chapters. The remainder of this chapter will be devoted to more information about malignant tumors, and detailed discussions of the four most common cancers. The branch of medicine devoted to the prevention, diagnosis, and treatment of malignant disease is called **oncology**.

Diagnosis of Malignancy

The signs and symptoms of malignant disease are highly variable. Many kinds of cancer (lung, pancreas) cause no symptoms until they have invaded surrounding tissues or spread by metastasis and are essentially untreatable. The seven warning signals publicized by the American Cancer Society (see box) are all potential indicators of malignancy. They are, however, highly nonspecific, and in any given instance, a benign explanation for one of these signs or symptoms is far more probable than a malignant one.

Cancer's Seven Warning Signals
(American Cancer Society)

- **C** Change in bowel or bladder habits
- **A** A sore that does not heal
- **U** Unusual bleeding or discharge
- **T** Thickening or lump in breast or elsewhere
- **I** Indigestion or difficulty in swallowing
- **O** Obvious change in a wart or mole
- **N** Nagging cough or hoarseness

Cancer screening is the testing of apparently healthy persons for subtle indications of malignant disease. The following screening procedures are currently advised for all persons, at specified ages or intervals:

Breast: monthly breast self-examination, yearly examination of the breasts by a physician, and mammography.

Uterine cervix: Pap smear.

Prostate: digital examination of the prostate.

Colon and rectum: digital examination, sigmoidoscopy or colonoscopy, and fecal blood testing.

When cancer is suspected, prompt and vigorous diagnostic evaluation is in order, unless the age or general health of the patient makes this inappropriate. Imaging techniques (x-ray, MRI, CT, ultrasound, nuclear imaging) can provide highly specific information about the nature, location, and extent of malignant disease. Blood studies for detection or measurement of immunologic or biologic markers (abnormal tumor products, immunoglobulins) can provide valuable further information.

But the diagnostic procedure par excellence for malignant disease is **biopsy**: removal of a specimen of tissue from the patient's body for microscopic examination. Punch or shave biopsies are used to obtain skin specimens. Specimens from the interior of the digestive tract and the urinary tract can be obtained through endoscopes. **Needle biopsy**, performed with a specially designed instrument that passes through the skin and removes a sliver of tissue from the area of interest, enables the diagnostician to assess internal structures without performing open surgery. Laparoscopy permits sampling of tissue in the abdominal or pelvic cavities. In many instances, however, an adequate biopsy can only be obtained at exploratory surgery. Sampling of tissue by biopsy may include removal of numerous or extensive specimens—for example, regional lymph nodes or areas of suspicious tissue change.

A biopsy specimen is examined **grossly** (with the naked eye) and then (after fixation, embedding in a medium such as paraffin, thin sectioning, and staining) **microscopically** by a pathologist to determine whether it contains malignant cells, from what type of normal cells they have arisen, how undifferentiated they are, what tissue abnormalities they show (cyst formation, abortive attempts at organization, tissue death), and how far they have extended or invaded. For certain types of cancer (breast cancer), pathologic examination of surgically removed material can be performed immediately (before the surgical wound is closed) by the **frozen section** technique, which substitutes freezing of tissue for the more time-consuming paraffin process.

Diagnostic information obtained about a cancer is generally formulated according to a rigorous and highly specific scheme. The **type** of a cancer is its histologic nature: what kind of cells (squamous epithelium, gland tissue, duct tissue) have undergone malignant change? The **grading** of a cancer is a measure of its degree of malignancy, based on histologic evaluation of its cells. Higher-grade malignancies contain more primitive cells, showing a higher amount of undifferentiation (**anaplasia**). The higher the grade, the greater the probability of invasion and metastasis. The **Broders classification** of squamous-cell carcinomas is an example of a simple grading system:

Grade I: 25% of cells undifferentiated
Grade II: 50% of cells undifferentiated
Grade III: 75% of cells undifferentiated
Grade IV: 100% of cells undifferentiated

Grading a tumor often permits a fairly accurate estimate of its future behavior, the likelihood of spread by invasion or metastasis, and the probable response to radiation or chemotherapy.

Staging is a measure of the extent of a malignant disease at the time of evaluation, expressed in arabic numerals (1, 2, 3 . . .) with or without qualifying letters. Staging takes into account the type, size, and extent of the primary tumor; the degree of lymph node involvement, if any; and the number and location of any distant metastases. The presence of associated symptoms, such as weight loss and fever, may be relevant to the staging of certain malignancies. A basic framework used in expressing the staging of a wide variety of malignancies is the **T-N-M** (tumor, nodes, metastases) **classification**, mentioned in Chapter 1. In this system, subscript numbers indicate the extent of involvement, according to criteria that are specific for each type of tumor. Thus, T2 might represent a primary tumor that is larger than 5 cm in diameter but has not invaded locally; N2, involvement of lymph nodes at two distinct sites; M0, no evidence of distant metastasis.

Arriving at an accurate prognosis for a malignant tumor depends on precise typing, grading, and staging; on other diagnostic information (imaging and laboratory studies); and on due consideration of the patient's age and general health. The compilation of cancer statistics by national and international tumor registries has made possible the publication of survival information for each type of tumor depending on grade and stage. The five-year survival rate is a familiar index of prognosis. If a given type, grade, and stage of tumor has a five-year survival rate of 56% with a given treatment, that means that 56% of persons with such a tumor who undergo such a treatment will still be living after 5 years.

Treatment of Malignancy

The goal of treatment in malignant disease is to effect a cure when possible and to conserve the patient's comfort, hydration, and nutrition in all cases. **Surgery** has always been the principal method of treating cancer. Complete resection of a primary tumor that has not spread or metastasized usually proves to be **curative**. But adequate resection may involve damage to or removal of much normal tissue, with resulting functional impairment or disfigurement; on the other hand, conservative surgery may fail to remove all cancer cells. Moreover, metastases may only be discovered months or years after surgery has been performed. When curative surgery is not feasible, a **palliative** procedure may be undertaken to reduce the volume of the tumor (**debulking**) or to remove devitalized, necrotic, bleeding, or infected tissue. In certain types of malignancy, a palliative effect may be achieved by surgical removal of certain endocrine glands: the testes in metastatic carcinoma of the prostate, the ovaries in breast cancer.

During the past generation, **chemotherapy** of cancer with a wide variety of agents has become firmly established as a valuable and often curative resource. Useful cancer drugs include alkylating agents (nitrogen mustard, chlorambucil, busulfan), antimetabolites (methotrexate, 5-fluorouracil, 6-mercaptopurine), antibiotics (doxorubicin, dactinomycin, mithramycin), plant alkaloids (vinblastine and vincristine from periwinkle), hormones (adrenal corticosteroids, estrogens, androgens), and others (enzymes, platinum complex).

Most of these agents are toxic to cancer cells, and most of them can also damage normal cells and tissues. Because cancer is a life-threatening disease, a higher risk of severe side effects is tolerable. Most cancer chemotherapy must be administered by injection and continued over a period of weeks. During and after treatment, red and white blood cell counts and other diagnostic tests are performed regularly to monitor drug effects and detect severe bone marrow depression or other toxic effects of the drugs on normal tissues.

A course of chemotherapy typically includes three or more drugs given according to a precise regimen or **protocol**. The drugs used in such combinations are represented by their first letters in initialisms such as MOPP (mechlorethamine, Oncovorin, procarbazine, and prednisone); note that Oncovorin is a brand name for vincristine.

Because rapidly proliferating tissue is particularly subject to damage by ionizing radiation, x-ray and other forms of radiation have long been used as an adjunct to surgery and chemotherapy in the treatment of many malignant tumors. The dose and delivery site of **radiation therapy** must be carefully adjusted to ensure maximal therapeutic response with minimal side effects and risk of delayed complications.

Cancer Statistics

Reporting of malignant disease to local and regional **tumor registries** enables the American Cancer Society to publish highly accurate statistics on the incidence and mortality of various types of cancer. Such statistics do not include data on skin tumors other than melanomas, since these typically respond to local treatment and do not cause death.

In a given year in the United States, about 1,400,000 new cases of cancer are diagnosed, and about 560,000 persons die of cancer. The relative incidence of the four commonest cancers, by gender, is as follows:

Men	**Women**
Prostate, 41%	Breast, 31%
Lung, 13%	Lung, 13%
Colon & Rectum, 9%	Colon & Rectum, 11%

Of all cancers causing death, the relative frequency with which these four cancers prove lethal is as follows:

Men	**Women**
Lung, 32%	Lung, 25%
Prostate, 14%	Breast, 17%
Colon & Rectum, 9%	Colon & Rectum, 10%

The remainder of the chapter is devoted to a discussion of these four malignancies.

Bronchogenic Carcinoma

A malignant tumor of the lung arising from bronchial epithelium. Bronchogenic carcinoma ranks first as a cause of cancer death in both men and women in the United States.

Causes: Cigarette smoking is by far the most common cause of bronchogenic carcinoma. Inhalation of industrial carcinogens, particularly asbestos, and exposure to radon are other known causes.

History: Gradual onset of cough, dyspnea, hemoptysis, anorexia, and weight loss.

Physical Examination: May indicate weight loss, muscle wasting, or signs of bronchial obstruction, pneumonia, atelectasis, cavitation, or pleural effusion.

Diagnostic Tests: Chest x-ray or CT scan demonstrates a mass infiltrate, atelectasis, cavitation, or pleural effusion. Cytologic examination of bronchial washings or pleural fluid or histologic examination of tissue obtained by biopsy shows malignant tissue arising from bronchial epithelium.

Course: Bronchogenic carcinoma is typically advanced and inoperable when first diagnosed. The 5-year survival rate is 10-15%. Obstruction of airways commonly leads to atelectasis and pneumonia. Obstruction of the vena cava (superior vena cava syndrome) and various neurologic complications (phrenic nerve palsy, Pancoast's syndrome due to involvement of the brachial plexus), and paraneoplastic syndromes (Cushing syndrome, hypercalcemia) due to production of hormone-like agents by tumor cells.

Treatment: Surgery, radiation, and chemotherapy.

Other diseases of the lung are discussed in Chapter 10.

Breast Cancer

A malignant tumor of the female breast, arising most frequently from ductal epithelium. The commonest cancer in women, and the second-commonest cause of cancer death (after lung cancer) in women. One in eight or nine women will develop breast cancer.

Cause: Women who have no children, or whose first pregnancy occurs late in the childbearing years, are at increased risk of breast cancer. So are women who have a family history of breast cancer, particularly cancer occurring at an early age in one or more female relatives. A supposed association between increased dietary fat and increased risk of breast cancer is not well supported by statistical studies. Several oncogenes enormously increase the risk of early-onset breast cancer.

History: A solitary, firm, nontender mass in the breast, usually discovered by the patient accidentally or during breast self-examination. (All women over 20 should practice breast self-examination monthly.) Sixty percent occur in the upper outer quadrant of the breast. Occasionally nipple discharge is the presenting symptom. With advancing disease, swelling and local pain. Bone pain, weight loss, and jaundice are symptoms of systemic spread through metastasis.

80 • *Human Diseases*

Physical Examination: There may be enlargement or abnormal contour of one breast on inspection. The tumor is felt as a hard, ill-defined, nontender solitary mass. There may be skin or nipple retraction, fixation of the tumor to the underlying chest wall or the overlying skin, and signs of local inflammation (swelling, redness, ulceration). Axillary lymph nodes may be found enlarged if cancer cells have spread to them.

Diagnostic: Mammography (a specialized x-ray procedure) can identify changes indicative of breast cancer (calcification, mass, or both) as much as 2 years before a tumor becomes palpable, and is therefore a valuable screening procedure for asymptomatic women over 50 and for younger women at increased risk. Ultrasound examination can supply valuable additional information. Biopsy is required for confirmation of malignancy and precise identification of tumor type. A biopsy can be obtained through the skin by either a large-needle or fine-needle technique. Excisional biopsy (removal of the tumor followed by frozen-section examination before closure of the surgical site) is the method usually chosen when clinical and mammographic evidence supports a diagnosis of cancer.

Course: An untreated breast cancer typically enlarges, invades surrounding and underlying tissues, and causes extensive cutaneous ulceration. Breast cancers spread to axillary and mediastinal lymph nodes, liver, bone, and brain. For a solitary, localized tumor, the 5-year survival rate is 95% and the 10-year survival rate is 90%. The figures for disease that has become systemic before treatment is instituted are 5% and 2%. Five-year and even 10-year rates do not adequately reflect the long-term mortality of breast cancer, which is eventually the cause of death in most patients, except when cancer is discovered very early by screening procedures.

Treatment: The basic treatment of breast cancer is surgical removal of the tumor. Various further procedures, including radical mastectomy (removal of the entire breast as well as surrounding and underlying tissues and axillary lymph nodes) may be appropriate with certain types and stages of cancer. Both radiation treatments and chemotherapy are usually administered after surgery. Radiation is not usually needed after radical mastectomy, but the procedure is mutilating and psychologically devastating. In metastatic disease, elimination of estrogen stimulation through either oophorectomy (removal of the ovaries) or tamoxifen, a chemical anti-estrogen, delays progression of disease and mitigates symptoms.

Other diseases of the breast are discussed in Chapter 8.

Adenocarcinoma of the Prostate

A malignant tumor arising from glandular epithelium of the prostate gland.

Cause: Adenocarcinoma of the prostate is the most common cancer in men (41% of all cancers diagnosed). The incidence of prostatic cancer found at autopsy in men over 50 is about 40%. However, prostate cancer causes only 14% of all cancer deaths in men. The risk of developing prostatic carcinoma is higher in men with a family history of it and in those who have undergone vasectomy. The tumor is testosterone-dependent (that is, it does not occur in men who have undergone orchidectomy). Adenocarcinoma of the prostate does not arise from benign prostatic hyperplasia.

History: There may be no symptoms. Diminished urine flow, urinary frequency, nocturia, and dribbling of urine may occur as in benign prostatic hyperplasia. The first symptom may be bone pain due to metastasis.

Physical Examination: The prostate, as palpated on digital rectal examination, may be unusually firm, nodular, or asymmetric.

Diagnostic Tests. The level of prostate specific antigen (PSA) or acid phosphatase or both in the serum is elevated in many cases of prostate carcinoma, particularly when metastasis has occurred. Transrectal ultrasound may detect abnormally dense areas within the prostate gland, representing tumor. Transrectal biopsy discloses zones of malignant tissue. The **Gleason grading** system gives a histopathologic estimate of malignancy and likely future behavior. X-ray studies and radionuclide bone scans may show metastases to bones of the spine or pelvis.

Course. Progression of disease is typically slow, and many patients die of other causes before the prostatic cancer has reached a lethal stage. Metastasis to lymph nodes and to the spine or pelvis eventually occurs. Urinary obstruction may lead to urinary tract infection and even renal failure.

Treatment. Surgical excision (usually radical prostatectomy), radiation; in advanced (metastatic) disease, castration or administration of estrogen (or an anti-androgen such as flutamide) to suppress tumor growth.

Other diseases of the prostate are discussed in Chapter 7.

Adenocarcinoma of the Colon and Rectum

A malignant neoplasm arising from glandular epithelium in the large intestine. In both men and women, colon cancer ranks second as a cause of cancer deaths in the U.S. One-half of all colon cancers are situated in the sigmoid colon or rectum. These tumors tend to grow slowly, but may eventually become bulky; they may encircle and constrict the bowel.

Causes: Most colon cancers arise by malignant transformation of benign polyps (adenomas). Several oncogenes are associated with heightened risk of developing primary cancer in the colon; some of these predispose to formation of multiple malignant tumors, which may involve organs other than the bowel. Risk factors for developing colon cancer include age over 40, a history of adenomas (benign polyps) of the colon, a family history of colon cancer, and a history of ulcerative colitis.

History: Depending on the location of the tumor, crampy abdominal pain, change of bowel habits, bloody stools, weakness, fatigue.

Physical Examination: A mass may be felt on abdominal or digital rectal examination. The liver may be enlarged or irregular if hepatic metastases are present.

Diagnostic Tests: The red blood count may be low as a result of hemorrhage. Chemical examination of the stool may show blood. The carcinoembryonic antigen (CEA) titer in the serum may be elevated. This is not a reliable diagnostic indicator of colon cancer, but is useful in watching for recurrence or metastatic disease after surgery. With extensive hepatic metastases, liver function tests become abnormal. Barium enema demonstrates mucosal defects, a space-occupying lesion, or an encircling obstruction. Abdominal CT scan may provide additional information. Endorectal ultrasound is valuable in distal lesions. Chest x-ray may show pulmonary metastases. Colonoscopy with biopsy provides definitive diagnosis.

Course: The overall survival rate in treated colon cancer is about 35%. If complete resection of primary tumor can be carried out, the survival rate is about 55%.

Treatment: The procedure of choice is surgical resection. **Rectal carcinoma** may require abdominoperineal resection with sigmoid colostomy. Tumors higher in the colon may be able to be resected with simple anastomosis of normal bowel above and below the surgical site. Chemotherapy and radiation therapy are valuable adjuncts to surgery in colon carcinoma.

Other diseases of the colon and rectum are discussed in Chapter 11.

Glossary

adenoma: a benign tumor arising from glandular epithelium.
anaplastic: referring to tumor tissue containing primitive, undifferentiated cells, unlike the structurally differentiated cells of normal tissue.
anorexia: loss of appetite.
atelectasis: deflation (collapse) of a segment of lung tissue due to blockage of air passages leading to it.
clone: a colony or family of cells that are all derived from a single ancestor cell.
colostomy: a surgically created opening from the colon to the abdominal wall, through which feces are passed rather than by the rectum; may be temporary or permanent.
dyspnea: shortness of breath.
endorectal: inside the rectum; said of diagnostic or therapeutic instruments or procedures.
effusion: abnormal formation of fluid in a tissue space.
  pleural effusion: accumulation of fluid in the pleural space.
hemoptysis: coughing up blood.
hepatic: pertaining to the liver.
hormone: a chemical messenger produced by glandular tissue and released into the bloodstream to stimulate or inhibit cells or tissues at remote sites.
hyperplasia: an increase in the number of cells in a tissue or organ.
mediastinal: pertaining to the mediastinum, the space between the lungs.
melanoma: a highly malignant tumor arising from pigment cells in the skin.
necrosis: death of tissue due to damage by physical or chemical injury or loss of blood supply.
nocturia: the need to arise from bed at night to urinate.
palliative: directed to the relief of symptoms rather than the elimination of their cause.
palpable: able to be felt (palpated).
paraneoplastic syndrome: a group of symptoms caused by paraneoplastic hormone-like products of neoplastic tissue.
polyp: a tumor protruding from the surface of a mucous membrane.
resection: surgical removal.
transrectal: said of a diagnostic or surgical procedure that is performed through the rectum.

Topics for Study or Discussion

1. Give a general definition of neoplasia, and state three differences between benign and malignant neoplasms.

2. What kind of cancer causes the largest number of cancer deaths in men? In women?

3. Define: carcinogen, debulking, grading, oncology, (chemotherapy) protocol, staging.

4. What are the three principal types of treatment used in cancer? Distinguish curative and palliative therapy.

5. List some of the physical, social, occupational, financial, and psychologic implications of a diagnosis of cancer.

Chapter 6

Trauma and Poisoning

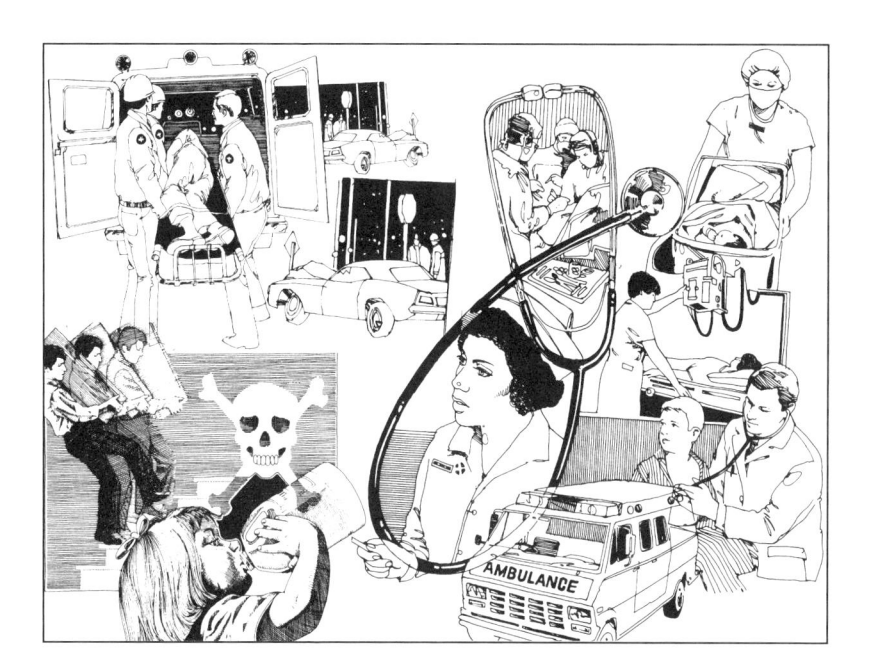

Learning Objectives

Upon completion of this chapter, the student should

- have a general understanding of the various kinds of trauma to which the human body is subject;

- know how physicians examine, diagnose, and treat victims of trauma;

- have basic information about chemical poisoning and its treatment.

This chapter surveys a broad variety of injuries to which the human body is subject. Most of these injuries are due to direct force or violence, but a few result from heat, cold, or radiant energy of various kinds. The chapter ends with a brief consideration of chemical poisoning.

Trauma

Trauma is a general term for an injury of any kind (see box). In this section, the subject of trauma will be discussed under three broad classifications: blunt, closed, or nonpenetrating injuries due to force; penetrating injuries due to force; and injuries of special types, or affecting special body parts or regions.

The Greek noun *trauma* (which Hippocrates, the Father of Medicine, spelled *troma*) comes from the verb *titrosko*, which means 'to wound'. In classical Greek it generally refers to wounds sustained in hand-to-hand combat or in other contact sports.

In modern medicine the word has a wider application. When physicians speak of repetitive trauma syndrome, emotional trauma, microtrauma, and chemical trauma, they are obviously taking the word in the sense of any assault on the integrity of the human organism from outside.

The Latin word *injuria*, from which our **injury** derives, is a compound of *in* (with the sense of 'against' or 'not') and *jus* 'legal right, law'. The original sense was something like 'any violation of a right'; often the term meant simply 'insult' or 'infringement on personal freedom'.

As in the case of *trauma*, the English word **injury** has undergone a considerable shift of meaning. Nowadays it almost always refers to direct physical violence, while the legal sense of 'crime against the person' has largely died out; we speak of accidental injury and of injuring oneself.

Finally, we often hear the phrase ***traumatic injury***, which may seem redundant, since both words mean roughly the same thing. But the sense of this expression is 'injury (gross damage to tissue) that is due to violent application of physical force (rather than to heat, radiant energy, or chemical agents)'.

Closed (Blunt, Nonpenetrating) Injuries

Nonpenetrating injuries result from a wide range of deliberate or accidental applications of force to the body: falls, automobile accidents, mishaps with bulky loads or machinery, criminal assault with fist or blunt instrument, and athletic injuries.

The direct application of blunt force to the body surface usually leads to a **contusion**: bruising or crushing of cutaneous and subcutaneous tissues, muscles, and other structures, as manifested by local swelling, discoloration due to leakage of blood from the circulation, pain, tenderness, and reduced mobility. **Ecchymosis** is the bluish discoloration that appears under the skin at the site of extravasated blood—that is, blood that has leaked from damaged blood vessels. A large accumulation of extravasated blood in a tissue space (under a fingernail, under the skin) is called a **hematoma**.

Contusions vary in extent from mild to life-threatening, depending on the amount of force applied, the way in which it was applied, and the structures or area injured. A severe contusion of muscle, particularly in the thigh, can result in myositis ossificans, the formation of one or more painful lumps in the area of injury due to calcification of damaged muscle tissue or of slowly resolving hematomas. Treatment includes local ice; compression and immobilization as needed with elastic bandaging, padding, or splinting; elevation; rest of the injured part; analgesics (perhaps including narcotics), anti-inflammatory agents, and other drugs as dictated by special circumstances. Surgical drainage of hematomas or repair of damaged tissue is sometimes necessary.

Injuries to bones usually result from blunt force or from some violent twisting or straining action. Any break in a bone is called a **fracture**. A fracture usually causes severe pain and local swelling. There may be obvious deformity of the broken bone and marked impairment of function.

Hundreds of qualifying terms may be added to the noun "fracture"; the following are some of the more frequently used:

comminuted fracture: a fracture resulting in more than two fragments.

compound fracture: a fracture accompanied by an open wound, from which a bone fragment may protrude.

displaced fracture: a fracture in which the relative positions of the fragments are significantly different from what they were before the fracture.

hairline fracture: a fine crack in a bone, barely visible on x-ray examination.

impacted fracture: a fracture in which the end of a long bone is driven into the body of the bone rather than being broken away from it.

stress fracture: a crack in a bone induced by repetitive stress on the same bone (as in jogging or doing aerobic steps) rather than by a single violent force.

The basis of all fracture treatment is simply immobilization during the period of healing. This may be a few days to a few months, depending on the site of the fracture, its size and shape, and the general health of the patient. When a fracture is not immobilized, the result may be a **nonunion**—a failure of the fragments to join together in solid bony union. For many fractures, **external fixation** (plaster or fiberglass cast) suffices; for others, **internal fixation** (wires, screws, pins, or plates inserted through a surgical incision) must be used. Before immobilization is applied, the fracture may require **reduction**: manipulation of the bone fragments so as to bring them as nearly as possible into a normal anatomic relationship. Certain types of fracture (carpal navicular, femoral neck) may interrupt the blood supply to one of the bone fragments, with consequent delay or failure of healing. The **ischemic** (lack of blood supply) fragment may then undergo **avascular necrosis** (death of tissue due to lack of blood supply). Treatment may include a bone graft, in which the patient's own bone, taken from another site, is reduced to small chips and packed into the bony defect. Bone grafting is also used in injury or disease of the spinal column.

Joint injuries commonly result from forces that tend to separate the bones making up the joint, or to drive them into a positional relationship that threatens to crush or tear supporting structures (ligaments, cartilages, joint membranes). **Ligaments** are nonyielding bands of connective tissue that limit the direction and range of movement of a joint. A **sprain** is a stretching or twisting injury to one or more of the ligaments supporting a joint, by some force that tends to deform the joint. The ligaments may be completely divided (particularly in knee injuries), but usually ligament tears are only partial. A sprain usually causes pain, swelling, and restriction of movement of the joint. A severe sprain may lead to chronic or permanent deformity or disability.

Sprains are treated with rest and immobilization (usually by means of splinting or bandaging), compression and elevation of the injured part, ice, analgesics, and nonsteroidal anti-inflammatory agents. Severe ligament tears or damage to articular cartilage may require surgical repair.

When the relationship between two bones at a joint is radically altered by some violent force, the result may be a **dislocation**: a deformity of the joint persisting after the initial application of violence. Often the bones become locked in an abnormal relationship because of their shapes, the pull of ligaments, or muscle spasm. A dislocation is often associated with severe sprain or ligamentous tearing. A **subluxation** is a dislocation of minor degree, without severe deformity.

A dislocation or subluxation causes local pain and more or less evident joint deformity, often with marked restriction in the range of motion. Initial treatment is reduction of the dislocation—restoration of the normal anatomic relationship between the bones involved. Sometimes this requires an open surgical procedure. After reduction the injured joint is immobilized with splinting or bandaging while the supporting structures about the joint heal. Severe damage to joint structures can culminate in ankylosis, a rigid fusion of the tissues causing complete loss of joint mobility.

Violent stretching of a muscle or tendon may partially or completely disrupt its fibers. A **strain** is a muscle or tendon pull causing pain, spasm, and perhaps local swelling and discoloration. The injury usually heals promptly with rest, ice, support, and analgesics as needed. Complete tear or rupture of a muscle (such as the rotator cuff of the shoulder) or tendon (such as the calcaneal tendon of the heel) is less common. Disability can be severe, and surgical repair is often needed.

Open (Penetrating) Wounds

Wounds that break the body surface are usually due to a scraping type of injury or to forceful application of something sharp, such as a knife or broken glass. They may also result from blunt trauma (especially over a bony prominence), from a gunshot, or from a fracture in which a bony fragment tears its way out through the skin (compound fracture). With any penetrating injury there is a risk of infection due to pathogens introduced from outside, including Staphylococcus, Streptococcus, and a variety of other organisms including those that cause tetanus and gas gangrene. In addition, a **foreign body** (needle, bullet, wooden splinter) may be retained within the tissues.

Scraping away of the surface of skin or mucous membrane by violent contact with a rough surface (concrete, gravel) is called an **abrasion**. A severe abrasion can destroy all levels of the skin, resulting in scarring. Often particles of foreign material are embedded in an abrasion and contribute to the amount of damage and the risk of infection and scarring. A deep abrasion may injure tissues far below the skin.

A cutting injury caused by a sharp object is properly called an **incised wound**. (Many health professionals incorrectly call such a wound a laceration. Lacerations are discussed below.) In a cut, or incised wound, some or all layers of the skin are separated, and injury may extend to underlying subcutaneous tissues, muscles, tendons, nerves, blood vessels, and internal organs. When a penetrating injury is caused by a needle, nail, or similar sharp object of small caliber, it is called a **puncture**.

A **gunshot wound** results from penetration of the skin surface by a missile (or missiles, in the form of shot) driven at high velocity by expanding gases generated by the rapid combustion of a charge of explosive. The extent of damage depends on the type of firearm and ammunition, the distance between the firearm and the victim, the site of penetration, and the direction in which the missile is traveling. Gunshot wounds can penetrate or shatter bones, violently damage soft tissues, destroy internal organs, and tear open major blood vessels, with resulting hemorrhage that can be rapidly fatal.

A **laceration** is a tearing of tissue due to blunt violence (collision with wall, furniture, or floor; being struck with a hard ball, a bat, or someone's knee) rather than to something sharp. The skin bursts at the site of a laceration because it is crushed between the injuring object and an underlying bony prominence (chin, elbow, knuckle) or a broad flat bony surface without subcutaneous padding (scalp, shin). Generally there is contusion of the wound edges.

Open wounds are treated by cleansing with surgical soap, irrigation or scrubbing to remove foreign material, application of sterile dressings, and administration of tetanus toxoid or tetanus immune globulin, prophylactic antibiotics, and analgesics as needed. Cuts and lacerations that penetrate all levels of the skin usually require surgical closure. **Debridement** (a French term variously pronounced) refers to the excision of crushed, shredded, or devitalized tissue before surgical repair.

Special Types of Injury

Head Injuries

Blunt or penetrating wounds of the head can cause irreversible damage to the brain, and hemorrhage within the brain or between the brain and the skull. Such injuries are frequently lethal, or result in permanent impairment of mental function.

Cerebral concussion is defined as a violent blow to the skull that causes brief unconsciousness but does no permanent damage to the brain or its supporting structures. In **cerebral contusion**, there is local injury to brain tissue, but again without lasting consequences. **Cerebral laceration** is a still more violent injury in which part of the brain is torn. The outcome is often death or severe permanent impairment (paralysis, seizures, dementia).

Intracranial hemorrhage can be extradural or epidural (between the outermost covering of the brain, the dura mater, and the skull), subdural (beneath the dura mater), subarachnoid (under the arachnoid membrane covering the brain), or intracerebral (within the substance of the brain). **Extradural hemorrhage** usually results from arterial bleeding and often proves rapidly fatal. **Subdural hemorrhage** is often venous, with chronic signs and symptoms (gradually progressing headache, stupor, personality change, or neurologic impairment). **Subarachnoid hemorrhage** is less often due to trauma than to rupture of a **congenital aneurysm** (abnormal bulge or weakness in a cerebral artery, present from birth). Any intracranial hemorrhage is life-threatening because of the danger of irreversible damage from compression of brain tissue within the rigid, nonexpanding skull.

The treatment of head injury demands prompt and decisive action to conserve brain tissue and arrest hemorrhage.

Spinal Injury

Injuries to the spinal cord, particularly at the cervical level, usually result from automobile accidents, falls, or diving accidents. Fracture or dislocation of one or more vertebrae can compress or even sever the spinal cord, with permanent loss of sensation and motor power (including the ability to breathe) at levels below the site of injury. Treatment includes rigid immobilization of the spine until diagnostic evaluation is completed, surgical reduction of dislocation or freeing of compressed nerve tissue, supportive care (including maintenance of breathing function by various types of respirator), and physical therapy to preserve joint and muscle mobility and restore function when possible.

Thoracic Injury

Blunt injury to the chest can fracture ribs and produce severe contusion of heart or lungs. Rib fractures may be so painful that the patient is unable to breathe deeply enough to maintain normal oxygen levels in tissues. Extensive rib fractures can lead to **flail chest**, in which normal respiratory efforts fail because part of the chest wall has lost its normal stability.

Penetrating wounds of the chest, due to stabbing, gunshot wounds, or accidents, endanger the heart and great vessels, the lungs, the esophagus, and other structures within the thorax. Puncture of the heart or a main blood vessel can be almost instantly fatal. Hemorrhage into the pleural cavity is called **hemothorax**.

An open wound of the chest wall can result in **pneumothorax** (presence of air in the pleural cavity). Under normal circumstances, inspiration results when the chest wall moves outward and the diaphragm moves downward, making the lungs expand. With an opening in the chest wall, inspiratory efforts suck atmospheric air into the pleural space so that the lung collapses. If the chest wound acts as a valve, allowing entry of air but not its escape, the pressure of the air in the pleural cavity may rise high enough to displace the mediastinum (the structures between the two lungs) to the opposite side, compressing the normal lung and adding to respiratory compromise.

Management of chest wounds includes vigorous efforts to maintain circulatory and respiratory function and to identify the precise nature, location, and extent of internal injuries so that adequate procedures can be applied in timely fashion to restore structural integrity.

Abdominal Injury

Blunt injury to the abdomen can cause bruising, laceration, or severe hemorrhage of internal organs (liver, spleen, kidney, digestive tract, urinary bladder). In penetrating abdominal injuries, the risk of damage and particularly of hemorrhage is much increased. Puncture of the stomach or intestine releases digestive fluids into the peritoneal cavity and causes chemical **peritonitis**. Hemorrhage into the abdominal cavity is called **hemoperitoneum**.

The diagnosis of abdominal injury depends on careful physical examination, x-ray studies and scans, and peritoneal lavage (injection of fluid through a needle passed through the abdominal wall, followed by its withdrawal and laboratory examination). This procedure can detect blood, digestive fluids, urine, or other substances not normally present.

Management includes supportive care and prompt surgical intervention to repair leaking blood vessels or punctured organs.

Child Abuse (Battered Child Syndrome)

Child abuse is any action by an adult (parent, relative, caregiver, teacher, or other person) that jeopardizes the safety, mental and physical health, and general well-being of a child. This may include physical battering, harshly punitive actions, failure to provide a nurturing home life, inadequate attention to hygiene and nutrition, and gross neglect. Much child abuse results from impulsive or vindictive behavior by a parent, but it often becomes habitual. Often child abuse is just a symptom of personality or mental disorder or of family pathology; alcohol, drug abuse, and a history of having been abused oneself as a child increase the risk that one will abuse children.

Child abuse may appear in numerous forms: severe malnutrition; scars, infections, digestive disorders, and other evidences of neglect; bruises, burns, abrasions, dislocations and fractures, and other evidences of direct physical violence. A special type of child abuse is sexual abuse, which may take many forms. Sexual abuse generally leads to both physical and emotional trauma.

The treatment of child abuse depends on the nature of the injuries sustained. Recognition that abuse has taken place is crucial. Parents often lie about the way in which injuries have occurred, and the physician must constantly be alert to the possibility of abuse. Child abuse is a serious crime. In virtually all jurisdictions, healthcare personnel and others who report suspected child abuse to law enforcement authorities are immune to legal reprisals by the persons accused.

Rape

Rape is sexual intercourse, with penetration, that is against the will of the passive participant. The victim may be forced into submission by violence or intimidation, or may be rendered submissive (or even unconscious) by intoxication with alcohol or drugs. Intercourse with a minor (usually legally defined in this context as a woman under the age of 16) is rape even if the victim consents. Date rape is rape in the setting of a social engagement. Often the phrase is misapplied to seduction (inducement to sexual intercourse by persuasion and enticement, without the use of force or intimidation).

Rape is a felony in all jurisdictions. Many cases go unreported and untreated because the victim is ashamed, or unwilling to submit to questioning by law enforcement officers or to medical examination for diagnosis and collection of evidence. Management includes identification and treatment of all injuries sustained, prophylaxis against sexually transmitted infection and pregnancy, and emotional support and counseling as needed.

Cumulative Trauma Disorder (CTD)

This term refers to various painful or disabling injuries that result not from sudden violent application of force but from repeated stresses and strains on certain body parts, particularly ligaments, tendons, and joints. Currently about one-half of all reported occupational disease conditions are the consequence of repetitive trauma. Lateral epicondylitis (tennis elbow) is a good example. Repetitive activities (usually occupational) that strain the origins of the wrist extensors at the lateral epicondyle of the humerus can induce chronic and disabling pain about the epicondyle. Treatment is rest, immobilization, use of nonsteroidal anti-inflammatory drugs or adrenal steroids, and occasionally surgery. Recovery may be protracted.

Injuries Not Due to Direct Application of Force

Suffocation and Drowning

Suffocation is any stoppage of respiratory effort or obstruction to respiratory air flow. This can come about through chemical or drug effect or injury to the respiratory centers of the brain or from blockage of the airway by swelling, hemorrhage, foreign body, or severe injury. Drowning is suffocation due to filling of the airway and lungs with water. Suffocation is rapidly fatal, causing failure of both oxygenation of the blood and removal of carbon dioxide from tissues.

The treatment of suffocation must be applied promptly. Clearing of the airway is of paramount importance; this may require tracheotomy (cutting into the trachea to bypass the mouth, oropharynx, and larynx). Artificial ventilation must be provided if the patient's breathing efforts are ineffectual or absent. Underlying causes of respiratory arrest must be sought and corrected.

Thermal Burns

Thermal burns are caused by contact of skin or mucous membrane with hot objects, liquids, or vapors. The amount of injury depends on the degree of heat and the extent and duration of contact. High heat induces an intense inflammatory reaction with leakage of fluid into tissues. It also coagulates protein and destroys tissues by vaporization or carbonization. Skin burns are classified as **first degree** (redness of the surface without blistering), **second degree** (redness and blistering), and **third degree** (redness, blistering, and charring). First and second degree burns normally heal without scarring unless they become infected. In third degree burns, the nature and depth of injury usually lead to scarring. Deep burns can destroy tissues below skin level: subcutaneous fat, muscles, nerves, tendons, and even bone. Extensive burns, even when only first degree, typically cause severe biochemical imbalance, due to sequestration of fluid in the burned area with proportionate reduction of blood volume. Dehydration, shock, toxemia, and severe local or systemic infection may complicate any severe burn.

Treatment is aimed at correcting fluid and electrolyte imbalances, relieving pain, and preventing or treating infection. Third degree burns often require grafting.

Cold Injury

The harmful local effects of intense cold (**frostbite**) are similar to those of heat: local inflammation, often with blistering and tissue destruction. Treatment is similar to that for burns.

Exposure to atmospheric cold, or prolonged immersion in cold water, can induce systemic hypothermia, a drop in the rectal (core) temperature below 35°C. The basic treatment is rewarming. Severe hypothermia can lead to profound derangement of physiologic functioning, including cardiac and respiratory arrest. Vigorous resuscitation efforts may be necessary.

Electric Shock

Passage of electrical energy through body tissues (exposure to a source of direct or indirect current, lightning stroke) causes varying degrees of structural damage and functional impairment. At any given voltage, indirect current is much more dangerous than direct. Lightning stroke involves very high voltage exposure for a very brief period. Conduction of electrical energy by living tissue can result in surface or deep burns, extensive damage to skeletal and cardiac muscle with release of myoglobin into the serum and cardiac arrhythmias or arrest, or loss of consciousness. Treatment is dictated by the nature and extent of injury and is largely supportive. The patient must be observed for several days for delayed evidence of damage.

Injury due to Radiant Energy

Depending on the dose, **ionizing radiation** (x-rays, gamma rays) can cause mild or irreversible damage to skin and other tissues. It can alter the chemistry of cells and tissues and induce abnormal cell division and even malignant change. Rapidly proliferating cells, such as those of bone marrow, lymphoid tissue, and the lining of the digestive tract, are particularly vulnerable to damage by radiation. Damage to sex cells (gametes) can lead to abnormalities in future offspring. Anemia, gastrointestinal ulceration, and blood cell malignancies are common consequences of excessive radiation exposure. Total body exposure to high doses of ionizing radiation can lead to a systemic response (radiation sickness) with vomiting, dehydration, weakness, anemia, and heightened susceptibility to infection. Treatment is purely symptomatic and supportive.

Sunlight and ultraviolet radiation from sunlamps or other devices can cause acute cutaneous burns similar to thermal burns. Prolonged or repeated exposure leads to tanning (increased pigment in skin), accelerates aging and degenerative changes in skin, and often induces malignant change. Severe **sunburn** can cause systemic symptoms (fever, vomiting). Treatment is similar to that for thermal burns, but otherwise supportive.

Multiple Trauma

A person who has been injured in an automobile or other high-speed accident, a natural disaster (flood, tornado), an explosion, a fire, the collapse of a building, or a fall from a considerable height, or who has been the victim of criminal assault or warfare, often has extensive trauma of various types and involving various body parts and systems. Patients with multiple trauma are generally treated in hospital emergency departments or trauma centers.

When many victims of multiple trauma must be treated at one facility within a brief period (for example, after a low altitude plane crash or a pileup of many cars on a highway), a procedure called **triage** (literally 'sorting') is used to ensure that available resources will be used for the greatest good of the largest number. Basically, triage means dealing first with those persons who are expected to survive but are most severely injured and in need of immediate treatment, and then with less severely injured persons. Triage also means not expending supplies or personnel time in futile efforts to save persons who are obviously injured beyond any hope of recovery.

The treatment of multiple trauma requires the coordinated efforts of many health professionals—physicians, nurses, technicians, and practitioners of surgical specialties such as orthopedic, thoracic, neurologic, and plastic surgery. Diagnostic procedures are carried out simultaneously with initial resuscitation efforts.

The physician's first concern is to ensure that the patient has a clear airway, since suffocation is rapidly fatal. Secondly, if the patient is not breathing, artificial ventilation must be started at once. The third priority is heart action and the adequacy of blood flow to tissues. (These can be remembered by the mnemonic ABC, for Airway, Breathing, Circulation.)

When respiration and circulation have been stabilized, a full assessment of the patient is undertaken to find and manage all injuries. Intracranial, thoracic, and abdominal injuries are carefully investigated and intensively treated. Bleeding sites are identified and surgically repaired. Fractures, dislocations, contusions, and lacerations are examined and treated with the same diligence and thoroughness as if each injury were the only one the patient had.

Poisoning

A poison is any chemical substance that has a harmful effect on the body through contact with skin or mucous membranes, ingestion, injection, inhalation, or absorption by any other route. Poisoning can occur accidentally or with homicidal or suicidal intent. It may be due to inappropriate use of prescribed medicines; abuse of illicit drugs; exposure to insecticides, household chemicals, or industrial toxins or wastes; contamination of food or water; or inhalation of toxic gases, vapors, or dusts. A biologic poison is one that is produced by a living thing, such as snake or insect venom and plant irritants and toxins.

The effects of poisons on the body are extremely various. Strong mineral acids and alkalis have a rapid irritant or corrosive action on skin and mucous membranes. Benzene can impair the production of blood cells by bone marrow, but only after repeated or prolonged exposure. Inhalation of carbon monoxide interferes with the ability of red blood cells to carry oxygen. Some chemical poisons have broadly deleterious effects on many types of cells and tissues; others, particularly some drugs, cause highly specific injury or malfunction, such as paralysis, loss of vision, or abnormal heart rhythm.

The treatment of poisoning begins with recognition that poisoning has occurred and identification of the poison and the amount taken or absorbed. Resuscitative efforts may take priority over other activities. Intensive evaluation and monitoring, with blood and other studies as needed, must be continued until the patient's condition is stable. General measures are emptying the stomach by lavage or by inducing vomiting, administration of drugs to stabilize heart action and blood pressure, and use of oxygen and artificial ventilation when indicated. More specific measures are available for a limited number of poisons in the form of antidotes. For example, acetaminophen poisoning is treated with acetylcysteine; cyanide poisoning with sodium thiosulfate and sodium nitrite intravenously; lead poisoning with edetate calcium disodium; rattlesnake envenomation with antivenin.

Topics for Study or Discussion

1. In a patient with multiple trauma, what is the treating physician's first concern?

2. Point out some major differences between blunt and penetrating injuries to the trunk of the body.

3. Define: concussion, contusion, laceration, trauma, triage.

4. Mention some medical problems discussed in this chapter that may have psychiatric or legal implications.

5. Give examples of chemical and biological poisoning; of local and systemic effects of poisons; of specific and nonspecific treatment for poisoning.

Chapter 7

Diseases of the Skin

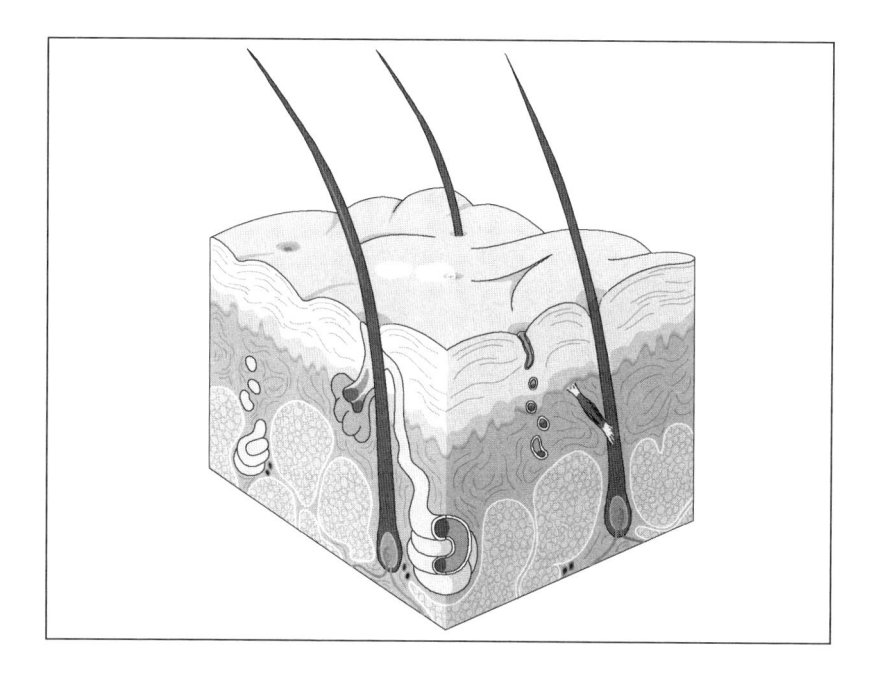

Learning Objectives

Upon completion of this chapter, the student should

- know the basic anatomy and physiology of the skin;

- have a general knowledge of the variety of symptoms of diseases of the skin, and diagnostic procedures used to assess them;

- understand signs, symptoms, and treatment of common diseases affecting the skin.

Anatomy and Physiology of the Skin

The **skin** is the largest "organ" in the body, and the most accessible for diagnosis and treatment. It covers the entire body and consists of two layers, the outer epidermis and the inner dermis or true skin.

The **epidermis** is a thin sheet of squamous (flat) epithelial cells, several layers thick, which are constantly renewed from the deepest layer, growing steadily outward to replace cells worn away. Most of the cells of the epidermis are keratinocytes, containing a horny material, keratin, that provides mechanical toughness to the outer skin surface. A few cells in the epidermis are pigment cells, containing melanin, which imparts to the skin its characteristic color, varying according to race, familial characteristics, age, sun exposure, and other factors. Pigment distribution is more intense in certain areas, such as around the nipples and in the anogenital region. At bodily orifices, the epidermis undergoes a transition to mucous membrane.

The **dermis** is a tough layer of connective tissue containing blood vessels, sensory nerves, hair follicles, and sebaceous and sweat glands. Hair protects the body surface and also provides some thermal insulation. Each hair follicle is accompanied by a sebaceous gland, which produces oil (sebum) that is discharged on the skin surface and exerts protective and moisture-retaining effects. Sweat glands secrete sweat, which helps in temperature regulation.

A Glossary of Cutaneous Signs and Symptoms

The skin is subject to numerous disorders, some local and others manifestations of systemic disease. Despite the wide variety of these disorders and their causes, the signs of skin disease can be reduced to a relatively small number of distinctive lesions. These are named and defined in the following glossary. A more general glossary appears at the end of the chapter, containing other new or unfamiliar terms that appear in the chapter.

Skin lesions are divided into **primary** (resulting from a skin disease) and **secondary** (resulting from complications of the basic disease, including the effects of scratching and infection).

Primary Skin Lesions

bulla (also, **bleb**): a blister; a thin-walled sac exceeding 1 cm in diameter and containing clear fluid.

comedo (plural, **comedones**): a papule consisting of a dilated sebaceous duct or gland plugged with keratin debris.

cyst: an abnormal thick-walled structure containing fluid or semisolid material.

ecchymosis: a broad zone of red or purple discoloration (more than 1 cm in diameter) due to hemorrhage under the epidermis.

macule: a clearly defined zone of skin, less than 1 cm in diameter, differing from surrounding skin in color but not in texture or elevation.

nodule: a firm elevation of the skin surface more than 1 cm in diameter.

papule: a clearly defined zone of skin, less than 1 cm in diameter, that is raised above surrounding skin, and may differ from it in color or texture.

petechia: a pinhead-sized, round, red or purple macule due to extravasation of blood under the epidermis.

plaque: a clearly defined zone of skin, more than 1 cm in diameter, that is raised above surrounding skin, and may differ from it in color or texture; a plaque may consist of many confluent papules.

purpura: a purple zone of hemorrhage in the skin, larger than a petechia but less than 1 cm in diameter; may be macular (flat) or papular (raised).

pustule: a thin-walled sac containing pus.

telangiectasis: dilatation of one or more small blood vessels visible through the skin.

vesicle: a small thin-walled sac containing clear fluid.

wheal (weal, welt): a hive; a small zone of edema in skin, which may be red or white; wheals are typically multiple and appear and disappear abruptly.

Secondary Skin Lesions

cicatrix (scar): a zone of fibrous tissue occurring at the site of a healed injury or inflammatory or destructive lesion extending into the dermis.

crust: a hard, friable, irregular layer of dried blood, serum, pus, tissue debris, or any combination of these adherent to the surface of injured or inflamed skin.

erosion: a surface defect in the epidermis produced by rubbing or scratching.

eschar: the crust that forms on a burn.

excoriation: abrasion of the epidermal surface by scratching.
fissure: a linear defect or crack in the continuity of the epidermis.
keloid: a firm, nodular, irregular, often pigmented mass of fibrous tissue representing a hypertrophic scar.
lichenification: thickening, coarsening, and pigment change of skin due to chronic irritation, usually scratching.
pit: a small depression in the skin resulting from local atrophy or scarring after trauma or inflammation.
scab: see *crust*.
scale: a flake of epidermis shed from the skin surface.
scar: see *cicatrix*.
ulcer: a cutaneous defect extending into the dermis.

Diagnostic Procedures in Disorders of the Skin

Inspection with good lighting, natural if possible, and magnification as needed.

Diascopy: inspection of red or purplish lesions through a transparent plastic or glass plate, which compresses the skin. If the color is due to dilated blood vessels, it blanches (fades) with compression; color due to deposition of pigment, including blood pigment, in tissues is not altered by surface pressure.

Wood light: an ultraviolet lamp with a filter that selects wavelengths under which certain funguses infecting skin or hair fluoresce brightly.

Microscopic examination of scrapings from the skin to identify fungal material, the mites of scabies, and distinctive kinds of scales; skin scrapings are usually treated with potassium hydroxide (KOH) and heat, which partially or completely dissolve human tissue but leave fungal elements unchanged.

Culture of exudate, pus, crusts, or scrapings for bacteria, fungi, or viruses.

Tzanck smear: a stained smear of material from an ulcer or vesicle. Changes in cells indicate viral infection but cannot distinguish varicella (discussed in Chapter 3) and herpes simplex (discussed below).

Blood studies may identify underlying, perhaps systemic, conditions, or provide additional information about the skin disorder.

Skin tests with various allergens (molds, pollens, medicines) administered by patch, scratch, or intradermal injection can identify and roughly measure skin sensitivity to these substances.

Biopsy: removal of a specimen of abnormal skin by shaving away the surface with a fine blade or removing a plug of skin with a round punch. Sometimes the lesion is completely excised and submitted for pathologic examination.

Dermatitis

Inflammation of the skin, a broad general term encompassing a variety of disorders. Three of the most common are discussed below.

Atopic Dermatitis (Eczema)

A chronic pruritic condition of the skin.

Cause: Unknown. Most patients have a personal or family history of allergy. May be exacerbated by irritants, emotional stress.

History: Recurrent itching, particularly affecting the back of the neck and the antecubital and popliteal areas, usually causing constant scratching.

Physical Examination: Patches of redness, sometimes with weeping, scaling, or vesiculation. Excoriations and lichenification from scratching. Sometimes evidence of secondary infection.

Diagnostic Tests: Scratch tests and RAST may be positive for many allergens.

Course: Chronic, with remissions and exacerbations. Secondary infection may result from scratching, and very chronic lesions may progress to fibrosis or pigmentation.

Treatment: Avoidance of known allergens, irritants, strong soaps, excessive wetting of skin and excessive bathing. Moisturizers to restore texture of skin, and topical adrenocortical steroids to reduce itching and inflammation.

Seborrheic Dermatitis

A scaly dermatitis of parts of the skin richly supplied with oil glands.

Cause: Unknown. There is a genetic predisposition. The response to treatment with antifungal medicine suggests that the disease may be an inflammatory reaction to normal skin fungi such as *Pityrosporum ovale*.

History: Itching, oiliness, scaling of scalp, face, and other areas.
Physical Examination: Erythema, dryness or oiliness, scaling of the scalp, face, eyelids (marginal blepharitis), and body folds.
Course: Secondary infection, bacterial or fungal, may occur.
Treatment: Seborrheic dermatitis of the scalp is treated with selenium sulfide shampoos. On the skin, topical adrenocortical steroids and topical ketoconazole, an antifungal, are about equally effective in controlling symptoms.

Contact Dermatitis

Dermatitis resulting from contact with an irritant or allergen.

Cause: Numerous substances, including industrial chemicals, cosmetics, toiletries, and household products, can cause either an irritant or allergic type of contact dermatitis. Irritant contact dermatitis results from direct chemical attack on the skin and typically produces symptoms within minutes of exposure. Allergic contact dermatitis occurs only in sensitized persons, and there may be a latent period of 2-5 days between exposure and appearance of symptoms.

History: Itching, burning, stinging, with variable amounts of swelling, redness, and other physical signs, on parts of the skin that have been exposed to the causative agent.

Physical Examination: Redness, swelling, vesicles or bullae, weeping, crusting. Signs of damage from scratching or of secondary infection may be present.

Course: Secondary infection may occur.

Treatment: Avoidance of the cause, soothing applications, topical or even systemic adrenocortical steroids.

Infections and Infestations of the Skin

The skin, being the first line of defense against bodily invasion, is exposed to numerous physical, chemical, and biological assaults. Many types of skin infection (bacterial, viral, and fungal) occur, some of them largely limited to the skin. In addition, the skin and hair are subject to parasitic infestation. Only the more common cutaneous infections and infestations are discussed here.

Impetigo

A spreading bacterial infection of the skin causing itching and crusted sores.

Cause: Staphylococci, sometimes streptococci. Infection may begin in a trivial cut or abrasion. Impetiginization refers to the development of impetigo in an area of skin already damaged by a noninfectious dermatitis. Scratching and poor personal hygiene, particularly among children, lead to rapid spread of lesions and often transmission to household contacts, schoolmates, or playmates.

History: Itching and crusted sores, especially on the face.

Physical Examination: Macules, vesicles, bullae, pustules, and copious gummy purulent exudate forming honey-colored crusts on an erythematous base. In severe infection there may be fever.

Diagnostic Tests: Smear and culture can identify the causative bacteria.

Course: Without treatment, increasing spread often occurs. Systemic effects (toxemia, dehydration) may occur in children, particularly those already debilitated by disease or malnutrition. A severe form of impetigo known as ecthyma may leave scars.

Treatment: Strict attention to personal hygiene; isolation may be appropriate. For most cases of impetigo, the antibiotic mupirocin applied as an ointment is curative. In the presence of extensive disease, fever, or toxemia, antibiotics are administered systemically.

Folliculitis

Bacterial infection in hair follicles.

Cause: Invasion of hair follicles (the weak point in the body's armor) by bacteria, usually staphylococci. Factors that tend to reduce the resistance of the skin to infection (prolonged pressure, friction, excessive perspiration, chemical irritation, diabetes mellitus) predispose to folliculitis. Any severe bacterial infection of the skin may spread to surrounding hair follicles (satellite folliculitis). Infection beginning in just one follicle can be widely propagated by shaving (face in men, legs in women). Hot tub folliculitis is often due to *Pseudomonas aeruginosa*. Folliculitis without demonstrable infection occurs in persons exposed to oil (industrial lubricants, cosmetics) and in those treated with adrenocortical steroids.

History: Itching and burning of hairy skin, with tiny painful lumps at the bases of hairs.

Physical Examination: Pustules in hair follicles. Occasionally generalized erythema and crusting. Distribution of lesions provides clues as to underlying cause.

Course: May become chronic. Abscess formation may occur, and even bacteremia and septicemia.

Treatment: Topical mupirocin is generally effective. Shaving of affected areas should be discontinued until infection resolves. Systemic antibiotics may be needed for severe infections or those contracted from hot tubs. Hot tub water should be chlorinated.

Other Bacterial Infections of the Skin

Bacterial infections of the skin can take a number of other forms. **Pyoderma** is a general term for any purulent (pus-forming) infection of the skin. An **abscess** is a sharply localized bacterial infection, usually due to staphylococci, in which pus forms in a tissue space walled off from surrounding tissues by fibrin, coagulated tissue fluids, and eventually fibrous tissue. A **furuncle** is a deep, solitary abscess; a **carbuncle** is a spreading lesion made up of furuncles communicating by subcutaneous passages.

Cellulitis refers to a type of infection occurring in soft tissues, including the skin, whose cardinal features are diffuse and spreading tissue swelling, redness, pain, and fever. Cellulitis is usually due to streptococci; a particularly severe form, with a sharply circumscribed border, bulla formation, and often septicemia, is called **erysipelas**. Abscesses, furuncles, and carbuncles are treated by surgical incision and drainage. Cellulitis and erysipelas respond to antibiotics given orally or by injection. Antibiotic treatment is guided by results of cultures of pus, tissue fluid, or blood.

Fungal Infections of the Skin

Tinea Corporis (Tinea Circinata, Ringworm of the Body)

Superficial fungal infection of the skin (see box).

Cause: Fungi of the genera *Epidermophyton, Microsporum,* and *Trichophyton*. Transmission from infected persons or animals sometimes occurs. Moisture and friction favor invasion of skin.

Diseases of the Skin • 109

History: One or more slowly expanding round or oval patches of red, scaly skin, usually on exposed surfaces, with a variable amount of itching. There may be a history of recent new exposure to domestic animals or to persons with similar lesions.

Physical Examination: Lesions are pink, red, or tan, round or oval and sharply circumscribed, and covered with fine scales. The outer border of a lesion is raised slightly, and with continuing expansion of the margin, the skin near the center of the lesion gradually clears and assumes a normal appearance.

Diagnostic Tests: Scrapings of scales heated with potassium hydroxide (KOH) often show fungal material on microscopic examination. Culture on Sabouraud's medium may be required to confirm the presence of fungi. Examination with Wood light shows characteristic fluorescence only when infection is due to species of *Microsporum*.

Course: Tinea may become chronic and widespread, with extension to scalp, hair, and nails. Secondary bacterial infection may complicate diagnosis and treatment. In some persons an autoimmune phenomenon called a **dermatophytid** or **id reaction** may cause eruption of vesicular lesions on areas not infected with fungus, particularly on the hands.

Treatment: Numerous antifungal medicines are effective in topical form. Topical adrenocortical steroids may also be used if inflammation and itching are severe. Systemic antifungal treatment may be needed when infection is severe or resistant to topical treatment.

Other Superficial Fungal Infections of the Skin

The fungal organisms responsible for tinea corporis can also cause more localized infections. In **tinea capitis** (ringworm of the scalp), infected hairs break off at the scalp surface, leaving patchy areas that

---

The long-established lay term *ringworm* causes much misunderstanding and consternation. Skin diseases known by this name are not due to worms, and physicians never thought they were. The word *ring* in *ringworm* refers to the circular shape of the lesions, with central clearing. Worm is just a metaphorical allusion to the "moth-eaten" appearance of skin infected by various superficial fungi, clothes-eating moth larvae being incorrectly called worms. *Tinea*, the Latin term for ringworm, also means 'moth'.

appear bald, often with black dots representing the roots of broken-off hairs. Mild itching and scaling may occur. Treatment is with oral antifungals such as griseofulvin and selenium sulfide shampoo. **Kerion** is a complication, with boggy edema and exudation of pus though hair follicle openings. **Tinea pedis** (athlete's foot) causes erythema, itching, scaling, fissuring, maceration, and vesicle formation of varying degree, particularly between the toes. **Tinea cruris** (jock itch) is a similar infection of the groin. **Tinea versicolor,** caused by *Malassezia furfur*, consists of variable numbers of white to tan macules with very fine scales. Patches are lighter than surrounding tanned skin, but darker than surrounding untanned skin, hence the name *versicolor* 'changing colors'. Tinea pedis, tinea cruris, and tinea versicolor usually respond to topical antifungals.

Tinea unguium (onychomycosis) is probably the most important chronic nail disease. Fungal infection of fingernails and toenails causes discoloration, deformity, splitting, crumbling of nails, and separation from nailbeds, generally without other symptoms. Oral antifungal treatment, usually for several months, is standard. Topical methods and even avulsion of infected nails are sometimes used.

Candidiasis (or candidosis; infection of skin and mucous membranes with the yeastlike fungus *Candida albicans*) causes shiny, sharply delimited patches of intense erythema with itching or burning. Infection is more common in diabetics, and typically occurs on areas where two skin surfaces are in apposition, with trapping of moisture: under the breasts, in the anogenital area, and in skin folds of obese persons. Diagnosis is confirmed by microscopic examination for hyphae or culture. Treatment is topical. Infections in the mouth (called thrush) and in the vagina are treated with antifungal formulations intended specifically for those areas.

Viral Infections of the Skin

Herpes Simplex

Local viral infection of skin or mucous membranes, causing vesicular lesions, typically recurrent.

Cause: Herpesvirus type 1 (oral, labial, facial herpes) and type 2 (genital herpes). Transmission is by direct contact with an infected person, not necessarily with visible lesions. Genital herpes is a sexually transmitted disease. The virus may lie dormant for months or years before causing symptoms. Viral activation, with ensuing skin eruption, may be triggered by physical or emotional stress, fever or respiratory infection (hence the lay terms "cold sore" and "fever blister"), sun exposure, and menstruation.

History: Clusters of small, painful vesicles about the nose or lips or on the genitals. These often recur in the same place, at greater or lesser intervals, in response to triggering factors mentioned above, or for no apparent reason. Vesicles may ulcerate. Women with genital herpes may have severe pain on urination. The first episode of infection is typically the most severe, and may be accompanied by fever.

Physical Examination: A cluster of 4-6 small vesicles or ulcers on an erythematous, edematous base. With a first infection there are often fever and regional lymphadenitis. Secondary infection may cause pustule formation, crusting, and even impetigo (discussed above).

Diagnostic Tests: Tzanck smear of material from lesions shows multinucleated giant cells with cytoplasmic inclusions, confirming viral infection but not specific for herpes. Viral culture yields more specific proof of herpes infection.

Course: An episode of infection typically runs its course in about a week, somewhat longer when it is the patient's first infection. Secondary bacterial infection may lead to exacerbation of symptoms. Intrauterine infection is associated with abortion or fetal damage. A child delivered through an infected birth canal may acquire localized or widespread neonatal infection, typically severe. Ocular infection with herpes simplex virus causes herpetic (dendritic) keratitis, a severe ulcerative disorder of the cornea that can lead to visual impairment.

Treatment: Analgesics and topical applications to control pain. Topical or (preferably) systemic treatment with antiviral drugs (acyclovir, valacyclovir).

Warts (Verrucae)

Virally induced coarse papules of the skin and mucous membranes.

Cause: **Human papillomavirus** (**HPV**), of which about 80 types have been identified by immunologic means. Most types preferentially affect particular areas (plantar warts on soles of the feet, genital warts on the external genitalia or uterine cervix). Transmission is by direct contact. Genital warts are transmitted sexually. Scratching and picking at lesions causes autoinoculation (implantation of infective viral material at new sites, with spread of lesions).

History: One or more papules on skin surface, or on anogenital mucosa. Mild itching may occur, and occasionally bleeding.

Physical Examination: One or more coarsely textured papules, varying from flat (on the sole of the foot or the face) to elevated (on the hands or the genitals). Typical genital warts are narrow-based, raised, and tend to come to a point; lesions of this type are called **condylomata acuminata** (singular, **condyloma acuminatum**). There may be evidence of excoriation or damage from scratching, picking, or crude attempts at removal. Secondary infection may occur.

Diagnostic Tests: Diagnosis is usually clinically evident, but biopsy can provide histologic confirmation. Wart virus cannot be cultured. Cervical infection produces characteristic changes on Pap smear, but the Pap smear is not an adequate screening test for HPV infection. Suspicious lesions treated with dilute acetic acid become chalky gray or white (acetowhitening) if they are warts. These areas are examined with a colposcope (a low-power microscope with light source, adapted for viewing the cervix through a vaginal speculum) and biopsies are taken.

Course: HPV infection is chronic and difficult to eradicate. Infection may resolve spontaneously after a time, but meanwhile other lesions may have developed, or the condition may have been transmitted to others. Genital infection with certain types of HPV is now recognized as a leading cause of cervical carcinoma, and is probably also associated with genital cancers in men.

Treatment: Numerous treatments are available, none of them perfectly satisfactory. Choice of treatment depends partly on the site of infection. Surgical excision, electrocautery, laser ablation, and cryotherapy (freezing with liquid nitrogen or a cryoprobe) are currently the most popular methods. Others include destruction with caustic chemicals such as salicylic acid, bichloracetic acid, and podophyllin, and injection of interferon directly into lesions.

Parasitic Infestations

Scabies

A chronic, pruritic eruption due to burrowing of mites in the skin.

Cause: The itch mite, *Sarcoptes scabiei*, a microscopic parasite that burrows under the skin surface and lays eggs. Transmission is from person to person by direct contact, probably also by indirect contact (sharing of toilets, showers, towels, clothing, bedding). Itching is due not to the mere presence of mites but to a sensitivity reaction to foreign mite protein; hence symptoms may not appear for about a month after infection.

History: Chronic itching, more intense at night, associated with formation of reddish papules and linear raised lesions.

Physical Examination: Reddish papules and burrows, found most often on the hands (finger webs), wrists, elbows, nipples, buttocks, and genitalia, never on the face or scalp. There may be evidence of excoriation, lichenification, or secondary infection.

Diagnostic Tests: The diagnosis is usually clinically evident. Microscopic examination of scrapings from lesions may show mites.

Course: Relentlessly chronic without treatment: an older name for scabies is "seven-year itch." In debilitated persons, especially children, secondary infection may cause extensive weeping and crusting.

Treatment: Topical treatment with permethrin, lindane, or crotamiton is generally curative. Itching may be treated with oral or topical antipruritics.

Pediculosis (Phthiriasis)

Human cutaneous infestation with lice.

Cause: The body louse (*Pediculus corporis*), the head louse (*Pediculus capitis*), and the pubic louse (*Pthirus pubis*; see box). These six-legged arthropods, visible to the naked eye, live and reproduce on the body surface and derive their sustenance from the host's blood, which they obtain by puncturing the skin. They remain in position by grasping body or scalp hairs, and also attach their nits (eggs) to hairs. Eggs hatch in about two weeks and females become sexually mature in another two weeks; hence a single louse (if a pregnant female) can grow to a substantial colony in about a month. Transmission is from person to person; pubic louse infestation is a sexually transmitted disease. Indirect transmission (from sharing bathroom facilities, clothing, hats, bedding) also occurs.

History: Itching in the infested area. Visible, mobile lice on body or scalp hairs, possibly along with nits. Minute dark spots may be noted on underwear; these are deposits of louse feces.

Physical Examination: With adequate illumination, lice and often nits are plainly visible on hairs. Fine blue patches may be noted on skin at sites where lice have fed. There may be indications of excoriations or secondary infection.

Course: Without treatment, colonies can become very large. Lice do not burrow under the skin or penetrate body orifices. *Pthirus* does not transmit diseases. *Pediculus* is a vector of typhus and plague in parts of the world where these diseases are endemic.

Treatment: Topical pyrethrin or lindane, left on the skin long enough to kill both adult lice and eggs, are curative.

The genus name *Pthirus* was derived incorrectly from *phtheir*, the Greek word for 'louse'. Although writers and editors constantly "correct" the spelling to *Phthirus*, the "wrong" spelling *Pthirus* is officially "right."

The next time you use the expression "lousy" or "nit-picking" in a metaphorical sense, stop and think what you are saying.

Acne Vulgaris

A chronic eruption of **comedones**, papules, pustules, and cysts occurring primarily in adolescence.

Causes. The ultimate cause is unknown. There may be a genetic predisposition (identical twins are equally affected). The disease tends to be worse in males, but does not occur in castrated males. It comes on about the time of puberty and typically resolves within 5-8 years, but may persist into the middle and late 20s or beyond. Acne or acneform lesions develop in Cushing syndrome, including the type induced by treatment with adrenocortical steroids; in women with hyperandrogenism of any cause; and in persons exposed to certain chemicals (chloracne, due to industrial exposure to chlorine; iodism, due to medicinal administration of iodide). Acne typically gets worse during times of emotional stress.

The lesions of acne develop in oil (sebaceous) glands, apparently as a result of heightened sebum production that leads to retention of sebum and plugging of gland ducts. Plugged, enlarged glands are called comedones (singular, comedo). These are colloquially called whiteheads when closed, and blackheads when the gland orifices are open, exposing sebum plugs, which darken as a result of chemical changes (not dirt). Very large comedones form cysts. Retained sebum is broken down by bacteria (*Propionibacterium acnes*) or spontaneous chemical changes to form fatty acids, which cause local inflammation and induce a foreign body reaction. Surface bacteria (staphylococci) invade inflamed tissue to produce pustules. Symptoms are aggravated by application of greasy or oily cosmetics and by repetitive picking or squeezing of lesions. Healing of pustules may be protracted, and may leave pits or scars.

History: Appearance of lesions varying in type (blackheads, whiteheads, papules, pustules, cysts), number, distribution, and severity on the face, upper back, and chest; rarely elsewhere.

Physical Examination: Essentially as above.

Diagnostic Tests: Culture may be useful to identify unusual organisms causing secondary infection. Other laboratory studies may disclose underlying or contributing causes.

Course: Eventually, spontaneous remission occurs. This can take years, however, and in the meantime the patient may suffer severe emotional distress. The course of cystic acne may be especially protracted, and any severe case of acne is likely to leave some scarring.

Treatment: Diet is no longer regarded as having an important influence on the severity of the disease. Numerous topical and systemic medicines are used in the treatment of acne. Vigorous skin hygiene with greaseless soaps and cleansers is the foundation of treatment. Topical drugs include benzoyl peroxide, tretinoin, and antibiotics (clindamycin, erythromycin). Antibiotics such as tetracycline, minocycline, and erythromycin may also be used by mouth for long periods. Expression of sebum from comedones with a comedo extractor by a physician may reduce symptoms. Injection of adrenocortical steroid into lesions may also help by lessening local inflammation. Isotretinoin taken by mouth for 4-6 months induces lengthy, usually permanent resolution of acne, but it is reserved for severe cases because of side effects (peeling of lips in 90%; elevation of blood cholesterol in 15%; abnormal liver function tests; grave risk of fetal damage if taken by a pregnant patient).

Rosacea (Acne Rosacea)

A reddish facial eruption occurring in the middle-aged and elderly. **Cause**: Unknown. Occurs more commonly in persons with migraine headaches. Responds to antibiotic treatment. Prolonged application of potent topical adrenocorticosteroids to the face can induce a reaction similar to rosacea.

History: Burning and flushing of the face, with patchy or diffuse rosy tint, papules, and sometimes pustules or excessive sebum production.

Physical Examination: As noted above. The cheeks, nose, and chin show a faint to bright inflammatory blush. Papules, pustules, telangiectases (visible patches of dilated skin vessels), and oiliness are usually present to some degree. Inflammation of the eyelids and even the cornea may occur. In some patients marked hyperplasia of the tissues of the nose (**rhinophyma**) eventually develops.

Course: Rosacea is highly chronic, but treatment provides a fair degree of control.

Treatment: Topical metronidazole or other antibiotics provide improvement in symptoms. Oral antibiotics and topical corticosteroids may be required. Lasers can obliterate telangiectases. For severe rhinophyma, plastic surgery is required.

Urticaria (Hives)

An acute, often transitory eruption of intensely itchy papules or wheals.

Cause: Urticaria is caused by a release of histamine from mast cells in the dermis, with resultant local edema, capillary dilatation, and stimulation of nerve endings. Many factors can incite this reaction: allergies to food (shellfish, strawberries), medicines (aspirin, penicillin), insect bites or stings (beestings), nonallergic sensitivity to medicines (atropine, codeine), parasitic infestation, sunlight, cold, heat (cholinergic urticaria), and even, in susceptible individuals. simple stroking of the skin (dermographism).

History: Sudden onset of a localized or generalized eruption of intensely itchy wheals or papules, which may be transitory.

Physical Examination: Wheals (raised white or red papules) surrounded by erythema. Wheals may be round or scalloped and confluent. Signs of scratching may be evident.

Diagnostic Tests: Blood studies and allergic screening may indicate the underlying cause, but usually do not.

Course: Urticaria often occurs in attacks at intervals of a few hours, but typically resolves within one or two weeks unless continued exposure to the causative agent occurs. Urticaria persisting beyond one month may point to occult infection or malignancy.
Complications: Secondary infection due to scratching.
Treatment: Severe urticaria responds to intramuscular epinephrine. Antihistamines such as diphenhydramine or hydroxyzine may be given orally or by injection to control an acute attack. Regular use of antihistamines prevents or mitigates further attacks. The nonsedating antihistamines terfenadine and astemizole may be useful prophylactically even though they are ineffective in other forms of pruritus. Doxepin, a tricyclic antidepressant, is also effective either orally or topically. In severe cases, topical and systemic corticosteroids may be used.

Vitiligo

Patches of depigmentation widely distributed over the skin, due to destruction of pigment cells. The condition is found in about 1% of the population, and occurs with increased frequency in persons with diabetes mellitus, hyperthyroidism, hypothyroidism, hypoadrenocorticism (Addison disease), and gastric carcinoma. PUVA (psoralen + ultraviolet A) treatment, using topical methoxsalen and ultraviolet light, may provide some improvement. The best method of management is often judicious use of cosmetics.

Psoriasis

A chronic skin disorder characterized by scaly plaques.
Cause: Increased proliferation of epidermal cells. Evidently an autoimmune disorder, to which some persons are genetically predisposed.
History: Plaques of scaly thickening of the skin, particularly the scalp, knees, and elbows, with moderate itching. Nails and joints may also be affected.
Physical Examination: Reddish-purple thickened plaques of skin covered with silvery, firmly adherent scales. Pitting or stippling of nails and inflammation of joints, particularly the distal interphalangeal joints, may also be noted. In guttate psoriasis the plaques are small and numerous. **Koebner phenomenon** (formation of lesions at sites of trauma) may be noted.

Diagnostic Tests: Skin biopsy (usually unnecessary) shows characteristic changes in the epidermis.

Treatment: Topical steroids, calcipotriene, tar ointments; tar shampoos to the scalp. UVB (ultraviolet B); PUVA (psoralen + ultraviolet A). Oral methotrexate, etretinate, cyclosporine.

Pityriasis Rosea

A mild, benign, self-limited scaly eruption.

Cause: Possibly viral. More common in spring and fall. The male:female attack rate is 2:3. Person-to-person transmission has not been demonstrated.

History: Appearance of a solitary scaly patch on the skin, followed in 1-2 weeks by a generalized eruption of similar but smaller lesions. Itching is mild or absent.

Physical Examination: A widespread eruption of oval fawn-colored macules with fine scales on the trunk and proximal extremities. The hands, face, and feet are typically spared. Trunk lesions follow a segmental distribution, especially on the back, giving a "Christmas tree" appearance.

Diagnostic Tests: Because pityriasis simulates secondary syphilis, a serologic test for syphilis is often done to rule out that possibility.

Course: Lesions disappear spontaneously in about 6 weeks.

Treatment: Ultraviolet treatments and topical or oral steroids may abolish symptoms, but treatment is seldom needed since itching is mild, affected body parts can easily be covered by clothing, and spontaneous resolution within weeks is virtually certain.

Malignant Neoplasms of the Skin

Basal Cell Carcinoma

A slowly growing, waxy or pearly papule with telangiectatic vessels, appearing usually on parts of the body exposed to sunlight, particularly the face. Most appear in the middle-aged or elderly. Ulceration and widespread erosion may occur if treatment is delayed, but metastasis is rare. Treatment is by surgical excision, including Mohs chemosurgery and cryotherapy.

Squamous Cell Carcinoma

A hard red nodule appearing on sun-exposed skin, usually in a middle-aged or elderly person. The lesion may develop in a pre-existing actinic keratosis and may rapidly ulcerate. Metastasis is uncommon. Treatment is by excision.

Malignant Melanoma

A pigmented malignancy of the skin that develops in persons of all ages, progresses rapidly, metastasizes widely, and is fatal without treatment. Among malignancies melanoma ranks ninth in incidence, and incidence is increasing. At least some cases are due to sun exposure. Melanoma can develop anew or in a previously benign nevus (pigmented spot). Features of a pigmented lesion that suggest malignancy are irregularity of shape or border, uneven distribution of pigment, pink, blue, or black color, bleeding or ulceration, and rapid enlargement. Treatment is by excision. Prognosis depends on the thickness of the tumor (Breslow classification) or the depth of invasion (Clark classification). In metastatic disease, radiation and chemotherapy may prolong survival.

Disorders of Hair

Although the visible part of scalp and body hair is not living tissue, the follicles in which hair is formed are subject to a number of disorders.

Alopecia (Baldness)

Hair loss leading to temporary or permanent, patchy or diffuse zones of baldness can result from scarring after trauma or after severe bacterial or fungal infection. It can also be a symptom of systemic disease (systemic lupus erythematosus, iron deficiency, pituitary deficiency). Male pattern baldness (affecting brow and vertex) is genetically determined; it may also affect genetically predisposed women with elevated blood levels of androgens from any cause. The condition often responds to topical minoxidil in persons of both sexes. Each hair follicle normally passes through cycles between anagen (active hair production, with increase in hair length), and telogen (resting phase). **Telogen effluvium** is a transitory generalized thinning of scalp hair due to a systemic condition that puts the growth of a large number of hairs into the telogen phase at the same time, with resultant increased shedding of hairs. Causes include pregnancy, oral contraceptives, excessive dieting, high fever, and any severe physical or emotional stress. Hair thinning becomes noticeable after a latent period of two to four months, and typically resolves spontaneously within a few months.

Hirsutism

Excessive or cosmetically objectionable hairiness (an excessive amount of hair; unusual darkness or coarseness of hair; abnormal distribution of hair—for example, on the face in women) is called hirsutism. In some cases it is a familial trait. Hirsutism in women is often due to increased levels of androgenic substances in the blood, generally as a feature of polycystic ovary syndrome, congenital adrenal hyperplasia, or functioning (hormone-producing) tumors of ovarian or adrenal tissue. In these disorders hirsutism is generally just one symptom of virilization, others being deep voice, male-pattern baldness, and hypertrophy of the clitoris. Treatment is with estrogens, often given as oral contraceptives, or antiandrogens (spironolactone, finasteride, flutamide).

Glossary

ablation: total removal of a part, normal or abnormal, by surgical or chemical means.

avulsion: the ripping or tearing away of a part.

blepharitis: inflammation of one or both eyelids.

cryoprobe: a cryosurgical instrument containing a circulating refrigerant, which can be rapidly chilled and can deliver subfreezing temperature to tissues with precision.

cryotherapy: local treatment of neoplasms or other lesions by freezing.

dermatitis: inflammation of the skin.

dermatosis: a general term for any abnormal condition of the skin, but usually excluding inflammatory conditions, which are called dermatitis.

dermographism: the property of abnormally sensitive skin by which strokes or writing with a pointed object are reproduced on the skin surface as raised red lines.

Diseases of the Skin • 121

exacerbation: an increase in the severity of a disease, particularly when occurring after a period of improvement (remission).

friable: crumbly; fragmenting or bleeding easily on touch or manipulation; said usually of diseased tissue.

hypertrophic: overgrown, usually as a result of increase in the size of cells.

keratitis: inflammation of the cornea of the eye from any cause.

dendritic keratitis: infection of the cornea by herpes simplex virus, causing a shallow, painful ulcer having a branching, treelike (dendritic) pattern.

nevus: 1) a pigmented lesion of the skin; 2) a skin lesion present since birth (birthmark).

occult: hidden; not obvious, but sometimes able to be inferred from indirect evidence.

plantar (NOT planter's): pertaining to the sole of the foot.

pruritus, pruritic: itching.

rhinophyma: enlargement and deformity of the external nose, usually as a result of rosacea.

telangiectatic: pertaining to telangiectasia.

telangiectasis: a permanent dilatation of small blood vessels (capillaries, arterioles, venules), visible through a skin or mucous surface.

vector: an animal (for example, a mosquito) that transmits a pathogenic organism from one host to another.

Topics for Study or Discussion

1. Sweat glands, oil glands, hair follicles, and nails are sometimes called dermal appendages. What beneficial functions, if any, does each of these serve? In what way can they be a liability?

2. Distinguish between a dermatitis and a dermatosis and give three examples of each.

3. Define or explain: alopecia, cicatrix, comedo, dermographism, macule, papule, telangiectasis, tinea corporis, urticaria, verruca.

4. Most cutaneous malignancies and many other skin problems occur primarily on sun-exposed skin. It is estimated that just one or two severe cases of sunburn in a lifetime increase the risk of skin cancer. Is there any such thing as a "healthy tan"?

5. Offer some examples to illustrate the saying that the skin is the mirror of the interior of the body. (What skin disorders are or can be symptoms of systemic disease?)

Chapter 8

Diseases of the Cardiovascular System

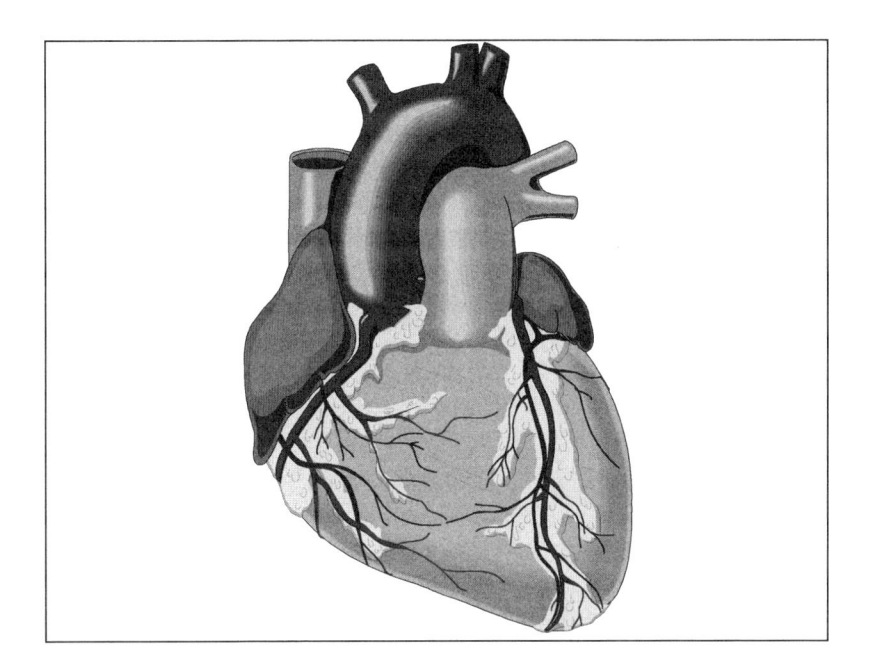

Learning Objectives

On completion of this chapter, the student should

- know the basic anatomy and physiology of the cardiovascular system;

- have a general knowledge of diagnostic procedures and treatments used in diseases of this system;

- understand signs, symptoms, and treatment of common diseases affecting this system.

Anatomy and Physiology of the Cardiovascular System

The **cardiovascular** or **circulatory system** consists of the heart and the blood vessels (arteries, capillaries, veins). The purpose of the system is to provide rapid delivery to the tissues of oxygen from the lungs, nutrients, minerals, vitamins, and water from the digestive system, hormones from glands, and white blood cells from bone marrow and lymphoid tissue, while removing waste products and delivering them to the lungs (carbon dioxide), liver (broken-down red blood cells), and kidney (nitrogenous wastes) for excretion.

The heart is a pump—actually two synchronized pumps each handling a different segment of the circulating blood at any given moment. The **right atrium** (antechamber) and the **right ventricle** receive venous blood from the systemic circulation and pump it into the lungs for gas exchange. The **left atrium** and **left ventricle** receive freshly oxygenated blood from the lungs and pump it through the arteries into the systemic circulation.

The contraction of a heart chamber is called **systole**; relaxation and refilling is called **diastole**. Valves in the heart (one for each of the four chambers) prevent backflow of blood from a chamber during systole. The heart is encased in a protective sac called the **pericardium**.

Glossary of Cardiovascular Terms

arrhythmia: irregular rhythm of the heartbeat, with or without an abnormally slow or fast rate.

ascites: swelling of the abdomen due to effusion of fluid into the peritoneal cavity.

auscultation of the heart: Each beat of the heart normally produces two sounds or tones, traditionally called "lub-dup." The first heart sound (Sl) corresponds to the beginning of ventricular systole and is due chiefly to closure of the mitral and tricuspid valves. It is lower in pitch, louder, and longer in duration than the second heart sound. The second sound (S2) corresponds to the beginning of ventricular diastole and is due chiefly to closure of the aortic and pulmonic valves. The physician notes the quality and loudness of sounds heard at the four valve areas (areas where valve sounds are best heard, not corresponding to the exact locations of the valves): aortic (A), mitral (M), pulmonic (P), and tricuspid (T).

M2: the second heart sound as heard at the mitral valve area. A2=P2: the second sounds as heard at the aortic and pulmonic valve areas are approximately equal in intensity. A **third heart sound (S3)** may be heard immediately after the second, during ventricular diastole, in young patients or in older patients with cardiac disease. A **fourth heart sound (S4)** may be heard immediately before the first heart sound. It is due to atrial systole and is seldom noted except in the presence of cardiac disease. See *gallop rhythm*.

bradyarrhythmia: a pulse that is both irregular and abnormally slow.

bradycardia: abnormal slowness of the heartbeat (pulse less than 60/min).

bruit: a rough vascular sound, synchronous with the heartbeat, heard on auscultation over a narrowing in an artery.

cardiac catheterization: a diagnostic procedure in which a catheter is introduced through the skin into a peripheral vein or artery and advanced into the heart to measure pressures and oxygen saturation in the great vessels and cardiac chambers, particularly useful in identifying structural disorders of the heart such as valvular disease and shunts.

commissurotomy: surgical enlargement of the aperture of a stenotic heart valve, particularly the mitral, by stretching or cutting.

diaphoresis: sweating.

dilatation, cardiac: enlargement of a heart chamber due to stretching of its muscular wall, without increased muscular development.

diuresis: an increase in the production of urine by the kidneys as a result of renal or systemic disease, toxic substances, or drugs administered to reduce body water, sodium, or both.

dyspnea: shortness of breath.

  paroxysmal nocturnal dyspnea: sudden attacks of labored breathing awakening the patient from sleep.

echocardiography: a noninvasive diagnostic procedure in which an ultrasonic beam is directed at the heart and the returning echoes are recorded and analyzed; valuable for the measurement of cardiac chambers (wall thickness and cavity volume), assessment of ventricular function, and identification of valvular malfunction.

edema: swelling due to the presence of fluid in tissue spaces.

  dependent edema: edema of the lower extremities, aggravated by the dependent (downward hanging) position.

peripheral edema: edema of the extremities.

pitting edema: edema that retains the mark of the examiner's fingers after release of pressure.

ejection fraction: the percentage of the blood contained in a ventricle at the end of diastole that is ejected from the heart during the succeeding systole, normally 65% or higher.

embolism: obstruction of a blood vessel by a detached bood clot, air, fat, or injected material.

exudate: a material deposited in or on tissues as a result of inflammation or degeneration and consisting of protein-rich fluid, inflammatory cells, and tissue debris.

fibrillation: rapid, random, ineffectual twitching of cardiac muscle, instead of normal regular systolic contractions, due usually to metabolic or coronary vascular disease; whereas atrial fibrillation can continue for years without serious impairment of health, ventricular fibrillation is rapidly fatal.

gallop rhythm: a cardiac rhythm that simulates the sound of a galloping horse on auscultation, usually due to the presence of a third or fourth heart sound, or both.

hemoptysis: coughing up blood.

hepatojugular reflux: increase in jugular venous distention when the examiner applies pressure to the liver.

hepatomegaly: enlargement of the liver.

hypertrophy, cardiac: enlargement of a heart chamber due to increase in the thickness of its muscular wall.

infarction: death of tissue due to interruption of its blood supply.

ischemia: inadequate blood supply.

Keith-Wagener changes: abnormal signs in the retina and retinal vessels due to hypertension and arteriosclerosis.

lumen: the hollow interior of a vessel or other tubular structure.

murmur: an abnormal sound, synchronous with the heartbeat, due to flow of blood through a valve or other passage in the heart. Murmurs are distinguished as to sound quality (harsh, blowing, high-pitched); timing (systolic, mid-systolic, late diastolic); loudness (grade 1 to 6 in one system, 1 to 4 in another; 1/6=grade 1 on a scale of 1 to 6, a barely audible murmur); radiation (to apex, carotids, left axilla); where best heard (left sternal border, aortic valve area); effect of position (squatting, standing, recumbency); and effect of respiratory movements (inspiration, expiration, breath-holding).

nocturia: the need to rise from bed to urinate during the night.

palpitation(s): various abnormal sensations accompanying heartbeat; unduly rapid heartbeat; noticeably irregular beat; a feeling that some or all heartbeats are unusually strong; a sense of missed beats; or intermittent flip-flop sensations in the heart.

paroxysmal: occurring in sudden attacks or seizures (paroxysms).

perfusion: delivery of oxygen and nutrients to tissues by the circulatory system, with removal of carbon dioxide and other wastes.

petechia (plural, **petechiae**): a very small spot of hemorrhage under the surface of skin or mucous membrane, usually multiple, due to a local or systemic disorder.

point of maximal intensity (PMI): the point on the chest wall where the impulse of the beating heart is most distinctly felt by the examiner's fingers.

precordial: in front of the heart.

pulse: the heartbeat, and by extension the rate of heartbeat, as measured at the wrist (radial pulse), the cardiac apex (apical pulse), or elsewhere.

rale: a crackling or bubbling sound heard on auscultation of the breath sounds.

    crepitant rale: a fine crackling rale.

rhonchus: a whistling or humming sound caused by passage of air through narrowed parts of the respiratory tract.

shock (precordial): an abnormally strong thrust applied to the chest wall by the beating heart, as detected by the examiner's fingers.

splitting: separation of the first or second heart sound, or both, into two distinctly audible components.

stigma (plural, **stigmata**): a structural or functional peculiarity or abnormality that is characteristic of an inherited or acquired condition, and may be useful in its diagnosis.

syncope: sudden loss of consciousness; fainting.

tachyarrhythmia: a pulse that is both irregular and abnormally rapid.

tachycardia: rapid heart rate (over 100/min).

thrill: an abnormal sensation felt by the examiner over the heart when blood jets through an anomalous or narrowed orifice.

(tunica) intima: the innermost layer or lining of an artery.

vascular: pertaining to one or more blood vessels.

venipuncture: insertion of a needle into a vein for the purpose of removing blood for testing, or to inject fluids, medicines, or diagnostic materials.

Congenital Heart Disease

A large and various group of structural abnormalities present at birth and involving the heart chambers, valves, associated great vessels, or some combination of these. Congenital heart disease can be genetically determined, or can result from interference with normal embryonic development by intrauterine exposure to maternal infections, medicines, drugs of abuse, or toxins. It can occur as an isolated problem or be part of a more extensive failure of normal development.

Some congenital heart disorders are incompatible with life; others cause few or no symptoms. Congenital heart diseases are divided into two large classes: **cyanotic**, causing obvious impairment of oxygenation of the blood in early life; and **acyanotic**, with delayed or absent symptoms. Cyanotic heart disease is a specialized topic within pediatric cardiology. Only a few types of acyanotic congenital heart disease can be discussed here.

Coarctation of the Aorta

Narrowing of the aortic arch, just beyond the origin of the left subclavian artery, often associated with abnormality of the aortic valve.

History: Usually no symptoms until evidence of cardiac failure or consequences of hypertension become evident.

Physical Examination: Arterial pulses prominent in the neck, weak or absent in the lower extremities. Blood pressure elevated in the arms, normal or low in the legs. A systolic murmur at the site of narrowing.

Diagnostic Tests: Chest x-ray may show left ventricular hypertrophy (LVH) and notching of ribs by dilated collateral vessels. Electrocardiogram confirms LVH. Cardiac catheterization shows the pressure differential across the narrowing, and aortography depicts the narrowing.

Course: Congestive heart failure, early death due to hypertension, aortic rupture, or endocarditis.

Treatment: Surgical correction of the narrowing. Balloon dilatation sometimes successful.

Patent Ductus Arteriosus

Persistence of the fetal communication between the aorta and the pulmonary artery, which shunts blood around the (unexpanded and nonfunctioning) lungs until birth; clinical significance depends on the amount of shunting that persists after birth.

History: No symptoms, or symptoms only with development of left ventricular hypertrophy or failure.

Physical Examination: Widened pulse pressure, reduced diastolic pressure. Accentuated second heart sound; continuous "machinery" murmur along the left sternal border.

Diagnostic Tests: Chest x-ray may be normal or may show left ventricular hypertrophy and dilatation of the pulmonary and aortic silhouettes. ECG may show left ventricular hypertrophy.

Course: Depends on shunt size; may be benign or lead to heart failure.

Treatment: Intravenous indomethacin may induce closure of the ductus in infancy. Surgical ligation is effective; placement of a plug by catheter may be successful.

Atrial Septal Defect

Persistence of communication through the interatrial septum after birth. The passage may appear at various sites on the septum and may be associated with valvular anomalies. Symptoms and prognosis depend on the size of the shunt.

History: There may be few or no symptoms unless pulmonary hypertension or right ventricular failure occurs.

Physical Examination: Right ventricular pulsations may be prominent, with a right ventricular heave. A systolic murmur is heard at the left sternal border.

Diagnostic Tests: Chest x-ray may show right ventricular dilatation and prominence of pulmonary vasculature. ECG, echo Doppler, radionuclide studies, MRI, and especially cardiac catheterization confirm the diagnosis and measure the degree of cardiovascular functional impairment.

Course: No serious problems with small shunts. Large shunts may lead to pulmonary hypertension, cardiac arrhythmias, and heart failure in middle age.

Treatment: Surgical closure of the shunt, if necessary.

Ventricular Septal Defect

Persistent communication between the right and left ventricle after birth, with shunting of blood from left to right. Symptoms, signs, and prognosis depend on the extent of the shunt.

History: There may be no symptoms unless pulmonary hypertension or right ventricular failure occurs.

Physical Examination: A precordial thrill and a holosystolic murmur heard along the left sternal border. Chest x-ray may show hypertrophy of one or both ventricles and increased pulmonary vascular markings. More precise and quantitative information may be provided by MRI, radionuclide scanning, and cardiac catheterization.

Course: The defect may close spontaneously. Progressive strain on the right and left ventricle may lead to failure; endocarditis may occur at the site of defect.

Treatment: Surgical closure, if necessary.

Valvular Heart Disease

Structural abnormality of one or more **heart valves**, which may be congenital or acquired. Valvular defects consist of **stenosis** (abnormal narrowing of the valve opening), **insufficiency** (failure of the valve to prevent backflow during systole), or both.

Valvular stenosis causes reduction in the volume of blood ejected from the involved chamber during systole, and usually an audible systolic murmur. Valvular insufficiency causes regurgitation of blood through the valve during diastole of the chamber involved, and usually an audible diastolic murmur. Either stenosis or insufficiency places an abnormal strain on the chamber affected, with the risk of dilatation and failure.

Cardiac catheterization is the definitive procedure for diagnosing valvular disease and measuring pressure gradients across defective valves at various points in the cardiac cycle. This discussion is limited to the most common types of valvular disease.

Mitral Stenosis

Abnormal narrowing of the **mitral valve**.

Cause: Most cases are residuals of acute rheumatic fever. This is usually a childhood disease; symptoms of mitral stenosis typically do not appear until the 30s or 40s.

History: Dyspnea, orthopnea, paroxysmal nocturnal dyspnea, fatique, chronic cough, hemoptysis.
Physical Examination: The first heart sound at the mitral area (Ml) is accentuated. Early in (ventricular) diastole, a mitral opening snap may be heard, followed by an evanescent, mid-diastolic rumble, produced by passage of blood through the stenotic valve during left atrial systole.
Diagnostic Tests: Echocardiography and cardiac catheterization yield precise diagnostic information.
Course: Eventually, right ventricular failure. Atrial fibrillation frequently occurs, with risk of systemic arterial embolism.
Treatment: Supportive. Digitalis or other anti-arrhythmic agents for atrial fibrillation, and anticoagulant to prevent arterial emboli. For severe disease, surgical commissurotomy, balloon dilatation, or valve replacement.

Mitral Valve Prolapse
Abnormal bulging of mitral valve leaflets into the left atrium during left ventricular systole, due to structurally abnormal (floppy or billowing) valve leaflets.
Causes: May be inherited as an autosomal dominant trait. Often occurs in conjunction with other connective tissue abnormalities, particularly Marfan syndrome. Occurs in 1-5% of the general population, and is seen principally in women.
History: Usually there are no symptoms. A few patients experience nonspecific chest pain, palpitations with or without actual arrhythmia, dyspnea on exertion, fatigue, and syncope.
Physical Examination: Variable murmurs: usually midsystolic click and late systolic murmur. The patient may present other stigmata of connective tissue abnormality: thin body habitus, high palate, deformities of the chest wall (pectus excavatum, scoliosis).
Diagnostic Studies: Echocardiography confirms valve prolapse and indicates whether actual regurgitation occurs.
Course: Most patients have no symptoms and no complications. Rarely regurgitation may have serious hemodynamic consequences. Endocarditis may develop on the mitral valve. Atrial fibrillation may occur. Sudden death may result from ectopic ventricular rhythms (**ventricular tachycardia**).
Treatment: Antibiotic prophylaxis of endocarditis before dental work and surgery. Beta-blockers usually control chest pain and arrhythmias. Rarely, surgical valve replacement.

Aortic Stenosis

Abnormal narrowing of the aortic valve opening, with reduction of left ventricular ejection volume during systole.

Causes: May be a consequence of acute rheumatic fever, but usually results from calcification of the valve with aging. Most patients are men over 50.

History: Weakness, dyspnea, chest pain, palpitations, syncope.

Physical Examination: Carotid pulsations are reduced. A precordial thrill may be noted. The second heart sound is reduced or absent. There is a harsh "diamond-shaped" (crescendo-decrescendo) murmur heard at the base of the heart and transmitted to the carotids and cardiac apex.

Diagnostic Tests: Chest x-ray may show left ventricular dilatation and calcification of the aortic valve. Electrocardiogram, echo-Doppler studies, and cardiac catheterization provide more precise and quantitative information.

Course: Left ventricular failure, arrhythmias, angina, syncope.

Treatment: Surgical replacement of the valve. Balloon dilatation of the valve may be successful.

Endocarditis

Inflammation of the lining membrane of the heart (**endocardium**), particularly over cardiac valves, due to infection or as a complication of systemic disease (acute rheumatic fever, systemic lupus erythematosus). Only infective endocarditis will be discussed here.

Infective Endocarditis (Acute and Subacute Bacterial Endocarditis)

Bacterial infection of one or more heart valves.

Cause: Usually, pre-existing congenital or acquired valvular disease or abnormal communications (septal defects) and bacteremia (after dental or surgical procedures or in systemic infection or septicemia).

History: Fever, chills, dyspnea, cough, abdominal pain, muscle or joint pain.

Physical Examination: Fever, pallor. Audible cardiac murmur, or change in quality or loudness of a pre-existing murmur. Signs of peripheral embolization of infective material (vegetations) from heart valves:

petechiae of the palate and conjunctivae, splinter hemorrhages under fingernails, Osler nodes (tender purplish lumps in fingers, toes), Janeway spots (painless red spots of palms and soles), Roth spots (retinal exudates). Splenomegaly.

Diagnostic Tests: Anemia, leukocytosis, hematuria, proteinuria. Blood cultures may permit identification of the organism. Chest x-ray, electrocardiogram, echocardiogram supply diagnostic information.

Course: Valve leaflets may ulcerate and slough, with severe impairment of cardiac function. Fragments of infectious material (septic emboli) may be carried to brain, heart, kidney, and other tissues, or to the lung, causing local infective vascular lesions (mycotic aneurysms).

Treatment: Intravenous antibiotics for several weeks. Surgery may be undertaken in very severe cases.

Cardiac Arrhythmias and Conduction Defects

Disturbance of the rate or rhythm of cardiac action due to abnormalities in the structure or function of the heart. The following is a useful classification.

Disorders of Impulse Formation
Failure of impulse formation (asystole).
Ectopic focus (stimulus for heartbeat comes from an irritable or diseased zone of tissue rather than the normal pacemaker).
Supraventricular: atrial fibrillation; paroxysmal atrial tachycardia.
Ventricular: ventricular tachycardia, ventricular fibrillation.
Circus movement, reentry: Wolff-Parkinson-White syndrome.

Disorders of Impulse Transmission (Heart Block)
Atrioventricular (AV) block.
>First degree block: delayed conduction, but all impulses get through.
>Second degree block: some impulses not conducted.
>Third degree block: no impulses transmitted.

Bundle branch blocks (right and left).

Causes: Congenital anomalies in the impulse-forming or conducting system of the heart; coronary artery disease, including myocardial infarction, with ischemia of parts of the system; alcohol, tobacco, or drugs.

History: Intermittent or continuous palpitations, a sense of rapid, irregular, or violent heart action, dyspnea, heaviness in the chest, lightheadedness, syncope, diuresis.

Physical Examination: The pulse may be abnormally fast or slow, or irregular. The blood pressure is often below normal. Cardiac auscultation reveals irregularity in the rhythm or force of contractions, and there may be a difference between the apical and radial pulse rates (pulse deficit). Examination may disclose evidence of underlying or concomitant cardiac disease.

Diagnostic Tests: Electrocardiography delineates abnormalities of cardiac impulse formation, conduction, rhythm, and rate. Holter monitoring (ambulatory electrocardiography) for a 24-hour period may be useful in recording transitory arrhythmias. Electrophysiologic studies can often pinpoint the location and nature of electrical abnormalities.

Course: Risk of embolization from atrial fibrillation. Hemodynamic impairment may be mild or lethal.

Treatment: Correction of any underlying cardiac disorder and elimination of contributing factors (alcohol abuse, cigarette smoking, drug use or abuse) may suffice to correct a rhythm problem. Digitalis and calcium-channel blockers are used to treat supraventricular tachyarrhythmias. Ventricular arrhythmias are treated with quinidine, lidocaine, and other drugs related to local anesthetics. Ventricular fibrillation is treated with electric shock (defibrillation). Abnormal circuits in the conduction system (as in Wolff-Parkinson-White syndrome) can be interrupted with electrical or radiofrequency ablation. Complete heart block and other severe disorders of impulse formation are treated with a transvenous or implanted pacemaker.

Coronary Artery Disease (Arteriosclerotic Heart Disease, Ischemic Heart Disease)

Heart disease due to impairment of coronary artery blood flow. This subject is conveniently discussed under three headings: angina pectoris, myocardial infarction, and congestive heart failure.

Angina Pectoris

Paroxysmal chest pain due to myocardial ischemia, without permanent damage to heart muscle.

Cause: The primary cause is narrowing of one or more coronary arteries by arteriosclerosis. Arteritis, congenital vascular anomalies, emboli, severe anemia, cardiac hypertrophy, and cocaine intoxication can also lead to signs and symptoms of inadequate coronary blood flow. Risk factors for development of coronary arteriosclerosis include a family history of the disease, male gender, elevated cholesterol, hypertension, cigarette smoking, diabetes mellitus, overweight, and a sedentary lifestyle.

History: Angina pectoris is a syndrome of anterior chest pain coming on abruptly and resolving spontaneously in less than 30 minutes. Pain is typically precipitated by physical exertion, strong emotion, exposure to cold, or eating a meal, and is relieved by rest or by taking nitroglycerin. The pain is described as a tightness, squeezing, or pressure; the patient often expresses this by holding a clenched fist in front of the chest. The pain may radiate into the neck, jaw, or arm, particularly the left. A variant, Prinzmetal's angina, occurs at rest and is more common in women and younger patients than typical angina.

Physical Examination: There may be no abnormal findings, but the blood pressure is often elevated by pain and anxiety. Examination may disclose signs of underlying cardiovascular or systemic disease.

Diagnostic Tests: The electrocardiogram may be normal during an attack, but usually shows ST segment depression and flattened or inverted T waves, indicating myocardial ischemia. There may also be evidence of conduction defects or ventricular hypertrophy. Holter monitoring allows recording of the ECG continuously for 24 hours. Stress testing records the electrocardiogram during standardized and closely supervised physical exertion. Angiography demonstrates narrowing of coronary vessels. Other studies (myocardial perfusion scintigraphy, radionuclide angiography, and echocardiography) can supply further information about the location and extent of coronary disease.

Course: Gradual progression to more severe disease (myocardial infarction, congestive heart failure) usually occurs, even with treatment. Unstable angina, which worsens with time despite treatment, has a less favorable prognosis.

Treatment: The standard treatment for an anginal attack is sublingual (under the tongue) nitroglycerin, which promptly abolishes pain of coronary ischemia by producing dilatation in the coronary arteries. Nitroglycerin can also be taken prophylactically before physical exertion.

Longer-acting nitrate preparations, beta-blocking agents, and calcium-channel blockers taken regularly can prevent or mitigate attacks. Most patients are advised to take aspirin daily for its effect in inhibiting platelet aggregation and reducing the risk of myocardial infarction. Coronary artery bypass graft (CABG) uses veins or other materials to conduct blood past narrowed places in coronary arteries. Percutaneous transluminal coronary angioplasty (PTCA, balloon angioplasty) dilates narrowed places with a balloon passed into the circulation through an arterial catheter.

Myocardial Infarction (Heart Attack, Coronary Thrombosis)

Damage to a segment of heart muscle by severe impairment of coronary blood flow.

Causes: The underlying causes are the same as for angina pectoris. Myocardial infarction is usually due to thrombosis in a coronary artery already narrowed by arteriosclerosis. Arteritis, vasospasm, embolism, sudden hypotension, or cocaine can also precipitate infarction.

History: Anterior chest pain, similar to angina but generally more severe and lasting more than 30 minutes. Pain often comes on at rest and is not relieved by nitroglycerin. Typically, males experience sweating, weakness, restlessness, shortness of breath, and nausea. Rarely, infarction occurs without pain (silent infarction). Females may experience the same symptoms or may perceive jaw or shoulder discomfort and/or chest tightness or discomfort without actual crushing pain.

Physical Examination: The pulse and blood pressure may be increased, normal, or decreased. Mild fever often develops after the first 12 hours. The heart sounds may be soft or distant. An atrial gallop (fourth heart sound) is often heard. A seagull murmur of mitral regurgitation indicates rupture of a papillary muscle. The cardiac rhythm may be abnormal. A pericardial friction rub is often heard. Jugular venous distention and rales of pulmonary edema are seen in heart failure.

Diagnostic Tests: The electrocardiogram shows ST segment elevation (changing later to depression) and inversion of T waves in leads pertaining to the area of infarction. Q waves indicate severe myocardial damage and a graver prognosis. The white blood cell count may be slightly elevated. Serial determination of the serum levels of the cardiac enzymes LDH (lactic dehydrogenase), CK-MB (the MB isoenzyme of creatine kinase), troponin C, and troponin T show a characteristic rise. Fluoroscopy or other imaging techniques may show segmental wall motion at the site of infarction. Scintigraphy with technetium-99m pyrophosphate shows a hot spot at the site. Doppler echocardiography may also confirm the extent and location of infarction.

Course: About 20% of persons who sustain myocardial infarction die before reaching a hospital. With intensive therapy, the prognosis for the other 80% is good. During the acute phase, arrhythmia, shock, and congestive heart failure are serious possibilities. Other dangerous complications include papillary muscle rupture with resulting serious valvular malfunction, **cardiorrhexis** (bursting of the ventricle), left **ventricular aneurysm** (extreme dilatation and thinning of the ventricle, with loss of contractile power), pericarditis, and formation of a **mural thrombus** (a localized clot adjacent to the infarcted area of ventricular wall).

Treatment: The standard treatment protocol includes hospitalization, administration of oxygen by inhalation and of narcotics for pain relief by injection, and continuous electrocardiographic monitoring. Administration of thrombolytic agents (tPA [tissue plasminogen activator], streptokinase, or anistreplase) is standard. Anticoagulants (aspirin, IV heparin) may also be administered. Beta-blocking agents are started early. In some centers, balloon angioplasty is performed during the acute phase of myocardial infarction.

Myocarditis

Local or generalized inflammation of heart muscle (myocardium).

Causes: Infection, drugs, chemical or biological toxins, autoimmune disorders. Infectious myocarditis may be due to viruses (coxsackievirus, Rocky Mountain spotted fever, HIV), parasites (Chagas disease, toxoplasmosis, trichinosis), or other organisms. Onset often follows an upper respiratory infection.

History: Chest pain, dyspnea, fatigue, palpitations.

Physical Examination: Tachycardia, sometimes gallop rhythm.

Diagnostic Tests: Chest x-ray shows cardiac dilatation. Electrocardiogram may indicate nonspecific electrical abnormalities. Scintigraphy and myocardial biopsy may provide more specific indications. Testing for antibodies in serum may identify a causative organism.

Course: Complete resolution often occurs spontaneously, but in other cases there is progressive deterioration of cardiac function and eventual circulatory failure.

Treatment: Largely supportive and symptomatic. Specific antimicrobial treatment may be available. Immunosuppressive agents may be used in autoimmune myocarditis. Heart transplant in end-stage (terminal) disease.

Pericarditis

Inflammation of the pericardium. **Acute pericarditis** can result from numerous causes but is often idiopathic. In **pericarditis with effusion**, fluid within the pericardium threatens to impair cardiac function. **Constrictive pericarditis** is scarring or calcification of the pericardium as a late consequence of inflammation, with the risk of hemodynamic compromise. Only the first two will be discussed here.

Acute Pericarditis

Causes: Often occurs after a viral respiratory infection. Frequently the exact cause cannot be determined. Infection can spread from the lungs or pleura in bacterial pneumonia and pulmonary tuberculosis. Pericarditis may complicate acute myocardial infarction. Systemic diseases that can cause pericarditis include acute rheumatic fever, systemic lupus erythematosus, uremia, malignancy, and myxedema. Exposure to radiation and certain drugs and toxins can also cause pericarditis.

History: The onset is often sudden. Sharp, dull, or intermittent anterior chest pain, aggravated by coughing or deep inspiration and relieved by sitting up or leaning forward. Fever. Dyspnea, weakness.

Physical Examination: Fever, tachycardia. A pericardial friction rub, often faint, transitory, or changing, may be heard along the left sternal border with the patient leaning forward.

Diagnostic Tests: The white blood cell count is elevated. The ECG shows widespread elevation of ST segments; later sometimes flattening or inversion of T waves.

Course: Spontaneous resolution usually occurs in 1-3 weeks. Recurrences are common after recovery.

Treatment: Rest and supportive therapy. Aspirin may be prescribed to combat pain; in severe cases, adrenal steroids. The underlying disease must be treated as well.

Pericarditis with Effusion

Causes: Same as for acute pericarditis.

History: In addition to symptoms of pericarditis, other symptoms include severe dyspnea, orthopnea, palpitations, cough, and difficulty swallowing.

Physical Examination: Pallor, diaphoresis, tachycardia, **hypotension**, **pulsus paradoxus** (drop in systolic blood pressure of 10 mm or more during inspiration), distention of neck veins. Heart tones distant, cardiac borders indistinct on percussion.

Diagnostic Tests: Chest x-ray and MRI confirm the effusion. The electrocardiogram shows reduced voltage and sometimes T wave inversion.

Course: Spontaneous resolution may occur. A large effusion carries the risk of cardiac tamponade (compression of the heart chambers, with failure of circulatory function).

Treatment: With a substantial effusion, **pericardiocentesis** (puncture of the pericardium with a needle or catheter and withdrawal of fluid). Any underlying disease must be treated.

Congestive Heart Failure

A syndrome of impaired **hemodynamics** due to inability of the heart to maintain normal circulation.

Causes: Any condition that impairs the contractile force of the heart (or that overtaxes a normal contractile force) may induce congestive heart failure. Coronary artery disease (particularly myocardial infarction), hypertensive cardiovascular disease, myocarditis, valvular heart disease (particularly aortic stenosis), hypo- or hyperthyroidism, and severe anemia can precipitate failure.

History: Shortness of breath, particularly on exertion; orthopnea, paroxysmal nocturnal dyspnea, cough; fatigue, nocturia; anorexia and right upper quadrant fullness due to hepatic engorgement; ankle edema.

Physical Examination: Dyspnea, cyanosis, tachycardia, hypotension. Jugular venous distention. Left ventricular dilatation and hypertrophy. Diminished first heart sound. Expiratory wheezes and rhonchi. Crepitant rales at bases; reduced breath sounds and dullness to percussion may indicate pleural effusion. Hepatomegaly, hepatojugular reflex. Pitting edema of the lower extremities, ascites.

Diagnostic Tests: The red blood count may be diminished. The electrocardiogram may indicate myocardial infarction, arrhythmia, or left ventricular hypertrophy. Echocardiography gives more precise information about ventricular size. Chest x-ray shows cardiomegaly, signs of pulmonary venous congestion (**Kerley B lines**), and sometimes pleural effusion. Radionuclide angiography allows estimation of ventricular ejection fraction.

Course: Congestive heart failure indicates a serious impairment of cardiovascular dynamics, and even with treatment the course is often steadily downhill. The prognosis for long-term survival is poor, and death often occurs suddenly.

Treatment: Rest, salt restriction, and early correction of identifiable precipitating factors. Diuretics (thiazides, loop diuretics, potassium-sparing diuretics) and ACE inhibitors are used to reverse biochemical imbalances that lead to sodium retention and circulatory volume overload. Digitalis glycosides increase the force of cardiac contraction.

Acute Pulmonary Edema

An extreme form of left ventricular failure in which respiratory symptoms predominate. It can be precipitated by acute myocardial infarction or by any factors that increase the severity of existing cardiac failure. There are severe dyspnea, cough, and wheezing, with frothy pink sputum. The pulse is rapid and weak, the lips and nail beds cyanotic. Auscultation reveals rales and rhonchi in the lungs. The arterial oxygen is low. Chest x-ray shows cardiomegaly, increased vascular markings, **Kerley B lines**, pleural effusion. Treatment is oxygen by inhalation, morphine, and intravenous diuretics.

Disorders of Blood Pressure: Shock and Hypertension

Shock

A condition in which the systemic blood pressure is too low to maintain adequate tissue perfusion.

Causes: Hypovolemia (reduced blood volume due to hemorrhage, dehydration, severe burns, ascites); cardiogenic (impairment of cardiac function by arrhythmia, myocardial infarction, myocarditis, acute valvular failure); vascular obstruction (pericardial tamponade, pulmonary embolism); dilatation of the circulatory system (septic shock, anaphylactic shock, toxic shock syndrome, neurogenic shock, drugs).

History: Weakness, palpitations, thirst, sweating, anxiety, loss of consciousness.

Physical Examination: The blood pressure is low and the pulse rapid. Peripheral pulses are weak or absent. The **tilt test** is positive (rise in pulse and drop in blood pressure when patient is moved from recumbent to erect position). In hypovolemic shock the skin is pale, cold, and clammy. In septic shock there may be high fever and flushing. Agitation, confusion, and deteriorating level of consciousness.

Diagnostic Tests: Procedures used during early treatment to assess the degree of shock include blood tests (complete blood count, electrolytes, arterial blood gases), urine flow, cardiac monitoring, and central venous pressure or pulmonary wedge pressure with Swan-Ganz catheter.

Course: Without treatment shock may lead to irreversible damage: cerebral ischemia and infarction, myocardial infarction, renal failure.

Treatment: Vigorous treatment is required to maintain tissue perfusion and prevent irreversible consequences. The patient is placed in the **Trendelenburg position** (head lower than feet), and oxygen is administered. Morphine sulfate is given for pain (unless there is respiratory depression or head injury). Volume replacement with blood, plasma, or artificial plasma expanders in hypovolemic shock. Treatment of underlying conditions. Compression of the arms, legs, and abdomen by an inflatable garment (military antishock trousers, MAST) can maintain cerebral, coronary, and renal blood flow until bleeding or other underlying condition is controlled and blood volume restored. Dopamine, adrenal steroids, and other drugs may be administered.

Hypertension

Sustained elevation of arterial blood pressure above 140 mmHg systolic or 90 mmHg diastolic.

Cause: Unknown in more than 90% of cases, which are thus called essential hypertension. Essential hypertension shows a genetic pattern, running in families and being much commoner in African-Americans. Its development may depend on environmental factors, excessive dietary salt, sodium retention by the kidney, abnormalities of the renin-angiotensin system, obesity, alcohol abuse, cigarette smoking, and use of NSAIDs. Secondary hypertension is due to a demonstrable cause: renal parenchymal disease, renal ischemia, Cushing disease, primary aldosteronism, pheochromocytoma, or estrogen use in the form of oral contraceptives.

History: There may be no symptoms whatsoever until complications develop.

Physical Examination: Elevated blood pressure and accentuation of the second heart sound; otherwise there may be no findings. Retinopathy is indicated by detection of **Keith-Wagener changes** on ophthalmoscopic examination. Left ventricular hypertrophy may be indicated by precordial heave or by a systolic ejection murmur.

Diagnostic Tests: Laboratory studies may be normal. The search for a cause of secondary hypertension may include examination of urine for signs of renal disease and testing of serum or urine levels of hormones.

Course: Some hypertensive patients experience a return of blood pressure to normal after a few weeks, months, or years. In most, however, elevation of blood pressure remains throughout life. Hypertension causes several forms of damage to the cardiovascular system (hypertensive cardiovascular disease), including left ventricular hypertrophy and dysfunction, arteriosclerosis, dilatation and dissecting aneurysm of the aorta, hypertensive encephalopathy, and hypertensive renal disease. In accelerated or malignant hypertension there is sustained high blood pressure responding poorly to treatment, and rapid progression of cardiovascular damage.

Treatment: Therapy of essential hypertension ideally includes lifestyle modification (cessation of smoking and alcohol abuse, increased physical exercise), restriction of dietary salt, and control of overweight. Drug therapy is tailored to the severity of the disease, and typically starts with a single drug (a thiazide diuretic or a beta-blocker), others being added as needed: ACE inhibitors, calcium channel blockers, methyldopa, alpha-receptor antagonists, guanethidine, and drugs of other classes.

Peripheral Arterial Disease

Chronic disease of systemic arteries causing compromise of circulation.

Atherosclerosis

Hardening and even calcification of arterial walls, with narrowing of their lumens.

Cause: Degeneration of arterial walls, with diffuse or plaque-like deposition of cholesterol crystals in the (tunica) intima of systemic arteries. Various inborn metabolic abnormalities in lipoproteins may predispose to abnormal elevation of serum cholesterol level and abnormal deposition of cholesterol in arterial walls. (Involvement of coronary and cerebral arteries in the same process is a principal cause of coronary artery disease and cerebral vascular disease.)

History: Intermittent claudication: cramping muscle pain in calves, thighs, buttocks (depending on site of arterial obstruction) that is brought on by walking and relieved by rest.

Physical Examination: Weakness or absence of femoral, popliteal, or pedal pulses. Bruit over aorta, iliac or femoral arteries. Trophic changes (loss of hair, thinning of skin, pigmentation).

Diagnostic Tests: Evidence of reduced blood flow can be obtained by Doppler ultrasonography, transcutaneous oximetry, or other measures.

Treatment: Physical therapy and treatment with pentoxifylline or other agents may improve exercise tolerance slightly. Surgical treatment (endarterectomy or arterial grafting) yields much better results. Percutaneous transluminal angioplasty (balloon dilatation) is effective in selected cases.

Aneurysm

A local dilatation of an artery due to congenital anomaly, degenerative disease, or trauma.

Aneurysm in a systemic artery can produce local swelling and pain with reduction of distal blood flow, manifested by pallor, cyanosis, pain, numbness, or **intermittent claudication**. Treatment is by surgical excision and insertion of a graft. Aortic aneurysm usually results from degenerative disease; surgical grafting is performed to avoid aortic rupture, which can be rapidly fatal.

Dissecting Aneurysm

Burrowing of blood between layers of the aorta.

Cause: Hypertension and abnormality or degeneration of the aorta (as in Marfan syndrome).

History: Sudden onset of severe chest pain radiating to the back, abdomen, or extremities; weakness, paralysis, collapse.

Physical Examination: The blood pressure is elevated despite clinical appearances of shock. Peripheral pulses are reduced or unequal. There may be loss of reflexes in the extremities.

Diagnostic Tests: Electrocardiogram may show left ventricular hypertrophy as a reflection of chronic hypertensive cardiovascular disease. Chest x-ray may show an abnormal aortic silhouette. CT scan, MRI, and angiography can provide more specific information.

Course: About 20% of patients die within the first 24 hours. More than 90% will eventually die without treatment.

Treatment: Reduction of blood pressure with IV nitroprusside, beta-blockers, or other agents, followed by surgical repair of the dissection.

Raynaud Phenomenon

A vasomotor disorder of the circulation affecting principally the fingers.

Causes: Various connective tissue disorders (rheumatoid arthritis, CREST syndrome, systemic lupus erythematosus), drugs. When no underlying cause can be found, the disorder is called **Raynaud disease**. Most patients are young women.

History: Sudden attacks of pallor, coldness, numbness, stiffness, and pain in 1-8 fingers, precipitated by exposure to cold or emotional upset. The thumbs are rarely involved. Pallor resolves spontaneously after a few minutes, and is succeeded by rebound erythema, warmth, throbbing, and swelling.

Physical Examination: During attacks, pallor and coldness of fingers; at other times, no abnormalities.

Course: Generally benign. When severe, Raynaud phenomenon may lead to atrophy of finger tissue, ulceration, or gangrene.

Treatment: Avoidance of cold exposure. Nifedipine to prevent vasospasm. In severe cases, cervical sympathectomy to block autonomic impulses causing vasospasm.

Thrombosis and Embolism

Thrombosis is the formation of a clot (**thrombus**) within the circulatory system. Thrombosis is usually due to injury of a blood vessel, prolonged immobilization with reduction of blood flow through a part, increased coagulability of the blood, or some combination of these. Most thrombi form in veins of the pelvis and lower extremity. A **mural thrombus** is a clot adherent to the wall of a heart chamber; this may occur in myocardial infarction or chronic atrial fibrillation. A thrombus may completely obstruct the vessel in which it develops. Eventually most thrombi are reabsorbed and replaced by scar tissue, usually with reestablishment of a passage (recanalization).

While venous obstruction is of some concern in thrombosis, a far greater danger is that of **embolization**—release of a clot from its point of origin, and travel to a remote site in the circulation where it can obstruct a large capillary zone. An embolus originating in a systemic vein can travel through the right atrium and right ventricle to block a portion of the circulation of a lung (**pulmonary embolism**, discussed in Chapter 10). An embolus released into the systemic arterial system from the left atrium or left ventricle can block the blood supply to part of the brain, kidney, a limb, or any other tissue. Any foreign substance in the circulatory system (air, fat, amniotic fluid, injected material) can act as an embolus.

Thrombophlebitis

Inflammation in the wall of a vein associated with clotting of blood within the vein. Thrombophlebitis generally affects the superficial or deep veins of the lower extremities.

Superficial Thrombophlebitis

Causes: Local trauma, venous catheter, venous stasis (pregnancy, varicose veins). Rarely, pancreatic carcinoma.

History: Soreness, redness, and swelling along the course of a vein, usually at the site of injury or recent venipuncture.

Physical Examination: Erythema, edema, induration, tenderness along the course of a superficial vein. No edema distal to the site of inflammation.

Diagnostic Tests: Doppler ultrasonography, impedance plethysmography, and venography confirm, localize, and quantify venous obstruction.

Course: Spontaneous resolution generally occurs. There is a very small risk of thromboembolism.

Treatment: Elastic wrapping of the leg and thigh, elevation, application of warm compresses, nonsteroidal anti-inflammatory medicines.

Deep Thrombophlebitis

Causes: Congestive heart failure, recent surgery or immobilization, oral contraceptives, malignancy.
History: Pain or tightness in the calf or thigh, with edema distally. There may be no symptoms until pulmonary embolism occurs.
Physical Examination: Distal edema may be the only objective sign. There may be pain or tenderness on calf rocking, or a positive **Homans sign** (calf pain or tightness on passive dorsiflexion of the foot).
Diagnostic Tests: As for superficial thrombophlebitis.
Course: There is considerable danger of pulmonary embolism. Healing may be followed by deep venous insufficiency, with chronic edema.
Treatment: Hospitalization. The same measures as for superficial thrombophlebitis. In addition, intravenous or low-dose intramuscular heparin.

Topics for Study or Discussion

1. Trace the path of a drop of blood from the aorta through the circulatory system and back to its point of origin. How many cardiac chambers did it pass through? How many cardiac valves?

2. Shock and congestive heart failure are both forms of circulatory failure. In what ways are they similar and in what ways different?

3. Define: arrhythmia, embolism, hypertension, infarction, thrombosis.

4. Mention three preventable or controllable risk factors for coronary artery disease and three noncontrollable risk factors.

5. List five potentially serious cardiac disorders in which the pulse rate and rhythm may be normal.

Chapter 9

Diseases of the Ear, Nose, and Throat

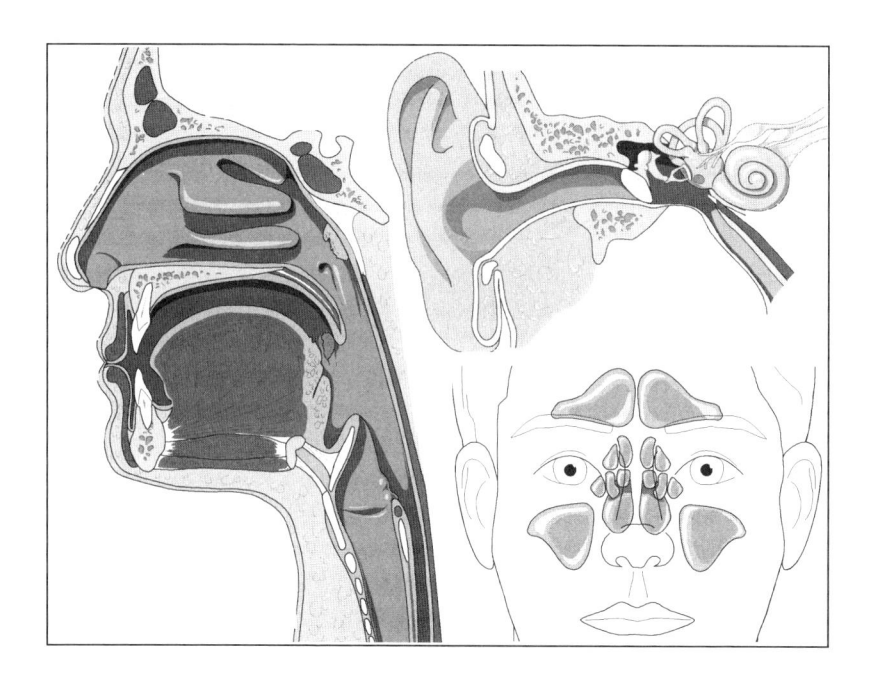

Learning Objectives

Upon completion of this chapter, the student should

- know the basic anatomy and physiology of the ear, nose, and throat;

- have a general knowledge of diagnostic procedures and treatments used in diseases of these organs;

- understand signs, symptoms, and treatment of common diseases affecting them.

148 • Human Diseases

The ear, nose, and throat are adjacent to one another anatomically, similar in histologic structure, and subject to many of the same diseases. Diseases, injuries, and abnormalities of the ear, nose, and throat (ENT) are the special field of the **otorhinolaryngologist**. This chapter briefly surveys the more common disorders to which these parts of the body are subject. If you encounter unfamiliar terms, look them up in the glossary at the end of the chapter.

The Ear

Anatomy and Physiology
Each ear has three parts:

1. The **outer ear**, consisting of the **pinna** (the cartilaginous appendage on either side of the head, which collects sound waves like a funnel) and the **external auditory meatus** (a tube that conducts sound waves from the pinna to the middle ear). The meatus is lined with skin that secretes **cerumen** (earwax), a mildly antimicrobial substance that traps dust and other particulate foreign material.

2. The **middle ear**, a cavity in the temporal bone separated from the external auditory meatus by the **tympanic membrane**, which vibrates in response to sound waves and imparts the vibration to a series of very small bones (**malleus**, **incus**, and **stapes**), which in turn transmit them to the inner ear.

3. The **inner ear**, consisting of the **cochlea** (an organ shaped like a snail shell, in which sound vibrations are converted to nerve impulses to be sent through the eighth cranial, or **vestibulocochlear**, **nerve**) and the vestibular system, the organ of balance (containing minute position sensors in a fluid medium, which send information about head position to the balance center in the brain, also through the eighth cranial nerve).

The middle ear communicates with the pharynx by a minute passage called the auditory (**eustachian**) **tube**, which serves to equalize air pressure between the middle ear and the atmosphere (see box). It also communicates with epithelium-lined air cells within the skull, called **mastoid air cells**.

The auditory tube between the middle ear and the pharynx was discovered by Bartolomeo Eustachio (1524-1574), an Italian anatomist who also made important studies of the heart, the kidney, and the nervous system.

It has been suggested that when William Shakespeare wrote *Hamlet*, he had in mind the then recent discovery of this passage. In Act I, Scene 5, the ghost of Hamlet's father tells Hamlet how he was murdered by his brother Claudius, who poured "juice of cursed hebona . . . in the porches of my ears."

According to Nomina Anatomica (NA), the name of this tube is *tuba auditoria* (or *auditiva*), usually rendered auditory tube in English.

Many health professionals nonetheless cling to the traditional name, *eustachian tube*, and most of them pronounce it with the soft French *ch* sound (as in champagne) rather than the more appropriate hard Italian *ch* (as in Chianti).

Diagnostic Procedures in Disorders of the Ear

The following are the principal methods of examining the ear:

Inspection and palpation of the pinna:

Otoscopy: inspection of the external auditory meatus and tympanic membrane with an **otoscope**, an instrument that directs a light into the ear through a conical speculum, and is equipped with a magnifying lens; mobility of the tympanic membrane can be assessed when the subject swallows or performs the **Valsalva maneuver** (or when, in children, the examiner blows a puff of air into the ear).

Measurements of hearing: 1) simple tests with ticking watch or tuning fork; 2) **audiography**, a precise measurement of the faintest loudness (in decibels) that the subject can hear, each ear tested separately at each of several pitches (for example, 250, 500, 1000, 2000, 3000, 4000, 6000, and 8000 Hz); this can be performed by a trained technician with carefully calibrated testing equipment, or by automated machinery activated by the subject; 3) more elaborate testing of the subject's ability to discriminate spoken words.

Weber test: a vibrating tuning fork placed against a bony surface of the head at the midline sends vibrations through the bones of the skull. These should be heard equally in the two ears; if there is hearing loss due to blockage of the external auditory meatus or to injury or disease of the middle ear, the tone of the fork will be heard louder in the affected ear; in hearing loss due to damage to the inner ear or acoustic nerve, however, the tone will be heard louder in the more normal ear.

Rinne test: the sound of a vibrating tuning fork positioned so that the tines are near the pinna (**air conduction**) and should be heard by the subject even after the sound sensed when the tuning fork is placed on the mastoid process behind the ear (**bone conduction**) can no longer be heard; when bone conduction is heard longer than air conduction in an ear with reduced hearing, the hearing loss is due to obstruction of the meatus or disease of the middle ear.

Tympanocentesis: puncture of the tympanic membrane and withdrawal of fluid from the middle ear for examination, including culture.

Pneumotympanometry: assessment of the mobility of the tympanic membrane by applying pressure to its outer surface with a device fitting tightly in the external meatus.

Infections of the Outer and Middle Ear

Otitis Externa (Swimmer's Ear)
Infection of the external auditory meatus.

Causes: Infection with bacteria *(Proteus, Pseudomonas)* and sometimes fungi *(Aspergillus)*. Predisposing causes include water exposure (swimming, showering), excessive cerumen, mechanical trauma (probing with paperclip), foreign body (cotton, pencil eraser), diabetes mellitus, and immune compromise.

History: Earache, itching in the external auditory meatus, purulent discharge. Hearing loss if the meatus is occluded by swelling or exudate.

Physical Examination: Redness and swelling of the meatus, sometimes with complete occlusion; purulent exudate, perhaps with excessive cerumen or foreign body visible. Tenderness on manipulation of the pinna.

Course: Generally benign, but in diabetes mellitus and AIDS an external ear infection may resist conservative treatment and become chronic, perhaps invading the skull or brain, with resulting neurologic damage.

Treatment: After gentle cleansing and removal of any foreign material, cerumen, or exudate, topical antibiotics (ear drops), often with hydrocortisone to combat local inflammation, are instilled several times a day. Sometimes a gauze wick is inserted to facilitate penetration of ear drops when edema of the meatus is extreme. In invasive infections, intravenous antibiotics and even surgery may be required.

Otitis Media

Bacterial infection of the **middle ear** and adjoining **mastoid air cells**.

Cause: Infection by *Streptococcus pneumoniae, Haemophilus influenzae, Streptococcus pyogenes,* and other bacteria. Otitis media commonly occurs as a sequel to a viral upper respiratory infection. Obstruction of the auditory tube by edema leads to pressure changes within the middle ear and secretion of mucus and serous fluid, which becomes infected by bacteria already present in the tissues. Otitis media is often bilateral. It is commoner in infants and small children than in adolescents and adults, accounting for one-third of all pediatric office visits.

History: Pain and pressure in one or both ears, hearing loss, sometimes fever.

Physical Examination: Redness of the tympanic membrane, sometimes with formation of bullae. Immobility of the tympanic membrane, reflecting malfunction of the auditory tube. Occasionally bulging of the membrane. If spontaneous rupture occurs, blood or purulent exudate in the external auditory meatus.

Course: It is estimated that 20-80% of all cases of otitis media will resolve spontaneously without treatment. However, all diagnosed cases are treated because of the risk of serious complications in a few patients. Neglect of the infection, its failure to respond to standard initial treatment, or a series of recurrent infections can lead to chronic otitis media, typically due to different organisms (*Proteus, Pseudomonas,* staphylococci) than acute infection. Complications of chronic otitis media include spontaneous rupture of the tympanic membrane, with chronic purulent drainage; destruction of the bones within the middle ear that transmit sound; invasion of mastoid air cells (**mastoiditis**), skull bones, and even the central nervous system by infection; formation of **cholesteatoma**, a benign but locally invasive growth of the tympanic membrane caused by prolonged negative pressure (partial vacuum) in the middle ear. Chronic otitis media can lead to permanent conductive hearing loss and, in small children, speech defects because of inability to hear speech sounds properly.

Treatment: Systemic antibiotics (amoxicillin with or without clavulanic acid, erythromycin, trimethoprim-sulfamethoxazole), decongestants, analgesics. If tympanic membrane rupture threatens, **myringotomy** (surgical puncture of the membrane, with release of pus). In children with recurrent or refractory infections, polyethylene tubes may be placed in the tympanic membrane(s) to aerate the middle ear(s) and allow for escape of purulent secretion. Cholesteatoma and mastoiditis are treated surgically. Chronic perforation of the tympanic membrane requires surgical repair (**tympanoplasty**).

Disorders of the Inner Ear

Tinnitus
Perception of abnormal sounds in the ear(s) or head. When pulsatile (simultaneous with heartbeat), it may result from vascular disease (arterial stenosis, aneurysm). **Tinnitus** is generally a humming or squealing noise heard constantly or intermittently in one or both ears, especially at night when external sounds are at a minimum. It is generally due to degenerative disease of the inner ear, and frequently accompanies **sensorineural hearing loss** (discussed below). Common causes are excessive noise exposure and certain medicines. Aspirin and other salicylates at higher doses cause tinnitus lasting only as long as they remain in the body. Other drugs (certain antibiotics) can cause permanent tinnitus. Treatment of tinnitus is generally unsatisfactory but includes masking with other sounds (music, "static" on a radio).

Vertigo
A sense of motion (spinning, falling, floor tipping) when no such motion is occurring.

Causes: Labyrinthitis, often following respiratory infection and hence often called viral. Degenerative changes in the balance-sensing mechanism of the inner ear. Increased pressure within the endolymphatic sac (**Ménière disease**). Vascular or neoplastic disease of the inner ear or temporal lobe of the cerebral cortex. Diplopia, head injury, multiple sclerosis, drugs, alcohol.

History: A feeling of spinning or falling to one side, or a sense that the floor is tipping or rotating, coming on suddenly, often with head movement, and lasting seconds, minutes, hours, days, weeks, or months. When severe, vertigo may make it impossible for the patient to stand or walk, and may be accompanied by nausea and vomiting. There may also be tinnitus and hearing loss.

Physical Examination: May be essentially normal. The **Romberg test** (patient standing with eyes closed) may indicate inability to maintain equilibrium. Eyes may show nystagmus.

Treatment: May be limited to treatment of the underlying cause. In **Ménière disease**, salt restriction and diuretic therapy may help by reducing the pressure of the endolymph. Medicines such as meclizine and dimenhydrinate may diminish or abolish vertigo temporarily. In some cases of positional vertigo, head manipulation can reduce symptoms by promoting reorientation of the balance mechanism.

Hearing Loss

Reduction, often permanent, in the acuity of hearing in one or both ears. Hearing loss is divided into three types depending on the location of the abnormality.

Conductive hearing loss: Disease or abnormality in the outer or middle ear: cerumen impaction, otitis media with effusion, hardening of the tympanic membrane (otosclerosis), injury or disease of the ossicles.

Sensory hearing loss: Disease of the cochlea: acoustic trauma, ototoxicity (aminoglycosides, loop diuretics, cisplatin), aging.

Neural: Eighth nerve lesions; cerebrovascular disease.

Hearing loss is assessed by audiometry and the Weber and Rinne tests. Treatment is that of the underlying cause, if possible.

Generally no treatment is effective.

The Nose

Anatomy and Physiology

The external nose is supported by a framework of cartilage and covered by skin. The **nostrils** (anterior **nares**) open into paired passages lined with **mucous membrane**, which is rich in serous and mucous glands and blood vessels. The lining membrane of these passages is closely attached to convoluted ridges of bone called **turbinates** (three on each side), which increase the surface area of membrane that is exposed to inspired air. Adjacent to the nasal passages, and communicating with them by narrow orifices, are the **paranasal sinuses**. These are cavities within the bones of the skull, somewhat variable in size and shape, and lined with mucosa like that of the nose. The nasal passages end at the **choanae**, or posterior nares, where they enter the **nasopharynx**, the uppermost part of the pharyngeal cavity. The nasal passages warm and moisturize inspired air, and particulate matter in the air is trapped in the mucous film lining them.

Diagnostic Procedures in Disorders of the Nose

Direct inspection with nasal speculum or **rhinoscope**.

Posterior rhinoscopy: inspection of posterior nares with angled mirror placed in the oropharynx.

Nasal smear: examination of a stained smear of scrapings from the nasal mucosa for evidence of infection (neutrophilic leukocytes) or allergy (eosinophilic leukocytes).

Culture of nasal secretions to identify bacterial pathogens.

Diseases of the Nose

Coryza (Common Cold)

A common, mild rhinitis caused by viruses.

Causes: Any of numerous viruses spread readily from person to person. Susceptibility to colds may be heightened by exposure to severe winter weather (especially whole-body chilling), drying of indoor air by heating systems, or crowding indoors during the winter.

History: Headache, nasal stuffiness, runny nose, sneezing, throat irritation, malaise. Occasionally fever, chills, anorexia, and muscle aching.

Physical Examination: Erythema and edema of nasal mucosa. Temperature may be slightly elevated.

Course: Generally self-limited. Sometimes complicated by sinusitis, otitis media, pharyngitis, bronchitis.

Treatment: Purely symptomatic. Oral decongestants are moderately effective. Aspirin, acetaminophen, or ibuprofen relieve discomfort. Rest, fluids. Antihistamines do not decongest, antibiotics do not kill cold viruses, and nasal decongestant sprays cause rebound congestion worse than the disease.

Allergic Rhinitis (Hay Fever)

A recurrent, often seasonal, inflammation of the nasal mucous membrane caused by allergy to inhaled materials.

Causes: Sensitivity to pollens, grasses, mold spores, dust mites, animal dander, second-hand cigarette smoke, and other inhalant allergens.

History: Recurrent or constant nasal congestion and irritation, with copious watery discharge, itching, sneezing (often many times in a row), and itching and watering of the eyes. Symptoms may occur consistently at certain seasons (spring, fall) or, especially when due to house dust, may be perennial.

Physical Examination: Watery, red eyes. Pale or bluish, markedly swollen nasal mucosa. **Polyps** (massive overgrowths of chronically inflamed mucosa) may be present.

Diagnostic Tests: Nasal smear shows eosinophils. Skin testing or RAST (radioallergosorbent testing) can identify causative allergens.

Treatment: Decongestants, antihistamines, nasal corticosteroid spray. Avoidance of known allergens when possible. Use of air filters as appropriate. Continued administration of desensitizing antigens often markedly reduces symptoms.

Sinusitis

Bacterial infection of one or more paranasal sinuses.

Cause: Usually occurs as a complication of viral or allergic rhinitis. Swelling of the nasal mucosa leads to blockage of the sinus openings, with accumulation of purulent secretion within the sinuses affected. Attacks may occur repeatedly in some persons, and sinusitis may become chronic.

History: Pain in one or more sinus cavities, often aggravated by bending forward. Pain may be manifested as a severe headache or may radiate into the teeth. Purulent nasal or postnasal discharge may be present. Occasionally fever, chills, and malaise. Sinusitis is enormously overdiagnosed by patients (who are misled by inaccurate advertising for nonprescription cold medicines) and even by physicians (who find it

easier to accept patients' self-diagnoses of sinusitis than to explain that the problem is a self-limited viral cold requiring no specific treatment).
Physical Examination: Edema and erythema of nasal mucosa. Purulent discharge in nasal passages or oropharynx (postnasal drip).
Diagnostic Tests: In chronic sinusitis, x-ray or other diagnostic imaging shows thickening of sinus membranes and often presence of fluid within cavities.
Treatment: Oral antibiotic (amoxicillin, trimethoprim-sulfamethoxazole), decongestant, analgesic. A short course of nasal decongestant spray may help to open and drain sinuses. Chronic sinusitis may respond to prolonged antibiotic therapy (ciprofloxacin). Surgical procedures can be used to correct anatomic lesions predisposing to sinusitis, or to improve drainage of a chronically infected sinus.

Epistaxis (Nosebleed)

Bleeding from the nose may be due to nasal trauma, irritation of the mucosa by dust or dry air, upper respiratory infection or allergic rhinitis, or coagulation defect. Treatment of acute nosebleed is by application of direct pressure and, if necessary, topical **vasoconstrictor**. If bleeding persists or recurs, **cautery** with silver nitrate or anterior nasal packing may be necessary. Rarely bleeding comes from the posterior nares (usually in middle-aged or elderly patients with hypertension or arteriosclerosis) and requires a posterior nasal pack. Prevention of further nosebleeds may include use of lubricating applications to the mucosa, humidification of air, and avoidance of dusts and other irritants.

The Throat

Anatomy and Physiology

The throat, or **pharynx**, is a cavity lined with mucous membrane that conducts air from the nose and mouth into the trachea, and food and drink from the mouth into the esophagus. It consists of three portions: the **nasopharynx**, on a level with the nasal passages and communicating with them; the oropharynx, on a level with the mouth and communicating with it; and the **hypopharynx** or **laryngopharynx**, which lies below the **oropharynx** and gives entry to the esophagus and the larynx.

The **tonsils** and **adenoids** are masses of lymphoid tissue surrounding the zone between the mouth and the oropharynx. At the boundary between the oropharynx and the hypopharynx lies the **epiglottis**, a flexible valve that closes the respiratory passage during swallowing of food or drink.

The lining of the pharynx secretes **mucus**, which keeps the surface moist, traps inhaled particles, and supplements the saliva as a lubricant for food. **Lymph glands** in the front and back of the neck receive lymphatic drainage from the throat and adjacent structures.

Diagnostic Procedures in Disorders of the Throat

Inspection of the throat with a focused light, often with the aid of a **tongue depressor** (tongue blade) to press the tongue out of the field of vision.

Palpation of **cervical lymph glands** and of masses, swellings, or other structures within the throat.

Throat culture to identify bacterial pathogens.

Strep screen (faster than culture, but detecting only beta-hemolytic streptococci).

Biopsy of masses or lesions suspected of being malignant.

X-ray or other imaging to identify foreign bodies, masses, or abnormalities of the airway due to injury or disease.

Acute Pharyngitis (Sore Throat)

Acute inflammation of the throat due to infection.

Cause: Usually viruses, including the Epstein-Barr virus, which causes infectious mononucleosis. Occasionally bacteria such as *Streptococcus pneumoniae* and Group A beta-hemolytic *Streptococcus pyogenes* ("strep throat"), or fungi such as *Candida*. Infection with cold viruses may predispose to bacterial infection. Sore throat is more prevalent in cold weather. It is often said to be the number one reason for visits to primary care physicians. In some practices (including my own) it actually accounts for the *majority* of patient visits during the winter.

History: Pain, irritation, or a sense of fullness or swelling in the throat, accentuated by swallowing and often radiating to the ears. Fever, painful glandular swelling in the neck.

Physical Examination: May be essentially normal. Fever is often present. Edema and erythema of the oropharynx, often involving the tonsils, soft palate, and uvula, occur in most bacterial and many viral throat infections. Severe infections, including streptococcal pharyngitis (strep throat) and infectious mononucleosis, cause formation of white or gray exudate (consisting of dead tissue, white blood cells, and bacteria) on pharyngeal walls and especially on the tonsils. A firmly adherent exudate is characteristic of *Candida* infection (thrush). The presence of vesicles or ulcers suggests viral infection (herpes simplex virus, **coxsackievirus**). Severe pain and swelling may cause a hollow or "hot potato" voice, and may make swallowing virtually impossible, so that the patient drools to avoid swallowing saliva, and becomes dehydrated from lack of fluid intake. Extreme swelling may compromise the airway. Cervical lymph glands may be swollen and tender. Some strains of beta-hemolytic streptococci cause a widespread red rash (**scarlet fever, scarlatina**).

Diagnostic Tests: Throat culture or **strep screen** may identify the causative organism. Blood studies (white blood cell count and differential, antistreptolysin O titer, heterophile antibodies) help to diagnose strep throat and infectious mononucleosis. Smears or scrapings of exudate can confirm presence of *Candida*.

Course: Viral sore throat runs its course within a week or two. Occasionally it becomes complicated by streptococcal infection, which may lead to acute rheumatic fever. It may also progress to otitis media, acute or chronic tonsillitis, or lower respiratory infection. **Peritonsillar abscess** (quinsy) is a severe bacterial infection developing above and behind one tonsil and causing extreme pain and swelling, with deviation of the uvula away from the affected side.

Treatment: Acute viral pharyngitis requires no treatment except analgesics, gargles, soothing lozenges, and perhaps a soft diet. Currently, however, most physicians treat acute pharyngitis with antibiotics. If streptococcal infection is diagnosed, a 10-day course of an antibiotic known to be able to eradicate streptococci (such as penicillin V, erythromycin or cephalexin) is mandatory. Candidal oropharyngitis (**thrush**) is treated with topical antifungal medicine. The treatment of **peritonsillar abscess** is surgical drainage.

Glossary

aneurysm: abnormal dilatation of a blood vessel.

bulla (plural, **bullae**): a blister or bleb.

decibel: a measure of the loudness of sound; one tenth of a bel (named for Alexander Graham Bell).

endolymph: the fluid medium contained in the inner ear.

Hz: abbreviation for hertz, a measure of the frequency of a vibration, particularly one producing sound; equivalent to one cycle (or double vibration) per second. The vibration rate of middle C on a piano tuned to standard concert pitch is about 262 Hz; the pitch of the highest C (four octaves above middle C and the top key on the piano) is about 4186 Hz. The normal human ear can detect sounds ranging in pitch from 20 to 20,000 Hz.

impaction: plugging of an orifice with a dense mass of some material, as cerumen in the external auditory meatus.

larynx: the voice box, containing the vocal cords and situated between the laryngopharynx (the lowermost part of the throat) and the trachea (windpipe).

malaise: a vague sense of being unwell.

nystagmus: rhythmic, involuntary, jerky movements of both eyes, usually from side to side.

purulent: containing or consisting of pus.

rhinitis: inflammation of the nasal mucous membrane.

rhinoscope: an instrument for examining the interior of the nose.

serous gland: one producing a thin, watery secretion, not containing mucus.

speculum: an instrument for inspecting a body cavity or orifice, often equipped with a light source, a magnifying lens, or both.

stenosis: abnormal narrowing of a passage or vessel.

topical: referring to a medicine applied directly to skin or mucous membrane.

Valsalva maneuver: attempt at forced expiration, with the lips and nostrils closed; this drives air into the auditory tubes unless they are obstructed.

vasoconstrictor: a medicine that constricts blood vessels, either when applied topically or through systemic action.

Topics for Study or Discussion

1. List and classify several reasons for hearing loss.

2. List some common causes of nosebleed.

3. Define: audiogram, auditory tube, cerumen, coryza, epistaxis, mastoiditis, pharyngitis, pinna, vertigo.

4. Point out some ways in which the ear, nose, and throat are related anatomically, physiologically, and with respect to diseases affecting two or more of them.

5. Discuss the inappropriate treatment of viral respiratory infections with antibiotics. State some objections to this practice. What share of the blame would you assign to patients, pharmaceutical manufacturers, and physicians respectively?

Chapter 10

Diseases of the Respiratory System

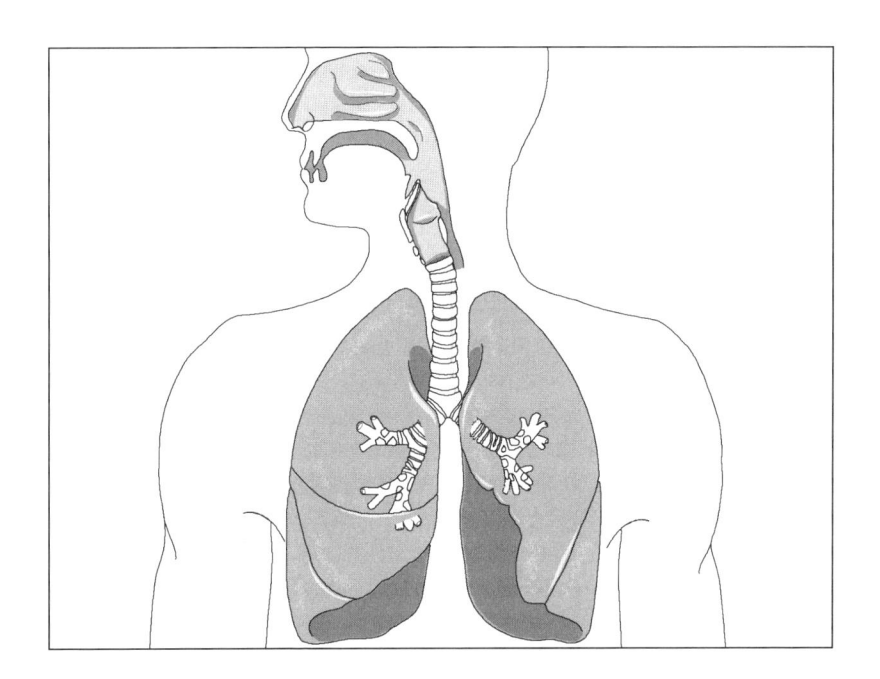

Learning Objectives

Upon completion of this chapter, the student should

- know the basic anatomy and physiology of the respiratory system;

- have a general knowledge of diagnostic procedures used in diseases of this system;

- understand signs, symptoms, and treatment of common diseases affecting them.

Anatomy and Physiology of the Respiratory System

The **respiratory system** comprises all the organs and tissues that serve to deliver oxygen to circulating blood and to remove carbon dioxide from it. The respiratory system consists of the nose, mouth, pharynx, larynx, trachea, bronchi, lungs, pleura, diaphragm, and chest wall (ribs and muscles).

Inspiration occurs when the diaphragm moves downward and the chest wall moves outward. This creates a slight vacuum within the chest cavity, causing the lungs to expand and draw air inward through the airway (mouth and nose, throat, trachea, and bronchi) into the lung tissue proper. At the end of inspiration, the diaphragm and chest wall relax, so that the lungs passively contract and expel air. This is known as **expiration**. During both phases of respiration, blood in pulmonary vessels takes up **oxygen** from the inspired air and releases **carbon dioxide** into the air that is about to be exhaled. Respiration is under involuntary control from a center in the brain stem. Respiratory rate varies with changes in the oxygen and carbon dioxide levels in the blood as well as in the composition and **pH** (alkalinity vs. acidity) of the serum.

The airway is lined by mucous membrane, which contains glands producing both mucous and serous secretions. The walls of the trachea and bronchi are reinforced by partial rings of cartilage, which prevent their collapse under negative pressure.

Lung tissue proper consists of numerous microscopic air sacs or **alveoli** (singular, **alveolus**), through whose extremely thin epithelial walls the respiratory gases can readily diffuse between the air within them and the blood in adjacent pulmonary vasculature. The lungs are protected by a delicate serous membrane called the **pleura**. The **visceral** layer of the pleura is closely applied to the surfaces of the lungs; the **parietal** layer lines the chest cavity. Normally the two layers are in contact, with a minute amount of serous fluid between them to serve as a lubricant as the lungs move with respect to the chest wall during respiration.

Symptoms and Signs of Respiratory Disease

Cough (dry or productive) or choking.
Production of sputum (watery, viscous, or purulent).
Hemoptysis (coughing up blood from respiratory passages).

Diseases of the Respiratory System • 163

Shortness of breath, tachypnea (increased respiratory rate).
Audible wheezing with respirations (inspiratory or expiratory).
Chest pain (constant, intermittent, or synchronous with breathing).
Cyanosis (blue color of skin, particularly lips and nail beds, due to presence of excess unoxygenated blood in the circulation).

Respiratory distress, indicated by increased effort to breathe, pursing of lips, use of **accessory muscles of respiration** (neck and upper chest muscles not needed for normal breathing), **intercostal retractions** (sucking in of muscles between ribs on inspiration).

Percussion of the chest may disclose **hyperresonance** due to a cavity within lung tissue or air in the pleural space; or **dullness** due to consolidation of lung tissue by infection, or neoplasm, or to fluid in the pleural space.

Auscultation may detect **rales** (crackling or bubbling sounds due to passage of air through fluid in respiratory passages); **rhonchi** (singular, rhonchus; whistling or honking sounds due to passage of air through respiratory passages narrowed by edema, secretions, or neoplasm); a **pleural friction rub** (due to inflammation or scarring of adjacent surfaces of visceral and parietal pleura); or reduction or absence of **breath sounds** (due to pulmonary consolidation, pleural air or fluid, collapse of a lung, or neoplasm).

Digital clubbing (enlargement of fingertips with elevation of proximal parts of nails, due to chronic pulmonary disease).

Diagnostic Procedures in Respiratory Disease

History and physical examination, with particular attention to skin color, respiratory effort, the fullness and symmetry of chest expansion during inspiration, respiratory noises heard with or without a stethoscope, and findings on percussion.

Examination of sputum for pathogenic organisms (by smear and culture), neoplastic cells, or other abnormal findings.

Pulmonary function tests, which measure the rate and volume of gas exchange in the respiratory system by means of finely calibrated instruments.

Arterial blood gas determination (measurement of partial pressures of oxygen and carbon dioxide in arterial blood).

Bronchoscopy (inspection of the interior of the trachea and main bronchi with a fiberoptic instrument). Specimens and biopsies can be taken through the instrument, and **bronchoalveolar lavage** (**BAL**; obtaining of material from lung tissue by washing) can be performed.

Imaging studies: standard PA (posteroanterior) and lateral chest x-rays, oblique or tomographic studies as needed; fluoroscopy; CT and MRI for various specialized diagnostic investigations; **ventilation-perfusion scan** (comparison of distribution of inspired radioactively tagged gas with distribution of injected radioactively tagged albumin, particularly useful in the diagnosis of pulmonary embolism).

Pleural or lung biopsy, either by percutaneous (needle) or open procedure.

Diseases of Respiratory Passages

Bronchitis

Inflammation of the bronchi, with mucus production and cough. Acute bronchitis is a common feature of respiratory infections. **Chronic bronchitis**, usually due to cigarette smoking, is a form of chronic obstructive pulmonary disease.

Acute Bronchitis

Acute, self-limited inflammation of the bronchial passages.

Cause: Usually viral in origin, as a complication of an upper respiratory infection. Sometimes due to bacterial secondary infection. Can also be due to irritation by smoke or dust.

History: Cough, usually productive, occurring as a complication of a respiratory infection. When severe it may be accompanied by fever, shortness of breath, and wheezing. Cough may be worsened by the recumbent position and may keep the patient awake at night.

Physical Examination: Often no physical findings other than frequent or spasmodic coughing. The breath sounds may be bronchial, or rhonchi may be heard, chiefly on inspiration.

Diagnostic Tests: Blood studies are normal. Smear and culture of sputum may indicate bacterial infection but usually do not. Chest x-ray may show increased bronchial markings.

Course: Cough may continue for weeks or months but resolution is eventually complete. Cough may result in rib fracture or other complications. Bronchitis lasting for three months and occurring in two successive years is termed chronic bronchitis.

Treatment: Largely symptomatic, with hydration, expectorants, and cough suppressants, at least for nighttime use. Many patients experience improvement when taking bronchodilator drugs either orally or by inhaler. Most patients are treated with antibiotics (erythromycin, trimethoprim-sulfamethoxazole, tetracyclines), even though the vast majority of cases of bronchitis are due to viral infection aggravated by cigarette smoking.

Chronic Bronchitis

Chronic productive cough lasting for at least three months in each of two successive years. Chronic bronchitis is one form of **chronic obstructive pulmonary disease**, the other being **emphysema**. The two forms may be combined in varying proportions.

Cause: Most cases occur in smokers. Air pollution, allergy, and infection may play a part in some cases. Obesity is a risk factor.

History: Severe, persistent cough with copious production of bronchial mucus, particularly on arising in the morning.

Physical Examination: Wheezes and inspiratory rhonchi on auscultation of the chest. When bronchitis is severe, cyanosis may be noted.

Diagnostic Tests: The hematocrit may be slightly elevated, reflecting polycythemia in response to diminished oxygen exchange in the lungs. Arterial blood shows reduction of oxygen and increase of carbon dioxide. Chest x-ray shows increased bronchopulmonary markings. Electrocardiogram may show right axis deviation and P pulmonale.

Course: Progressive deterioration of pulmonary function and heightened susceptibility to bacterial infection.

Treatment: Cessation of smoking and avoidance of respiratory irritants and infections are essential. Bronchodilators orally or by inhaler may improve bronchial air flow. Ipratropium by inhaler is particularly effective. Hydration, exercise, and postural drainage may assist in freeing the tract of secretions. When hypoxia is severe, home oxygen may be useful.

Bronchiectasis

An irreversible dilatation of large bronchi, due to chronic infection, obstruction, or autoimmune disease. About half of cases occur in persons with **cystic fibrosis**. Symptoms include chronic cough, production of copious purulent sputum, and hemoptysis. Most patients suffer weakness, weight loss, and recurrent pneumonia. Rales are heard at the lung bases, and x-ray, particularly CT scan, may show lung cysts and fibrous **cuffing** around affected bronchi. Treatment is with careful personal hygiene, postural drainage of chest secretions, antibiotics selected on the basis of sputum culture and sensitivity, and bronchodilators.

Emphysema

An abnormal and irreversible enlargement of air spaces in lung tissue due to breakdown of walls of air sacs.

Cause: Cigarette smoking is a principal cause. Some cases are due to infection, allergy, or respiratory irritants. In some patients, emphysema is linked to an inherited deficiency of alpha$_1$-antitrypsin in respiratory epithelium and other tissues.

History: The onset is usually after age 50. Shortness of breath, growing progressively worse, is the dominant symptom. Some patients experience weakness and weight loss.

Physical Examination: Tachypnea and dyspnea may be evident, with activity of the accessory respiratory muscles and pursed lips. The anteroposterior diameter of the chest is increased (**barrel chest**). There is hyperresonance of the thorax on percussion, and the breath sounds are reduced on auscultation. Weakness and wasting of the muscles of the extremities are often noted.

Diagnostic Tests: Chest x-ray typically shows hyperinflation of the chest cavity (low diaphragms, heart in vertical position), and hyperlucency of lung tissue. X-ray may also show bullae or blebs (air-filled cavities). Blood gas studies are usually normal but may show diminished partial pressure of oxygen. Pulmonary function tests show increased total lung capacity but reduced vital capacity and rate of air exchange.

Course: Recurrent respiratory infections, congestive heart failure (right ventricular failure, cor pulmonale), progressive respiratory failure.

Treatment: Smoking cessation, bronchodilators, oxygen inhalation, antibiotics as needed, physical therapy. For cardiac failure, sodium restriction and diuretics.

Asthma (Reactive Airways Disease, RAD)

A chronic or recurrent inflammatory disease of the trachea and bronchi characterized by recurrent narrowing of air passages with wheezing and shortness of breath.

Cause: Abnormal sensitivity of respiratory passages to a wide variety of triggering factors: emotional stress; dust, smoke, and other airborne irritants; physical exertion (exercise-induced asthma); respiratory infection; and drugs (aspirin, beta-blockers). Asthma affects about 5% of the population; there may be a genetic predisposition.

History: Paroxysms of wheezing, dyspnea, cough, and tightness in the chest. Severe asthma may result in physical exhaustion and symptoms of hypoxia.

Physical Examination: Tachypnea; labored, noisy respirations with prolongation of the expiratory phase. Sibilant (whistling) or sonorous (humming) rhonchi may be heard throughout the chest, particularly on expiration. In severe asthma, retraction of intercostal muscles may be noted on inspiration. The chest may be hyperresonant to percussion, and cyanosis may indicate hypoxia.

Diagnostic Tests: Pulmonary function tests indicate significant reduction in measures of air flow. When the diagnosis is in doubt, a provocative test (challenge of an asymptomatic patient with methacholine or histamine) will lead to reduction in air flow. During an asthmatic attack, administration of bronchodilator by injection or inhalation will lead to marked improvement in air flow measurements. In severe asthma, the blood level of oxygen may be reduced. The eosinophil count may be increased in allergic asthma, and eosinophils may be detected in sputum. Chest x-ray may show hyperinflation of the thorax.

Course: Many cases of childhood asthma are "outgrown." Asthma may persist and progress throughout life, depending on its underlying cause and triggering factors. Infection, cor pulmonale, and acute respiratory distress syndrome are possible complications.

Treatment: Avoidance of known inciting factors; smoking cessation. For intermittent symptoms and exercise-induced asthma, aerosolized bronchodilator administered by inhalation usually suffices to control symptoms. More severe or chronic disease is better treated with aerosolized corticosteroid, with bronchodilator treatment during exacerbations. Many patients become adept at manipulating the dosage of these agents on the basis of measurements made with a simple, portable peak flow meter. Other treatments include oral theophylline, mast-cell stabilizers (cromolyn, nedocromil), and the atropine-like drug ipratropium. In severe, refractory asthma (**status asthmaticus**), oxygen is administered by inhalation and bronchodilators and corticosteroids are administered by injection.

Adult (also Acute) Respiratory Distress Syndrome (ARDS)

Acute respiratory failure induced by severe respiratory or systemic illness.

Causes: Respiratory: pneumonia, inhalation of smoke or toxic gases, pulmonary injury, near-drowning, hanging, pulmonary embolism, aspiration of gastric contents. Systemic: septicemia, severe trauma (particularly burns and head injuries), shock, repeated blood transfusions, drugs, toxins.

History: Abrupt onset of severe dyspnea within 24-48 hours after the inciting event or condition.

Physical Examination: Obvious respiratory distress, tachypnea, intercostal retractions, coarse rales on auscultations. Signs of underlying disease are usually evident.

Diagnostic Tests: The arterial oxygen level is depressed. Chest x-ray shows diffuse infiltrates in both lungs.

Course: Most cases progress to multiple organ system failure. The mortality rate is over 50% and average survival time is about 2 weeks. Survivors usually regain full health eventually.

Treatment: Largely supportive. Identification and treatment of underlying condition. Oxygen, antibiotics, diuretics, and other agents as appropriate.

Pneumonia (Pneumonitis)

Inflammation of lung tissue, usually due to infection.

Cause: Infection by a variety of microorganisms, including *Streptococcus pneumoniae, Klebsiella pneumoniae, Mycoplasma pneumoniae, Chlamydia pneumoniae, Legionella pneumophila, Staphylococcus aureus, Pneumocystis carinii,* and various viruses. Symptoms, signs, and clinical course depend on the infecting agent. Predisposing causes are debility, impaired immunity, cigarette smoking, chronic pulmonary or bronchial disease, and advanced age. Pneumonia often occurs as a complication or extension of upper respiratory infection.

History: Fever, chills, cough, purulent or bloody sputum, pleuritic chest pain (stabbing, sharply localized pain with respiratory movements), dypsnea, myalgia, malaise.

Physical Examination: Most patients have fever. The pulse and respiratory rate may be markedly increased. Examination of the lungs reveals rales or evidence of consolidation (reduced or absent breath sounds, flat percussion note). In mycoplasmal or viral pneumonia, physical findings may be minimal.

Diagnostic Tests: The white blood count may be elevated. Examination of stained sputum shows white blood cells and the infecting organism, if bacterial. Sputum culture yields growth of bacterial agents. Bronchoscopy and bronchoalveolar washings may be necessary to obtain satisfactory sputum for examination. Chest x-ray shows evidence of pulmonary infiltrates or consolidation, atelectasis, pleural effusion.

Course: Some pneumonias, including most viral and mycoplasmal infections, resolve spontaneously. Lobar pneumonia due to *Streptococcus pneumoniae*, staphylococcal pneumonia, and (in immunocompromised hosts) *Pneumocystis carinii* pneumonia frequently progress to a fatal termination, even with treatment. Pneumonia ranks sixth as a cause of death in the U.S.

Complications: Pleural effusion, empyema, septicemia, endocarditis, arthritis, respiratory failure.

Treatment: Oral antibiotics may suffice in mild disease. Penicillins, cephalosporins, and erythromycin are the agents usually chosen. In more severe disease, hospitalization, intravenous antibiotics, and oxygen by inhalation may be necessary.

Pulmonary Tuberculosis

Cause: Infection of lungs and other tissues and organs by *Mycobacterium tuberculosis*. Person-to-person spread by respiratory droplets is the usual route of infection. Primary infection may be asymptomatic but leaves a focus of infective organisms in the lung and induces a state of hypersensitivity to the infecting organism. Postprimary infection, which may result from breakdown of a primary focus or from a new dose of organisms from without, typically leads to significant and chronic clinical disease. The infection can also be transmitted by unpasteurized milk from infected cows. Other species, notably those of the *M. avium-intracellulare complex* (MAI, MAC) may also cause tuberculosis, typically acquired through the gastrointestinal tract. Persons with AIDS are at particular risk of tuberculosis, including MAI tuberculosis.

History: Cough, purulent or bloody sputum, fever, night sweats, weakness, anorexia, weight loss.

Physical Examination: Fever, cachexia (wasting), evidence of rales, consolidation, or cavitation in the lungs.

Diagnostic Tests: The tuberculin skin test is positive. Sputum contains acid-fast organisms, and sputum culture is positive for *M. tuberculosis*. Chest x-ray may show a calcified primary focus, hilar lymphadenopathy, upper lobe infiltrates, pleural effusion, or cavitation.

Course: Prognosis with treatment is good. Complications include **phthisis** (wasting) and hemorrhage.

Treatment: Simultaneous treatment with three or four drugs (isoniazid, rifampin, pyrazinamide, streptomycin, ethambutol) for a protracted period is the standard.

Pneumoconiosis

A chronic fibrosis of lung tissue caused by prolonged inhalation of mineral dusts, including coal, silicates, and asbestos.

Cause: Chronic pulmonary exposure, usually occupational, to finely divided mineral materials.

History: Many patients have few or no symptoms. When lung damage is severe, particularly in **asbestosis**, there may be progressive shortness of breath.

Physical Examination: Auscultation of the chest may reveal crackling rales on inspiration. Severe disease may lead to digital clubbing and cyanosis.

Diagnostic Tests: Chest x-ray shows diffusely scattered fibrotic changes in the lungs. In **anthracosis** (due to inhalation of coal dust), nodular opacities are seen particularly in the upper lung fields. In **silicosis** (due to inhalation of silicates, particularly from sand and hard coal) there are also rounded densities in lung tissue, and egg-shell calcification may be noted in hilar lymph nodes. Asbestos causes interstitial fibrosis, with linear and nodular markings in lung tissue, pleural thickening, and calcified pleural plaques. Pulmonary function tests show reduced vital capacity and flow rates. Arterial oxygen is reduced, and so is arterial carbon dioxide because of hyperventilation.

Course: Although many persons are free of symptoms despite x-ray evidence of fibrosis, others experience progressive and disabling impairment of lung function. Pneumoconioses, especially asbestosis, tend to be worse in cigarette smokers. There is an increased incidence of pulmonary tuberculosis in persons with silicosis. Asbestos exposure can lead to a malignant tumor of the pleura (**pleural mesothelioma**). In addition, the risk of bronchogenic carcinoma in smokers is greatly increased by concomitant asbestosis.

Treatment: Purely supportive and symptomatic.

Bronchogenic carcinoma is discussed in Chapter 5.

Pulmonary Embolism and Infarction

Obstruction of parts of the pulmonary arterial circulation by one or more emboli.

Cause: Thromboemboli from the deep veins of the lower extremities or pelvis passing through the right ventricle are the principal cause. Emboli may also consist of tumor material, amniotic fluid, fat, air, or injected foreign material. Predisposing causes of pulmonary thromboembolism are prolonged immobilization, surgery, childbirth, injury to venous endothelium, hypercoagulable state (cancer, oral contraceptives), congestive heart failure, obesity, and advanced age. Trapping of an embolus in a pulmonary artery results in both reflex vasoconstriction, with extensive compromise of pulmonary circulation, and reflex bronchoconstriction, with impairment of pulmonary gas exchange.

History: Sudden onset of dyspnea, chest pain, anxiety, diaphoresis, collapse. If infarction occurs, chest pain may be pleuritic and there may be hemoptysis.

Physical Examination: Tachycardia, tachypnea, crackling rales or wheezes, pleural friction rub, cyanosis, fever.

Diagnostic Tests: The arterial oxygen tension is diminished. The electrocardiogram may show right axis deviation or right heart strain. Chest x-ray in acute pulmonary embolism may show an infiltrate or atelectasis. If infarction occurs, a wedge-shaped zone of opacification may be apparent. A **ventilation-perfusion scan** (radionuclide scan) shows areas of lung tissue that are normally ventilated (normal air flow) but not normally perfused (impeded blood flow). Pulmonary angiogram confirms and localizes pulmonary arterial obstruction. The source of the embolus may be discovered by venography, ultrasonography, impedance plethysmography, or other diagnostic modality.

Course: About 10% of patients die within the first hour, and the overall mortality rate is about 30%. Fatal outcome is usually due to right ventricular failure or cardiogenic shock.

Treatment: Vigorous supportive efforts, including oxygen and treatment for shock and cardiac failure. Thrombolytic therapy with streptokinase, urokinase, or tissue plasminogen activator (tPA) is often successful in dissolving the embolus. Intravenous heparin and oral warfarin are administered to prevent further thrombosis of deep veins. Passage of further emboli through the inferior vena cava may be prevented by surgical plication, ligation, or insertion of a filter. Prevention of pulmonary embolism includes use of compressive stockings in surgical and other bedfast patients, early ambulation after surgery, and use of low-dose heparin in selected medical and surgical patients.

Diseases of the Pleura

Pleural Effusion

Presence of fluid in the pleural space as a result of local or systemic disease.

Causes: **Pleural transudates** (fluid relatively low in protein) occur in congestive heart failure, cirrhosis with ascites, nephrotic syndrome, myxedema, and obstructive disorders of the pulmonary circulation (superior vena cava obstruction, pulmonary embolism, constrictive pericarditis). **Pleural exudates** (fluid higher in protein and also containing LDH) are due to pneumonia and other pulmonary or pleural infections including tuberculosis, malignant disease, and uremia.

History: There may be no symptoms. With large effusions, dyspnea. With local inflammation, pleuritic chest pain.

Physical Examination: Reduced breath sounds, dullness to percussion, reduced **tactile fremitus** (transmission of vocal sounds to the examiner's hand on the chest wall) over the effusion. In the presence of pleural inflammation, a pleural friction rub may be heard.

Diagnostic Tests: Chest x-ray, particularly **lateral decubitus films** (taken with patient lying on side), shows the effusion. Fluid obtained by thoracentesis is examined for protein and LDH (to distinguish between transudate and exudate) and for white blood cells, pathogenic microorganisms, and malignant cells to establish an underlying cause for the effusion. Pleural biopsy, closed (needle) or open, may be required for definitive diagnosis.

Treatment: Correction of the cause of effusion, if possible.

Spontaneous Pneumothorax

Sudden leakage of air from a lung into the pleural space.

Cause: Rupture of a bleb or bulla, which may be solitary or part of a generalized process. The condition is commoner in males and in smokers.

History: Sudden onset of chest pain and dyspnea, which may occur at rest or during sleep.

Physical Examination: Tachycardia; reduced breath sounds, hyperresonance, and reduced **tactile fremitus** over the pneumothorax.

Diagnostic Tests: Chest x-ray (inspiratory and expiratory films) shows pneumothorax.

Course: A small pneumothorax resolves spontaneously. Larger ones may severely compromise cardiopulmonary dynamics. The recurrence rate is 50%.

Treatment: Thoracostomy tube connected to a water seal bottle and suction, to withdraw air from the pleural space. **Thoracotomy** (open surgery) may be required for a continuing leak, or for recurrent pneumothorax.

Topics for Study or Discussion

1. List five pulmonary disorders that cause cough and shortness of breath.

2. Explain the results of arterial gas studies and pulmonary function tests in asthma, acute respiratory distress syndrome, and pneumoconiosis.

3. Define or explain: (pulmonary) alveolus, asthma, bronchiectasis, bronchoalveolar lavage, cyanosis, hemoptysis, pleura, pneumoconiosis, rhonchus.

4. In what diseases might bronchoscopy be of help in diagnosis? Sputum smear and culture? Ventilation-perfusion scan?

5. What is the single most important preventable cause of respiratory disease and death?

Chapter 11

Diseases of the Digestive System

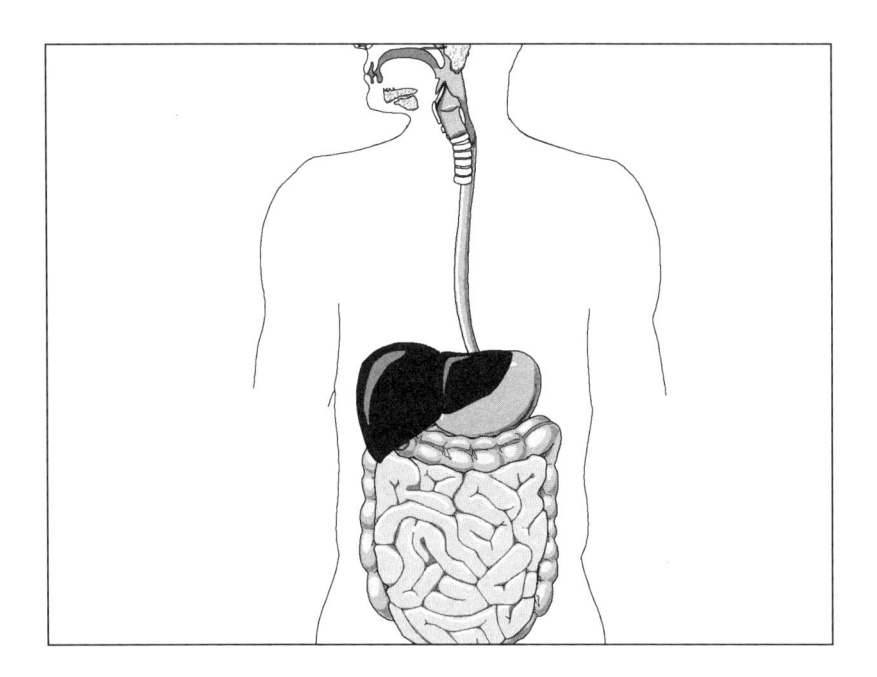

Learning Objectives

Upon completion of this chapter, the student should:

- know the basic anatomy and physiology of the digestive system;

- have a general knowledge of diagnostic procedures used in digestive and hepatobiliary disease;

- understand signs, symptoms, and treatment of common diseases affecting this system.

Anatomy and Physiology of the Digestive System

The **digestive system** includes all those structures concerned with the ingestion of solids and liquids, their mechanical and chemical breakdown into usable nutrients, the absorption of these into the circulation, and the excretion of solid wastes. The **alimentary canal** is a coiled but unbranched tube extending from the lips to the anus and divided into mouth, oropharynx, esophagus, stomach, small intestine (duodenum, jejunum, ileum), and large intestine (colon, rectum).

Numerous microscopic glandular structures occur in the walls of the digestive tract (gastric glands, intestinal glands), and in addition larger secretory organs (salivary glands, liver, pancreas) pour their products through **ducts** into parts of the **tract**. These secretions serve to liquefy and lubricate food and to break down fats, proteins, and carbohydrates to fatty acids, amino acids, and simple sugars, respectively.

Symptoms and Signs of Digestive Disease

Dysphagia (difficulty in swallowing), odynophagia (pain on swallowing).

Anorexia (loss of appetite), nausea, vomiting.

Hematemesis (vomiting of blood).

Constipation (firm, difficult stools), obstipation (total inability to pass stool).

Lientery (passage of undigested food in stools), diarrhea (abnormal frequency, urgency, and looseness of stools).

Hematochezia (passage of blood from the rectum), melena (black stools, often due to the presence of blood), pale or white stools (due to absence of bile flow into the intestine).

Abdominal pain (diffuse or localized; intermittent or constant; random or affected by body position, meals, certain foods, bowel movement, medicine). Sharp, crampy pains are often called colicky. Burning pain in the epigastrium or chest due to digestive disorders may be called heartburn.

Abdominal tenderness (local or generalized), rebound tenderness (additional stab of pain when pressure on abdomen is released, often indi-

cating peritoneal irritation), spasm of abdominal wall, palpable abdominal mass, enlargement of abdominal organs, abnormal bulge of abdominal wall.
Bloating, belching, flatulence (excessive intestinal gas).
Borborygmi (singular, **borborygmus**) (audible rumbling and gurgling sounds in the digestive tract).
Anal pain, itching, swelling, or bleeding.
Muscle wasting, pallor, fatigue.
Jaundice (discoloration of skin and sclerae by excessive bile pigment).

Diagnostic Procedures Used in Digestive Disorders

History and physical examination: observation of abdomen for surgical or traumatic scars, swellings, discolorations, asymmetry; palpation of abdomen for masses, palpable organs, tenderness, spasm, hernia; percussion for hyperresonance (indicating excessive or displaced gas or air), flatness or dullness (indicating an abnormal mass, enlargement or consolidation of an organ, or impacted stool); auscultation for diminished, hyperactive, or high-pitched bowel sounds.

External anal examination, digital rectal examination.

Examination of stool for occult blood, fat, pathogens (bacteria, fungi, parasites), abnormal constituents.

Absorption tests based on determination of blood or stool levels of substances that have been ingested in measured amounts.

Imaging studies: flat, upright, and (usually left) lateral decubitus films of the abdomen; fluoroscopic studies with swallowed or injected barium or other contrast medium (**barium swallow**, upper GI series, small bowel series, **barium enema**); CT or MRI for specific indications (for example, to assess gallbladder, masses).

Endoscopy: esophagoscopy, gastroscopy, gastroduodenoscopy, anoscopy, sigmoidoscopy, colonoscopy; biopsy specimens, washings, cultures, and other materials can be obtained through endoscopes.

Laparoscopy (inspection of abdominal cavity through an endoscope inserted through an incision in the abdominal wall), **exploratory laparotomy** (inspection of the abdominal and pelvic cavities through an incision in the abdominal wall).

Diseases of the Esophagus

Peptic Esophagitis (Gastroesophageal Reflux Disease, GERD)

Inflammation of the esophagus caused by backflow of gastric juice.

Cause: Structural or functional incompetence of the lower esophageal sphincter (LES), associated with disordered gastric motility and prolonged gastric emptying time. In a few cases, reflux of gastric juice may be facilitated by **esophageal hiatus hernia** (weakness or dilatation of the opening in the diaphragm where the esophagus passes through, with herniation of part or all of the stomach into the thorax; often asymptomatic). Reflux of acid gastric juice into the esophagus causes inflammation because the esophageal mucosa is not adapted to resist acid and digestive enzymes.

History: Recurrent epigastric and retrosternal distress, usually described as heartburn; belching, nausea, gagging, cough, hoarseness in varying proportions. There is a strong association with asthma, obesity, and diabetes mellitus. Symptoms are triggered or aggravated by recumbency (especially after a meal), vigorous exercise, smoking, overeating, caffeine, chocolate, alcohol, and certain drugs.

Physical Examination: Unremarkable.

Diagnostic Tests: Imaging studies confirm reflux of swallowed barium from the stomach and may identify ulceration or stricture. Twenty-four-hour monitoring of esophageal pH with a swallowed electrode proves a sustained abnormal acid state in the esophagus. Endoscopy gives direct visual proof of inflammation.

Course: The underlying disorder of the LES and of gastric motility is irreversible. Severe reflux disease can lead to peptic ulceration of the esophagus, with eventual stricture due to scarring. Another possible complication is **Barrett esophagus**, a metaplasia (transformation) of normal squamous esophageal epithelium into columnar epithelium; some cases of Barrett esophagus progress to adenocarcinoma.

Treatment: Avoidance of smoking, alcohol, caffeine, and large meals. Over-the-counter antacids may suffice to control symptoms. Otherwise acid production may require suppression by H_2 antagonists (cimetidine, ranitidine, famotidine, nizatidine) or proton pump inhibitors (omeprazole, lansoprazole). Prokinetic drugs (bethanechol, metoclopramide, cisapride) may improve sphincter function and gastric motility.

Diseases of the Stomach and Intestine

Peptic Ulcer Disease and Gastritis
Inflammation and ulceration of the stomach, duodenum, or both by acid gastric juice.

Cause: Most commonly, infection of the gastric mucosa by ***Helicobacter pylori***, a motile bacterium that survives in the acid environment of the stomach by secreting urease, an enzyme that converts urea to ammonia and bicarbonate, thus providing a protective alkaline medium for itself. *H. pylori* infection, which is spread from person to person by the fecal-oral route, results ultimately in a marked increase of acid production. Peptic ulceration can also result from regular use of prostaglandin-inhibiting drugs: adrenal corticosteroids and nonsteroidal anti-inflammatory agents such as ibuprofen and aspirin. In rare cases it is part of **Zollinger-Ellison syndrome**, in which a tumor of the pancreas produces excessive amounts of the hormone gastrin and thus causes hypersecretion of gastric acid. Severe stress, head injuries, and burns are sometimes complicated by peptic ulcer. Most peptic ulcers occur in the duodenum, but the stomach may be involved as well or instead.

History: Burning epigastric pain that comes on within an hour after meals and is relieved by taking antacids or food. Night pain is common. Tobacco, alcohol, caffeine, and certain foods aggravate symptoms, apparently by stimulating acid production. With complications: hematemesis, melena, early satiety (feeling that the stomach is full after only one or two mouthfuls of food), weight loss, severe abdominal pain, collapse.

Physical Examination: Unremarkable. Abdominal tenderness is variable and may be absent. With hemorrhage: pallor and tachycardia. With perforation: boardlike rigidity of the abdomen due to chemical peritonitis.

Diagnostic Tests: Upper GI studies with barium contrast medium can show ulceration, scarring, obstruction, or perforation. Endoscopy visualizes ulcers, bleeding sites, and scarring, and is important to rule out carcinoma in gastric lesions. Infection by *H. pylori* can be confirmed by culture, biopsy, serologic testing, or breath-testing for evidence of urease activity on orally administered, radioactively tagged urea.

Course: Without treatment, peptic ulcer disease tends to persist, with remissions and exacerbations, for many years. The most serious complications are hemorrhage (the principal cause of ulcer mortality), obstruction due to scarring, perforation of the digestive tract with release of gastric juice into the peritoneal cavity, and penetration into the retroperitoneal space.

Treatment: Smoking cessation, avoidance of alcohol and caffeine. Acidity may be adequately controlled by over-the-counter antacids, H_2 antagonists (cimetidine, ranitidine, famotidine, nizatidine) in over-the-counter or prescription strength, or proton pump inhibitors (omeprazole, lansoprazole). Proven *H. pylori* infection is treated with a course of therapy including bismuth subsalicylate and two antibiotics: tetracycline or amoxicillin, and metronidazole or clarithromycin.

Gastroenteritis

Inflammation of the stomach and intestine, manifested by abdominal pain, vomiting, and diarrhea; usually acute, infectious, and self-limited.

Causes: Infection with viruses (adenovirus, echovirus, coxsackievirus, rotavirus), bacteria (*Escherichia coli, Campylobacter, Yersinia, Salmonella, Shigella, Clostridium*), protozoa (*Entamoeba histolytica, Giardia lamblia*), fungi (*Candida albicans*). Most of these infections are acquired by the fecal-oral route. Some are much more likely to occur in immunocompromised persons. Outbreaks are usually due to contaminated food or water. "Food poisoning" is due to toxins produced by staphylococci, *Salmonella, Clostridium*, or other organisms. Gastroenteritis can also be a reaction to medicines, foods, poisonous plants, toxic chemicals.

History: Usually abrupt onset of abdominal distress or cramping, anorexia, nausea, vomiting, and diarrhea. Chills, fever, malaise. Hematemesis and bloody diarrhea are ominous signs. In severe or protracted disease, or in children or the elderly, dehydration and electrolyte depletion can lead to prostration, vascular collapse, and death.

Physical Examination: May be unremarkable. Abdominal tenderness, **tympanites** (hollow percussion note due to distention of bowel with gas), hyperactive bowel sounds. In severe disease, signs of dehydration and electrolyte depletion include dryness of mucous membranes, decreased **skin turgor** (loss of normal consistency and fullness), tachycardia, hypoactive deep tendon reflexes, and decreased urine output.

Diagnostic Tests: Stool examination for white blood cells and organisms, with culture for pathogenic bacteria. Blood studies may show hematologic abnormalities or fluid and electrolyte imbalance.

Course: Most cases of gastroenteritis, even those caused by bacteria such as *Salmonella, Campylobacter,* and *Yersinia,* resolve spontaneously without specific treatment. However, **cholera** (due to *Vibrio cholerae*; rare in the U.S.), **bacillary dysentery** (due to *Shigella* species), **typhoid fever** (due to *Salmonella typhi*), and **pseudomembranous enterocolitis**

(due to toxin-producing *Clostridium difficile*, often following treatment with antibiotics that kill normal intestinal flora) are all severe and potentially fatal infections requiring prompt, aggressive treatment. Any case of gastroenteritis in small children or in elderly or debilitated persons can lead to dangerous electrolyte and water depletion and vascular collapse.

Treatment: Largely symptomatic and supportive. Over-the-counter products may suffice to control nausea, cramping, and diarrhea. Water and electrolytes may be replaced orally or intravenously as indicated. Antibiotic treatment is indicated only in certain specific infections. Trimethoprim-sulfamethoxazole or ciprofloxacin are effective in bacillary dysentery (shigellosis), typhoid fever, and cholera; pseudomembranous enterocolitis is treated with metronidazole or vancomycin.

Appendicitis

Acute inflammation of the appendix.

Cause: Obstruction of the appendiceal lumen by a fecalith (stonelike mass of hardened feces), seed, or parasite, or by swelling due to infection or neoplasm. Obstruction is followed by inflammation, impairment of blood supply, necrosis, and rupture.

History: Gradual onset of generalized abdominal distress gradually becoming more severe and steady and localizing in the right lower quadrant. Anorexia, nausea, vomiting, fever, chills, constipation. Sudden spontaneous relief of pain suggests perforation.

Physical Examination: Slight fever and tachycardia, tenderness and rebound tenderness over **McBurney point** (about one-third of the distance from the right anterior superior iliac spine to the umbilicus), tenderness and rebound tenderness in the same area on rectal or pelvic examination. Diminished bowel sounds. After perforation, boardlike rigidity of the abdomen indicating peritonitis, signs of toxicity, vascular collapse. In infants, the elderly, and pregnant women the findings may be atypical or deceptively mild.

Diagnostic Tests: Moderate elevation of the white blood cell count, with left shift (increase of band or immature forms). Abdominal imaging may show a mass, ileus or other signs of peritonitis, or an opacity in the appendiceal lumen; barium injected by rectum fails to fill the appendix.

Course: Without treatment the condition has a mortality rate over 90%. Most cases progress to perforation within 12-36 hours, followed by generalized peritonitis, septicemia, and collapse.

Treatment: Surgical removal of the appendix (by open procedure or laparoscopy) is the only effective treatment. Perforation requires surgical repair, intravenous fluids, and antibiotics.

Irritable Bowel Syndrome

Intermittent or chronic abdominal distress and bowel dysfunction without any demonstrable organic lesion.

Cause: Unknown. More likely to occur with emotional stress, dietary irregularities, and heavy intake of caffeine. Lactose intolerance may be partly responsible.

History: Intermittent lower abdominal pain, often relieved by having a bowel movement; alternating diarrhea and constipation; flatulence.

Physical Examination: Essentially negative.

Diagnostic Tests: Stool examinations, barium enema, colonoscopy, and blood studies are all negative.

Course: Symptoms tend to wax and wane for many years, with intervals of complete remission.

Treatment: Regular eating habits, avoidance of coffee and other triggering factors. Antispasmodics may be prescribed to reduce bowel motility and cramping.

Inflammatory Bowel Disease

Crohn Disease (Regional Enteritis, Regional Ileitis)

A chronic inflammatory disease of the bowel that can lead to intestinal obstruction, abscess and **fistula** formation, and systemic complications.

Cause: Unknown. The disease shows a familial pattern of incidence.

History: Recurrent crampy or steady abdominal pain, nausea, diarrhea, steatorrhea (excessive fat in stool), hematochezia, weakness, weight loss, and fever.

Physical Examination: Abdominal tenderness, signs of complications.

Diagnostic Tests: The white blood count and erythrocyte sedimentation rate are elevated. There may be mild anemia and reduction of serum levels of potassium, calcium, magnesium, and other substances. Barium enema shows regional narrowing of the lumen ("**string sign**") alternating with normal caliber. Sigmoidoscopy and colonoscopy show local inflammation with skip areas. On biopsy, all layers of the bowel are seen to be involved, not just the mucosa as in ulcerative colitis.

Course: Complications include intestinal obstruction, formation of abscesses and fistulas, perforation of the bowel.

Treatment: Low-fiber diet, drugs to reduce intestinal motility, specific anti-inflammatory drugs (azathioprine, sulfasalazine, olsalazine). Surgery may be necessary to deal with perforation or fistula formation. In severe disease, segmental resection of the bowel, or colectomy with ileostomy, may be necessary.

Ulcerative Colitis

A chronic inflammatory disease of the colon, chiefly the left colon, causing superficial ulceration.

Cause: Unknown.

History: Bloody diarrhea, abdominal cramps, tenesmus, anorexia, malaise, weakness, hemorrhoids or anal fissures. Bowel movements may occur more than 20 times a day, and may awaken the patient at night.

Physical Examination: Fever, abdominal tenderness, signs of complications.

Diagnostic Tests: The white blood count and erythrocyte sedimentation rate are elevated. Anemia may be present. Stool examination reveals mucus, blood, and pus, but no bacteria or parasites. Serum electrolytes and protein may be depleted. Sigmoidoscopy and colonoscopy show erythematous, friable mucosa with superficial ulceration and sometimes polyp formation. Biopsy shows chronic inflammation and microabscesses of the crypts of Lieberkühn.

Course: The course is intermittent, with spontaneous remissions and exacerbations. Physical and emotional stress and dietary irregularities may increase symptoms. Possible complications include colonic hemorrhage, perforation, toxic dilatation; polyp formation with progression to carcinoma; arthritis, spondylitis; iritis; oral ulcers.

Treatment: General supportive treatment and control of diet (high protein, low milk) are crucial to long-term control of the disease. Sulfasalazine, mesalamine, and corticosteroids suppress colonic inflammation and reduce symptoms. In severe disease, hospitalization with intravenous alimentation and fluid replacement and antibiotic treatment to combat sepsis may be necessary. In intractable disease, colectomy and ileostomy may be necessary.

Diverticulosis and Diverticulitis

A **diverticulum** (plural, diverticula) is a blister, or bubble-like outpouching of a hollow or tubular organ. **Diverticulosis** of the colon is the formation of one or more such outpouchings of the colon. **Diverticulitis** means inflammation and infection of colonic diverticula.

Cause: Unknown; more common in middle-aged and elderly.

History: Most patients with diverticulosis have no symptoms. The diverticula may be discovered incidentally on routine examination (barium enema, colonoscopy). A few patients may experience irregular bowel habits or abdominal pain. Patients in whom diverticulitis develops experience acute abdominal pain, nausea, vomiting, constipation, and sometimes fever or blood in the stools.

Physical Examination: There may be mild fever, abdominal tenderness, and even the sensation of a mass, most often in the region of the sigmoid colon (left lower quadrant of the abdomen).

Diagnostic Tests: The white blood count and sedimentation rate may be slightly elevated. The stool may be positive for occult blood. Barium enema, sigmoidoscopy, or colonoscopy may be performed to identify and localize the lesion, but are contraindicated in the presence of acute inflammation because of the danger of perforation of the bowel. X-ray studies may be used to identify free air in the peritoneal cavity due to perforation, and CT scan to detect abscess formation. Diagnostic evaluation needs to be particularly thorough to rule out malignancy.

Course: Diverticulitis may lead to hemorrhage, perforation of the bowel, obstruction due to fibrous scarring, fistula formation, abscess formation.

Treatment: Patients with mild or no symptoms may require no treatment, but are often advised to follow a high-fiber diet. During the acute phase of diverticulitis, patients are kept at bed rest, with nothing by mouth, intravenous fluids and nutrition, and, if necessary, a nasogastric tube. Usually antibiotic treatment is used because of the risk of peritonitis and abscess formation. Metronidazole, ciprofloxacin, and trimethoprim-sulfamethoxazole are the drugs usually used. As many as one-third of patients with diverticulitis will need surgery to drain an abscess or to resect a segment of badly diseased colon.

Adenocarcinoma of the colon and rectum is discussed in Chapter 5.

Intestinal Obstruction

Blockage of the flow of digestive fluids through the small or large intestine.

Causes: Surgical adhesions, hernia, neoplasms, gallstones, **volvulus** (twisting of a loop of intestine), **intussusception** (passage of a segment of intestine into the segment distal to it), foreign body, fecal impaction. Obstruction due to causes outside the bowel (volvulus, hernia) are often complicated by strangulation (ischemia of the involved portion of bowel).

History: Crampy abdominal pain, nausea, vomiting, obstipation. Obstruction of the small intestine causes more severe and rapidly progressing symptoms than obstruction of the colon.

Physical Examination: Abdominal distention, borborygmi; increased bowel sounds, often high-pitched or in peristaltic rushes. A fullness or mass may be palpated at the site of obstruction. Tenderness in the presence of strangulation. The rectum is empty of stool unless fecal impaction is the cause of obstruction.

Diagnostic Tests: The white blood count is elevated, particularly in the presence of strangulation. Blood chemistries may show electrolyte imbalance and dehydration due to vomiting and sequestration of fluid above the obstruction. Abdominal x-rays show dilated loops of bowel containing fluid levels, and may demonstrate the cause (volvulus, gallstone). Barium enema may be necessary to identify an obstruction in the colon.

Treatment: A nasogastric tube with suction to decompress the bowel proximal to the obstruction. Intravenous fluids to correct dehydration and electrolyte imbalance. Surgery is often necessary to relieve obstruction and to resect infarcted areas of bowel in cases of strangulation.

Adynamic Ileus

Failure of normal flow of materials through the digestive tract because of atony or paralysis of the bowel.

Causes: Recent abdominal surgery, peritonitis, mesenteric ischemia or infarction, medicines (opiates, anticholinergics).

History: Nausea, vomiting, obstipation, abdominal distention. Pain mild or absent.

Physical Examination: Abdominal distention, little or no tenderness, bowel sounds diminished or absent.

Diagnostic Tests: X-ray of the abdomen shows distended loops of small intestine with fluid levels.

Treatment: Nasogastric tube and suction, intravenous fluids, correction of the underlying cause if possible.

Hemorrhoids

Dilated veins just above or just below the anus.
Cause: Unknown. Constipation with straining at stool, prolonged sitting, and local infection have been implicated.
History: Anorectal discomfort or pain, swelling or protrusion, and bleeding.
Physical Examination: Dilated veins externally or internally, as seen by endoscopy. Sigmoidoscopy or colonoscopy and barium enema may be performed to rule out malignancy.
Course: Symptoms are typically mild and intermittent. Bleeding is occasionally significant. Thrombosis of a hemorrhoid results in acute pain and swelling, but the problem resolves spontaneously in a few weeks.
Treatment: High-fiber diet, stool softeners, hot sitz baths, soothing applications or suppositories. With severe pain or bleeding, surgery is indicated. Band ligation is used for internal hemorrhoids; external hemorrhoids are treated by excision or cryosurgery.

Anal Fissure

A superficial longitudinal ulceration of the anal canal.
Cause: Probably trauma from a hard stool or hard, sharp material in stool. Chronic fissure may result from infection.
History: Anorectal pain and bleeding, chiefly with bowel movements.
Physical Examination: Fissure in anal canal. With chronic fissure a tag of anoderm (**sentinel pile**) may form below the fissure. Digital examination demonstrates anal tenderness and spasm.
Course: Acute fissures heal spontaneously in a few days. Chronic fissure may persist for weeks or months.
Treatment: High-fiber diet, stool softeners, hot sitz baths, anesthetic or anti-inflammatory ointments or suppositories. Severe chronic fissure occasionally requires surgical excision.

Disorders of the Peritoneum

The **peritoneum** is a delicate serous membrane that lines the abdominal and pelvic cavities (**parietal peritoneum**) and also covers the stomach, small intestine, and colon (except for the distal part of the rectum), as well as the liver, spleen, uterus, ovaries, ureters, and dome of the bladder (**visceral peritoneum**). Structures such as the pancreas and kidneys that lie behind the peritoneal cavity are called retroperitoneal.

Acute Peritonitis

Acute inflammation of the peritoneum.

Causes: Infection (penetrating abdominal wounds, surgery, peritoneal dialysis for renal failure, spread from digestive or urinary tract or from a systemic site); chemical irritation (leakage of gastric or intestinal contents, bile, pancreatic secretions from injured, diseased, or perforated structure); systemic disease, neoplasm.

History: Fairly abrupt onset of severe local or generalized abdominal pain, nausea, vomiting, fever.

Physical Examination: Elevated temperature and pulse. Boardlike rigidity of abdomen, tenderness and rebound tenderness. Diminished or absent bowel sounds and abdominal distention due to ileus.

Diagnostic Tests: The white blood count is elevated. Blood studies may also show electrolyte imbalances due to peritoneal effusion, vomiting, and dehydration. Anemia may occur. Fluid obtained by abdominal paracentesis may show amylase or lipase (indicating leak of intestinal contents or pancreatic juice), significant cellular abnormalities, or infecting microorganisms. Various types of imaging may be of use in confirming and identifying intra-abdominal catastrophe.

Course: Without treatment the outlook is poor. Septicemia and vascular collapse often occur within a few hours of onset. In some patients, peritonitis becomes localized, with **abscess** formation, particularly **subphrenic** (just below diaphragm) or pelvic. Peritonitis often results in eventual formation of fibrous adhesions that may produce intestinal obstruction.

Treatment: Hospitalization, nothing by mouth, gastrointestinal suction to decompress the bowel and draw off secretions, intravenous fluids, narcotics for pain, antibiotics for infection, surgery to repair underlying abnormality.

Abdominal Hernia

A localized weakness in the **musculoaponeurotic** wall of the abdomen, with protrusion of abdominal contents. Abdominal hernias are classified according to position as:

umbilical (at the navel): often congenital, seldom requiring surgical repair because they resolve during infancy.

inguinal (in the groin):
  direct inguinal: due to thinning and stretching of the lower abdominal wall, often with aging.
  indirect inguinal: (usually congenital) weakness and bulging in the inguinal canal, the passage through which, in the male fetus, the testicle descends from the abdominal cavity to the scrotum; a similar potential passage exists in women.

femoral: herniation into the femoral canal, through which the femoral artery and vein pass from the pelvis into the thigh.

Cause: Congenital weakness or malformation; thinning of the abdominal musculature by aging. Herniation may be precipitated or aggravated by vigorous or repeated straining of the abdominal wall (chronic constipation, urinary obstruction, heavy lifting, chronic cough).

History: A tender bulge in the abdominal wall that enlarges with straining. Intestinal obstruction may occur, with severe abdominal pain, nausea, vomiting, weakness, shock, and collapse.

Physical Examination: A fluctuant bulge in the abdominal wall that enlarges with straining and can be reduced with manipulation or recumbency. A defect in the abdominal wall at the site of the hernia can be palpated. Visible or palpable mass, tenderness. Evidence of strangulation or bowel obstruction.

Diagnostic Tests: Barium enema and other studies may be done to rule out obstructive disease of the bowel or urinary tract.

Complications: **Strangulation** (compromise of blood supply), **incarceration** (inability to reduce hernia), bowel obstruction.

Treatment: Surgical repair of the defect, sometimes with implantation of reinforcing mesh.

Diseases of the Liver

The **liver**, the largest gland in the body, lies in the right upper quadrant of the abdomen just below the **diaphragm** and is largely covered by peritoneum. The liver performs numerous vital functions and is intimately concerned with carbohydrate and nitrogen metabolism and with removal of certain waste products. **Bile**, the secretory product of the liver,

Diseases of the Digestive System

passes through a duct into the duodenum. Bile contains **bile salts**, which help in the digestion of fats, and bilirubin, a breakdown product of hemoglobin. Bile does not flow steadily into the duodenum, but is stored in the **gallbladder**, a bulb or pouch connected by the cystic duct to the common bile duct. Ingestion of a fatty meal stimulates contraction of the gallbladder and increased flow of bile into the intestine.

Hepatitis

Hepatitis is a general term referring to inflammation of the liver. Hepatitis can be caused by various drugs, toxic chemicals, and infections. Viral infections are the most important causes of hepatitis.

Hepatitis A

Cause: Hepatitis A virus. Transmission is by the fecal-oral route. Contaminated food and water are important means of infection.

History: Anorexia, nausea, vomiting, malaise, upper respiratory or flulike symptoms, fever, joint pain, aversion to tobacco, abdominal discomfort, diarrhea or constipation. Infection may be asymptomatic in children.

Physical Examination: Fever, **jaundice**, enlargement and tenderness of the liver, splenomegaly, cervical lymphadenopathy.

Diagnostic Tests: The serum bilirubin is elevated, and liver function tests are abnormal. Atypical lymphocytes may appear in the blood. Anti-HAV (IgM) antibody appears early in the course of the disease and disappears after recovery. IgG antibody develops later and persists indefinitely, indicating past history of, and immunity to, the disease.

Course: Symptoms characteristically resolve within 2-3 weeks. The mortality is very low.

Treatment: Supportive and symptomatic.

Hepatitis B (Serum Hepatitis)

Cause: Hepatitis B virus. Transmission is by blood (shared needles, needlestick injury in healthcare workers) or sexual contact. Maternal transmission to neonates occurs also.

History: Fever, anorexia, nausea, vomiting, malaise, joint pain and swelling, rash, aversion to tobacco, abdominal pain, bowel irregularities.

Physical Examination: Fever, **jaundice**, enlargement and tenderness of liver. Splenomegaly, cervical lymphadenopathy.

Diagnostic Tests: The serum bilirubin is elevated, and liver function tests are abnormal. Atypical lymphocytes may appear in the blood. Hepatitis B surface antigen (HB$_s$Ag) appears early in the disease and indicates presence of infection and infectivity of the patient. Antibody to surface antigen (AntiHB$_s$) indicates recovery, immunity to future infection, and lack of infectivity. Presence of HB$_s$Ag after the acute phase suggests chronic infection.

Course: The incubation period may be 6-12 weeks or longer, and acute illness may persist for as long as 16 weeks. The mortality rate is somewhat higher than that of hepatitis A. Some patients become carriers of the disease, able to transmit infection months or years after recovery. In some, a chronic phase occurs. **Chronic persistent hepatitis** is mild and generally asymptomatic, while **chronic active hepatitis** leads to gradual deterioration of liver function, cirrhosis, and an appreciable risk of hepatocellular carcinoma.

Treatment: Chiefly supportive. Chronic hepatitis is treated with interferon alfa-2b and lamivudine.

Hepatitis C

A mild or asymptomatic viral hepatitis usually transmitted by sharing needles or by blood transfusion. In about 50% of cases it becomes chronic, with risk of cirrhosis and hepatocellular carcinoma. Carriers can be identified by serologic testing. Treatment is with interferon alfa.

Hepatitis D (Delta Hepatitis)

Hepatitis due to a defective virus; it occurs only in persons already infected with hepatitis B, and is common among IV drug users. In itself a relatively mild illness, it may add to the severity of hepatitis B.

Hepatic Cirrhosis (Portal Cirrhosis, Laënnec Cirrhosis)

A chronic disorder of the liver characterized by inflammation of secretory cells followed by nodular regeneration and fibrosis.

Causes: The principal cause is chronic alcohol abuse. Other toxic, metabolic, nutritional, and infectious factors may play a part in the genesis of cirrhosis. The cirrhotic level contains various combinations of fatty change and fibrosis forming small and large nodules.

History: Usually gradual onset of anorexia, nausea, weakness, weight loss, abdominal swelling due to ascites (accumulation of fluid in the abdominal cavity), and often jaundice. Disturbance of sex steroid hormone metabolism causes impotence in men and amenorrhea in women.

Physical Examination: Fever, muscle wasting, pleural effusion, **ascites**, peripheral edema. The liver is usually enlarged and may be firm or even hard. The spleen may also be enlarged. Jaundice appears relatively late. Elevation of estrogen level causes gynecomastia in men, spider angiomas (spider nevi) on the face and upper trunk, and palmar erythema. The tongue may appear smooth, shiny, and inflamed. With advanced disease there may be coarse, flapping tremors (**asterixis**) and delirium due to hepatic failure, which may progress to hepatic coma.

Diagnostic Tests: Laboratory tests show elevation of bilirubin and enzymes such as transaminases, lactic dehydrogenase, and alkaline phosphatase, which rise in the presence of liver cell damage. Anemia may be present, and coagulation studies may yield abnormal results. Liver biopsy confirms presence of typical histologic changes. Imaging studies including radioactive liver scans provide further information. Esophagoscopy may show esophageal varices.

Course: Symptoms may wax and wane over a period of years, often in response to varying levels of alcohol consumption. Progressive hepatic failure often occurs. Fibrosis within the liver typically shuts off branches of the portal circulation and increases the pressure in the portal vein (**portal hypertension**). In consequence, other vessels (particularly the lower esophageal venous plexus) dilate and become varicose or tortuous. Hemorrhage from bleeding esophageal varices is often life-threatening, particularly when hepatic disease causes a coagulation disorder. There is an increased incidence of hepatocellular carcinoma in persons with cirrhosis.

Treatment: Abstinence from alcohol, attention to nutrition, particularly carbohydrate, protein, vitamins. Rest, sodium restriction, and diuretics for edema and ascites. Severe ascites may require abdominal paracentesis. Patients with portal hypertension and bleeding esophageal varices may need a **portacaval shunt** (surgical procedure allowing portal vein blood to bypass the liver and empty directly into the inferior vena cava).

Diseases of the Gallbladder and Bile Ducts

Cholelithiasis (Gallstones)

The formation of **gallstones** is a common disorder, generally due to some disturbance in the flow of bile from the gallbladder or in the composition of bile. Gallstones are more common in women and in elderly persons. Risk factors include pregnancy, diabetes mellitus, high serum cholesterol, Crohn disease, and sickle cell anemia. In the latter condition, stones consist primarily of bilirubin from hemolyzed red blood cells. In the other conditions, gallstones are composed primarily of cholesterol.

Gallstones are often asymptomatic ("silent"), but about 90% of persons with **cholecystitis** (inflammation of the gallbladder) have pre-existing **cholelithiasis**. Stones may be demonstrated on plain abdominal films, but ultrasound and imaging after injection of opaque medium are more sensitive and specific. Potential serious complications are blockage of the **common bile duct** by a stone with ensuing obstructive jaundice, blockage of the **cystic duct** with ensuing cholecystitis, and passage of a stone into the intestine with the potential for causing bowel obstruction (**gallstone ileus**). Treatment of symptomatic gallstones is surgical removal (along with the gallbladder), usually through a **laparoscope**. Oral bile salts (chenodeoxycholic acid, ursodeoxycholic acid) and extracorporeal shock-wave lithotripsy (ESWL) sometimes dissolve stones.

Acute Cholecystitis

Acute inflammation of the gallbladder.

Causes: As mentioned above, most patients with cholecystitis have pre-existing cholelithiasis. Impaction of a stone in the cystic duct leads to obstruction of the flow of bile from the gallbladder, with ischemia, acute inflammation, and sometimes abscess formation or perforation.

History: Fairly acute onset of severe epigastric and right upper quadrant pain, nausea, and vomiting.

Physical Examination: Fever and jaundice may be present. In the right upper quadrant of the abdomen, there are tenderness, rebound tenderness, and involuntary guarding (spasm of abdominal muscles on palpation). Bowel sounds are reduced or absent. Occasionally a mass can be felt below the liver edge, representing a distended gallbladder.

Diagnostic Tests: The white blood cell count, bilirubin, and levels of serum enzymes reflecting hepatic damage may all be elevated. Imaging studies (plain abdominal x-ray, ultrasound, scans with radiotagged media) may precisely identify the problem.

Course: Acute cholecystitis may resolve spontaneously. Often relapses occur, with gradual development of chronic cholecystitis. Inflammation may culminate in gangrene or perforation of the gallbladder, or may ascend into the liver via the biliary tract (ascending cholangitis).

Treatment: Chiefly supportive, with narcotics for pain, intravenous fluids, and close observation. Impending or actual perforation is treated by surgical (laparoscopic) decompression (drainage) of the gallbladder or, preferably, by removal of the gallbladder (cholecystectomy).

Disorders of the Pancreas

The **pancreas** is a flat retroperitoneal organ lying behind and below the stomach, with its right end (head) embraced by the sweep of the duodenum. It is composed of two types of glandular tissue: groups of cells that secrete enzymes for the digestion of carbohydrate, protein, and fat, which are poured through a duct into the duodenum near the orifice of the common bile duct; and other groups of cells that secrete hormones (insulin, glucagon, somatostatin) and release them directly into the bloodstream. The endocrine function of the pancreas is discussed in Chapter 14.

Acute Pancreatitis

Acute inflammation of the pancreas.

Causes: Most cases occur in alcoholics or in persons with chronic biliary tract disease (cholelithiasis, cholecystitis). In these instances, obstruction of the pancreatic duct by edema, or backflow of bile from the duodenum into the pancreatic duct, causes release of pancreatic enzymes into the substance of the gland, with resulting intense inflammation, necrosis, and often hemorrhage. Other causes are hypercalcemia (abnormally high level of calcium in the blood), hypertriglyceridemia (abnormally high level of triglycerides in the blood), abdominal trauma or surgery, certain medicines, and viral infection including mumps. An acute attack of pancreatitis is often precipitated by excessive alcohol consumption or by eating a large meal.

History: Abrupt onset of severe, persisting epigastric pain, worse on lying flat, and radiating to the flanks and back. Nausea, vomiting, sweating, prostration, restlessness.

Physical Examination: Pallor, tachycardia, fever, epigastric tenderness, reduced or absent bowel sounds. Jaundice or hypotension may occur. In the presence of severe pancreatic hemorrhage, a bluish discoloration of the skin may appear over the left flank (Turner or **Grey Turner sign**). There may be evidence of ascites or a left pleural effusion.

Diagnostic Tests: Blood studies may show leukocytosis, hyperglycemia, anemia, and **hypocalcemia** (drop in serum calcium). Blood levels of pancreatic enzymes (amylase, lipase) are typically elevated. Imaging studies may show gallstones, a mass representing the swollen pancreas, left atelectasis (collapse of part of left lung caused by shallow breathing at site of pain), or left pleural effusion.

Course: Acute pancreatitis has a high mortality rate and, among survivors, a high recurrence rate. Possible outcomes include abscess formation, splenic vein thrombosis, ileus, shock, renal failure, adult respiratory distress syndrome, severe hypocalcemia with tetany, formation of pseudocysts (pockets of imflammatory fluid and debris between the pancreas and surrounding tissues), and progression to chronic disease.

Treatment: Hospitalization, narcotics for pain relief, nasogastric suction, intravenous fluids with attention to water balance, nutritional needs, and replacement of calcium. Surgery may be required to control hemorrhage, correct underlying disease, or drain pseudocysts.

Chronic Pancreatitis

Chronic inflammation of the pancreas.

Causes: Essentially the same as for acute pancreatitis. With recurrent or chronic disease, fibrosis of the pancreas and its ducts leads to worsening disease, with loss of both endocrine and exocrine pancreatic function.

History: Recurrent bouts of left upper quadrant pain, anorexia, nausea, vomiting. Weight loss, flatulence, and steatorrhea (greasy stools) because of deficiency or absence of pancreatic enzymes.

Physical Examination: Epigastric and left upper quadrant tenderness, involuntary guarding, ileus.

Diagnostic Tests: Sugar may appear in the urine and blood sugar may be elevated as a result of diabetes mellitus due to destruction of pancreatic endocrine tissue. The serum levels of pancreatic amylase and lipase may be elevated. The proportion of fat in the composition of the stools is increased because of deficiency of lipase in the intestine.

Abdominal x-ray may show widening of the curve of the duodenum due to pancreatic edema. Retrograde injection of opaque medium into the pancreatic duct with a catheter placed endoscopically can clearly outline anatomic conditions (dilatation vs. narrowing of duct, stone formation).

Course: Without treatment, progressive deterioration of pancreatic function, with nutritional deficiencies, flatulence, steatorrhea, and diabetes mellitus. Pseudocyst formation.

Treatment: Avoidance of alcohol and fatty foods, oral supplementation of pancreatic enzymes. Surgery may be required to improve pancreatic drainage or remove pseudocysts.

Topics for Study or Discussion

1. Name three gastrointestinal disorders that are due to infection; three that may be precipitated or aggravated by alcohol abuse; and three that may be precipitated or aggravated by smoking.

2. Name three gastrointestinal disorders that can be complicated by life-threatening hemorrhage and result in intestinal obstruction.

3. Define or explain: anorexia, Crohn disease, dysphagia, flatulence, GERD, hematochezia, ileus, melena, pancreas, peritoneum.

4. Name three kinds of gastroenteritis that must generally be treated with antibiotics, and three kinds that do not respond to antibiotics.

5. State three important differences between Crohn disease and ulcerative colitis, and three important differences between hepatitis A and hepatitis B.

Chapter 12

The Excretory System, the Male Reproductive System, and Sexually Transmitted Diseases

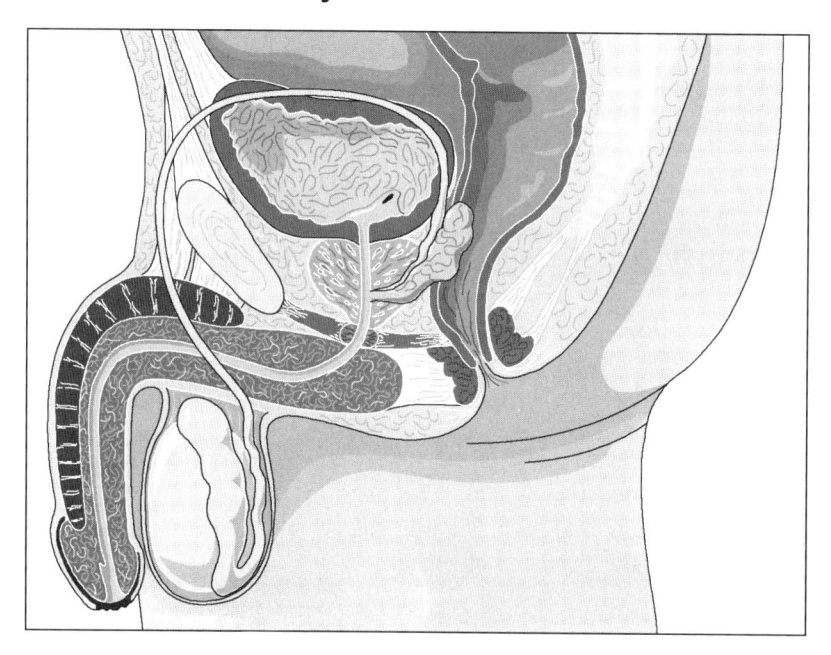

Learning Objectives

Upon completion of this chapter, the student should
- know the basic anatomy and physiology of the excretory and male genitourinary systems;
- have a general knowledge of diagnostic procedures and treatments used in these systems;
- understand signs, symptoms, and treatment of common diseases affecting these systems;
- know about some of the more common sexually transmitted diseases.

Disorders of the Excretory System

Anatomy and Physiology

The **excretory or urinary system** consists of the kidneys, the ureters, the bladder, and the urethra. The **kidneys** are paired, bean-shaped organs lying behind the abdominal cavity on either side of the aorta. The kidneys produce urine by filtering the blood through numerous microscopic units called glomeruli and then further processing the filtrate in the **renal tubules**. Most of the water that passes through the glomeruli is reabsorbed in the renal tubules. Other substances are reabsorbed as well, while still others are actively excreted by the tubules. The principal functions of the kidney are the excretion of water, waste materials (particularly nitrogenous wastes such as urea and creatinine), and other substances (potassium, extraneous chemicals including medicines), and the maintenance of water and electrolyte balance.

Urine formed by the glomeruli and tubules passes into the **renal pelvis**, a funnel-shaped collecting cavity, from which it flows downward through the **ureter** and into the **bladder**. The **urethra**, the outflow tract of the bladder, differs in the two sexes. The female urethra is short, emptying near the vestibule of the vagina but otherwise independent of the female reproductive system. The male urethra passes through the penis and in addition to its function in emptying the bladder it serves as the channel for the expulsion of semen.

Symptoms and Signs of Urinary Disorders

Pain, constant or intermittent, generally located at or near the site of disease.

Flank or costovertebral angle (CVA) pain (pain at the angle formed by the lowermost rib and the spinal column), usually accompanied by tenderness, suggests disease within the kidney (pyelonephritis).

Ureteral pain (**ureteral colic**) is intense pain, generally intermittent or with intermittent exacerbations, that originates in the flank or abdomen and radiates into the groin; it suggests ureteral obstruction by a stone.

Suprapubic pain, overlying the site of the bladder, suggests bladder distention or infection (cystitis).

Perineal pain (in the male) suggests prostatic disease.
Pain with voiding (dysuria) indicates urethritis or cystitis.

Urinary abnormalities:
Anuria: total cessation of urinary output.
Decreased force or caliber of the urinary stream.
Dribbling: uncontrollable passage of drops of urine, particularly just after voiding.
Hematuria: blood in the urine (gross hematuria is visible to the naked eye; microscopic or occult hematuria can be detected only by microscopic or chemical examination of the urine).
Hesitancy: difficulty in initiating urine flow.
Incontinence: involuntary passage of urine.
Oliguria: marked reduction in the volume of urine excreted in 24 hours.
Pollakiuria: increased frequency of urination, without an increase in the total volume of urine excreted in 24 hours.
Polyuria: increase in the 24-hour excretion of urine.

Diagnostic Procedures in Excretory Disorders

History and physical examination, with special attention to the external genitalia and abdominal, rectal, and pelvic examinations.

Urinalysis: a group of standard laboratory examinations of the urine, including determination of pH and specific gravity, chemical testing for sugar (normally absent), **albumin** (protein, normally absent), occult blood, **leukocyte esterase** (an enzyme indicating the presence of white blood cells), **nitrite** (a product of bacterial action), acetone, bilirubin, and other substances, and microscopic examination for red and white blood cells, renal tubular epithelial (RTE) cells, crystals, **casts** (plugs of material formed in renal tubules), and other materials.

Urine culture, usually with colony count and sensitivity studies, to identify urinary pathogens.

Catheterization of the bladder: insertion of a flexible or rigid tube into the bladder through the urethra to withdraw sterile urine; its principal diagnostic application is determination of **residual volume** (amount of urine remaining in the bladder after normal voiding).

Cystoscopy: insertion of an endoscope through the urethra and into the bladder to inspect its inner surfaces, including the ureteral orifices.

Imaging studies: plain or KUB (kidney, ureters, bladder) film; ultrasound or MRI studies to identify stones, neoplasms, cysts; **intravenous pyelogram (IVP)** (x-ray examination of urinary tract after intravenous injection of radiopaque contrast medium that is quickly excreted in the urine); **voiding cystourethrogram** (film of the act of voiding with contrast medium in the urine).

Disorders of the Kidney

Polycystic Kidney

A hereditary abnormality of both kidneys transmitted in an autosomal dominant pattern. Both kidneys are enlarged and cystic, and some patients also have hepatic cysts or cerebral aneurysms. Symptoms include abdominal or flank pain, hematuria, and a tendency to urinary tract infections and stones. On examination the kidneys are large and palpable through the abdominal wall. Ultrasound examination or CT scan confirms enlargement and cystic malformation. The urine contains protein and red blood cells. Progression to **renal failure** is the usual outcome. Many patients develop **renal hypertension** (high blood pressure due to disease of kidney cells). Treatment includes monitoring of renal function, vigorous treatment of infection and hypertension, and, with advancing failure of kidney function, **renal dialysis** or **renal transplant**.

Acute Renal Failure

An abrupt, severe decline in kidney function, with retention of nitrogenous waste products of protein metabolism (**azotemia, uremia**)

Cause: The abnormality may be **prerenal** (impaired blood supply to kidney), **renal** (also parenchymal or intrinsic; disease of the kidney proper), or **postrenal** (obstruction of the outflow of urine from the kidney). Prerenal azotemia can result from renal artery stenosis, hypotension, or the effects of certain drugs (NSAIDs, ACE inhibitors) on renal blood flow. Renal azotemia can result from any severe disease of kidney tissue, including **acute glomerulonephritis, vasculitis** affecting the intrinsic renal circulation, or **acute tubular necrosis**.

History: Malaise, weakness, anorexia, nausea, reduced urine volume (**oliguria**). In advanced disease, vomiting, hematemesis, diarrhea, drowsiness, seizures, pruritus, cardiac arrhythmias, peripheral edema, dyspnea.

Physical Examination: Essentially negative. A pericardial friction rub may be heard in uremic pericarditis. In advanced disease, pallor, peripheral edema, pulmonary edema, congestive heart failure, coma.

Diagnostic Tests: The levels of BUN and creatinine are markedly increased in the blood. The serum pH is low (**metabolic acidosis**). Serum potassium and phosphorus levels are elevated and calcium is depressed. Anemia may be severe.

Course: The case mortality rate is 20-50% depending on the cause and underlying diseases. If the inciting cause is reversible, the renal failure itself may completely resolve. Most patients with reversible disease recover completely within six weeks. Typically there is an oliguric acute phase, followed by copious diuresis as renal function improves, and at length a return to normal urine volume. Infection is a common complication.

Treatment: Largely supportive. Restriction of water, protein, and potassium intake, with high carbohydrate diet and vitamin supplementation. Close monitoring of water and electrolyte balance. Renal dialysis or intravenous administration of glucose, insulin, and sodium bicarbonate, and oral sodium polystyrene sulfonate, to reduce serum potassium.

Acute Glomerulonephritis

Acute inflammation of **renal glomeruli**, with failure to excrete nitrogenous wastes.

Causes: Poststreptococcal glomerulonephritis is an autoimmune disease that follows infection (usually pharyngitis) with group A beta-hemolytic streptococci, type 12. In **Berger disease** (IgA nephropathy), immune complexes form in the glomerulus, often after a respiratory or gastrointestinal infection or a flu-like illness.

History: Sudden appearance of tea-colored or Coca-Cola-colored urine, with reduction in urine volume and possibly peripheral edema.

Physical Examination: Blood pressure elevation (in poststreptocccal glomerulonephritis); peripheral edema.

Diagnostic Tests: The urine contains red blood cells, white blood cells, renal tubular epithelial cells, casts, and protein. Creatinine clearance and urinary sodium are reduced, and the 24-hour urinary excretion of protein is increased. In poststreptococcal disease, the ASO titer is elevated. Serum protein electrophoresis and antibody studies may indicate the presence of antibody to glomerular protein. Renal biopsy allows precise identification of tissue changes.

Course: Most patients with poststreptococcal glomerulonephritis recover without sequelae, but in a few the renal damage is rapidly progressive. About half of patients with Berger disease suffer progressive loss of kidney function.

Treatment: Largely supportive. Antibiotic to eradicate streptococci. Fluid restriction. Diuretics to reverse fluid retention. Attention to nutrition and control of hypertension. Renal dialysis if renal failure becomes severe.

Nephrotic Syndrome

A disorder of kidney function in which a large amount of protein is lost in the urine from damaged glomeruli

Causes: Various abnormalities of glomeruli due to systemic disease (diabetes, systemic lupus erythematosus, amyloidosis); other forms: minimal change, focal glomerular sclerosis, membranous nephropathy, membranoproliferative glomerulonephritis.

History: Gradual onset of peripheral edema, with weight gain, dyspnea.

Physical Examination: Edema, ascites, anasarca (generalized edema); pulmonary edema, pleural effusion.

Diagnostic Tests: Marked increase in 24-hour urinary excretion of protein. Reduction of total protein and albumin in the serum. Increase in serum cholesterol level. There may be no cellular elements in the urine and no evidence of nitrogen retention. Renal biopsy provides histologic identification of the underlying disease process.

Treatment: Limitation of protein and salt intake; diuretics, cholesterol-lowering agents.

Urolithiasis (Kidney Stones)

Formation of stonelike concretions (**calculi**) in the urinary tract, which may obstruct a ureter at a site of natural narrowing such as the **ureteropelvic junction** (UPJ) and **ureterovesical junction** (UVJ).

Causes: Changes in the concentration of dissolved minerals or other substances in the urine: uric acid in gout; cystine in cystinuria; calcium in disorders of calcium metabolism. Local infection may play a part. Men are affected 4 times more often than women, and the disorder tends to run in families.

History: Passage of a stone into a ureter causes severe flank pain radiating to the groin (ureteral colic), nausea, vomiting, restlessness, and often hematuria.

Physical Examination: There may be tenderness over the involved kidney in the flank or abdomen. Fever suggests infection resulting from urinary obstruction.

Diagnostic Tests: The urine shows microscopic or gross blood. X-ray or ultrasound examination identifies and localizes most stones, but about 15% are not radiopaque. Intravenous pyelography can be done to demonstrate obstruction of the tract. Examination of stones shows them to be aggregates of crystalline and organic materials. Chemical analysis of stones indicates which of five common types is present: calcium oxalate, calcium phosphate, ammoniomagnesium phosphate (struvite), uric acid, or cystine.

Course: Most stones pass spontaneously without treatment. Recurrences are common. Obstruction of a ureter can result in **renal failure** (obstructive uropathy), infection, or both.

Treatment: Strong analgesics are prescribed, and all urine is collected and strained to identify stones or fragments. If infection is present or renal function is compromised, obstruction may be relieved by passing a ureteral catheter endoscopically from the bladder, or by percutaneous nephrostomy. Stones lying low in a ureter may be extracted from below. **Extracorporeal shock wave lithotripsy** can be used to break stones into fragments, which then pass with the urine. A stone lodged in the renal pelvis or proximal ureter may be removed by percutaneous nephrolithotomy.

Acute Pyelonephritis

Acute inflammation of kidney tissue and the renal pelvis due to infection.

Cause: Bacterial infection with *Escherichia coli, Proteus, Pseudomonas, Klebsiella, Enterobacter*, or *Staphylococcus aureus*. Infection usually ascends from the lower urinary tract (bladder and urethra), but may be spread through the circulation from a remote focus. Obstruction to urine flow caused by prostatic enlargement, a ureteral stone, or pregnancy may be the underlying cause. **Vesicoureteral reflux** of urine or anomalies of the urinary tract (tortuous or duplicated ureter) are also risk factors.

History: Fever, chills, nausea, vomiting, flank pain, urinary urgency, pollakiuria, dysuria.

Physical Examination: The temperature and pulse are elevated. Tenderness at one or both costovertebral angles is usually noted on palpation.

Diagnostic Tests: The white blood cell count is elevated. Examination of the urine shows white blood cells, red blood cells, and bacteria. Urine culture identifies the infecting organism.

Course: Pyelonephritis resolves promptly with antibiotic treatment unless an underlying problem of septicemia or urinary obstruction remains unresolved.

Treatment: Antibiotics (trimethoprim-sulfamethoxazole, ciprofloxacin) are administered orally or intravenously. Urinary obstruction must be relieved by catheterization, nephrostomy (draining urine from the renal pelvis), or other procedure.

Acute Cystitis

Acute inflammation of the bladder, usually due to bacterial infection.

Cause: Usually infection due to *Escherichia coli* or other organisms ascending from the urethra. Cystitis is much commoner in women, in whom the urethra is short and straight, with its orifice in the vaginal vestibule where it is exposed to fecal contamination and trauma from sexual intercourse. Less commonly, cystitis may be due to urethral obstruction (principally in males), viral infection, bladder trauma, or spread of infection from adjacent pelvic organs. Pregnancy, diabetes mellitus, presence of an indwelling catheter, and advanced age are risk factors.

History: Fairly sudden onset of pollakiuria, urgency, urinary burning, and bladder spasms after voiding. Hematuria may occur. Often there is suprapubic or low back discomfort.

Physical Examination: Essentially unremarkable. Fever is absent. There may be suprapubic tenderness.

Diagnostic Examination: Laboratory studies of urine show white blood cells (sometimes clumped), red blood cells or occult blood, and bacteria. Tests for leukocyte esterase and nitrites are often positive. Urine culture identifies the causative organism. Colony counts and sensitivity studies are routinely performed also. Cystitis is so uncommon in men that aggressive evaluation is usually undertaken in the male to identify any serious underlying cause such as obstruction or malignancy.

Course: The response is rapid, but many sexually active women experience frequent recurrences.

Treatment: Antibiotics (trimethoprim-sulfamethoxazole, cephalexin) are often effective in courses of just 2-3 days. Urinary symptoms may be relieved by phenazopyridine (a bladder anesthetic taken orally) or antispasmodics. The frequency of recurrences in women can be drastically reduced by regularly voiding just after intercourse. Long-term low-dose antibiotic prophylaxis also helps to prevent recurrences.

Urinary Incontinence

Four distinct types of involuntary leakage of urine from the bladder are recognized. **Urge incontinence**, which occurs after a sudden, intense, irresistible urge to void, is the commonest type of incontinence in elderly persons. It is due to overactivity of the **detrusor muscle** of the bladder, and is best managed by behavioral therapy: instructing the patient to void frequently during waking hours. Drug therapy with a variety of agents including antidepressants and calcium channel blockers.

Stress incontinence, which is seen almost exclusively in women, occurs when mechanical stress is placed on the bladder, as by coughing, laughing, or changing position. It may result from structural damage to the bladder as in childbirth. Treatment with pelvic muscle exercises (Kegel exercises), adrenergic agents (phenylpropanolamine), or estrogens may help. Surgical correction of anatomic abnormalities is often necessary, and is highly successful.

Overflow incontinence is leakage of urine from an over-distended bladder, occurring almost exclusively in men with urinary obstruction due to prostatic disease. Treatment is correction of the obstruction.

Total incontinence is complete lack of control over voiding, usually due to neurologic disease, spinal cord injury, or radical prostatectomy. Continuous or intermittent catheterization may be the only effective means of controlling this type of incontinence. Incontinence is primarily a disorder of the elderly; besides the causes mentioned above it may be due to dementia, urinary tract infection, diuresis, drugs, diminished mobility, and, in women, atrophic vaginitis.

Disorders of the Male Reproductive System

The **male reproductive system** consists of the paired **testes** (**testicles**), each with its collecting system (the **epididymis**, a coiled tubular structure attached to the testicle; and the **spermatic duct** or **vas deferens**, a tube that conducts sperm to the prostate), the **penis**, the **scrotum** (a cutaneous sac containing the testicles), the **prostate** (a gland surrounding the urethra just below the bladder), and the **seminal vesicles** (small pouchlike glands adjacent to the vas deferens).

The testicle produces **spermatozoa** (singular, spermatozoon), the male **gametes** (sex cells). Each spermatozoon is capable of fertilizing a female ovum and carries the paternal contribution to the genetic makeup of the offspring. In addition, the testicles produce male hormones that are responsible for the development and maintenance of secondary sexual characteristics (facial and body hair, male body build, deep voice). The prostate contains secretory cells that produce the fluid component of semen. It also contains smooth muscle, and under sexual stimulation it closes off the bladder from the urethra and brings about ejaculation of **semen** (prostatic fluid + spermatozoa) through the urethra.

Epididymitis

Inflammation of the epididymis.

Causes: In younger men, typically due to sexually transmitted infection (gonorrhea or chlamydia); in older men, to spread of infection by gram-negative rods (*Escherichia coli*, *Proteus*, *Pseudomonas*, and others) from the urinary tract or prostate.

History: Pain and swelling in the scrotum adjacent to a testicle, urinary burning, fever.

Physical Examination: Fever, enlarged and tender epididymis, often enlargement of testicle and prostate as well.

Diagnostic Tests: Blood studies show leukocytosis. Stained urethral smear shows white blood cells and may show gonococci. The urine may show white blood cells, red blood cells, and bacteria.

Course: Complications include involvement of the testicle (**epididymo-orchitis**), abscess formation, and scarring of the epididymis with resultant infertility.

Treatment: An antibiotic, preferably selected on the basis of culture, and continued for 2-4 weeks. Scrotal support, ice, analgesics.

Testicular Torsion

Twisting of a **spermatic cord**. The condition runs in families, usually occurs before age 25, may follow strenuous activity, and may recur. Symptoms include pain, tenderness, and swelling in the affected cord. The affected testis lies higher than its fellow, because twisting shortens the cord. If spontaneous **detorsion** (untwisting) does not occur, the condition can lead to gangrene of the testicle within hours. Medical intervention is manual detorsion or, failing that, open surgery. Even when detorsion is accomplished without surgery, a procedure is eventually performed to anchor both testicles so as to prevent recurrence.

Prostatitis

Inflammation of the prostate, typically due to bacterial infection, which may be acute or chronic. In **acute prostatitis** the presenting complaints are fever, urinary frequency and burning, occasionally urinary retention, and pain in the perineum or back. On digital rectal examination the prostate is enlarged, warm, and exquisitely tender. The white blood count is elevated, and the urine contains white blood cells, red blood cells, and bacteria. Treatment is with oral or intravenous antibiotics. In **chronic prostatitis**, symptoms are milder but of longer duration. Fever is absent and prostatic tenderness not so marked. The urinalysis is normal. Treatment is with antibiotics, and must often be continued for a long time.

Benign Prostatic Hyperplasia (BPH)

Enlargement of the prostate accompanying aging, with varying degrees of urinary obstruction.

Cause: Some prostatic enlargement due to overgrowth of androgen-sensitive glandular elements occurs naturally with aging. Causes of severely symptomatic enlargement are unknown.

History: Gradual onset of urinary symptoms, which may be **obstructive** (decreased force and caliber of urinary stream, hesitancy, intermittency) or **irritative** (frequency, urgency, nocturia).

Physical Examination: The prostate is symmetrically enlarged on digital rectal examination, firm but not hard. Abdominal examination may indicate distention of the bladder. Catheterization after voiding may indicate residual urine.

Diagnostic Tests: Urinalysis may indicate evidence of infection (white blood cells) or of bladder irritation (red blood cells). The blood urea nitrogen may be elevated if obstruction is advanced (**obstructive uropathy**). Intravenous pyelography may show bladder distention and bilateral ureteral dilatation. Urinary flowmetry gives an objective measure of the rate of flow from the bladder. Cystoscopy and urethroscopy may be of value in confirming the benign nature of the disorder.

Course: Symptoms may remain relatively mild for years, even decades. Obstruction may lead to infection and even to kidney failure. Benign prostatic hyperplasia does not evolve into carcinoma.

Treatment: Medical treatment with finasteride (an alpha-reductase inhibitor) or terazosin or doxazosin (alpha-adrenergic blocking agents) can reduce obstructive symptoms. In more severe cases, surgical excision of prostate tissue is indicated. **Transurethral resection** (TUR) is the usual procedure, but in some cases suprapubic (open) resection is preferred. Balloon dilatation of the prostate and transurethral laser excision are alternative procedures.

Adenocarcinoma of the prostate is discussed in Chapter 5.

Sexually Transmitted Diseases

Diseases in this category are distinguished by being transmitted often, or almost exclusively, through sexual contact. Otherwise they have little in common: some are bacterial, some viral, some parasitic; some are trivial, some life-threatening or even uniformly lethal; some are easily cured, others are virtually unresponsive to treatment. The list of sexually transmitted diseases includes as many as 40 infections; only the more common and important are discussed in this book. Some sexually transmitted diseases are discussed in other chapters: AIDS in Chapter 4; genital warts, genital herpes, and pubic pediculosis in Chapter 7; hepatitis B in Chapter 11; and trichomoniasis in Chapter 13. Review these briefly before proceeding.

Syphilis (Lues)

A sexually transmitted spirochetal infection with widespread and life-threatening consequences.

Cause: *Treponema pallidum*, a spirochete that can enter the body through abraded skin or intact mucous membrane. Infection is usually transmitted sexually, but can also be spread by sharing needles. In addition, a woman infected with syphilis during the earlier months of pregnancy usually passes the infection along to her child, unless she is treated.

History: *Primary stage*: Appearance of a firm, painless papule or nodule (**chancre**), up to 2 cm in diameter, on the genitals or other site, 2-12 weeks after inoculation. The chancre eventually ulcerates and forms a crust, taking several weeks to heal and sometimes leaving a scar. Inguinal lymph nodes become swollen and tender. *Second stage*: Several weeks later, a generalized, nonspecific cutaneous rash may appear. Soft, moist plaques (**condylomata lata**) may occur on the skin of the genitals, perineum, perianal region, or groin, and ulcerations may also develop on oral or genital mucous membranes. There may be patchy hair loss. Symptoms of this stage may persist or recur over several weeks. *Tertiary (late) stage*: Years after the first two stages, damage to cardiovascular and nervous tissue may result in cardiac symptoms, congestive heart failure, dementia, ataxia (tabes dorsalis), or paralysis. (**Latent syphilis** refers to a condition in which spirochetes remain alive in the body, but no signs or symptoms of infection occur after the secondary stage.)

Physical Examination: Findings are highly variable. *Primary stage*: The chancre and enlargement of inguinal nodes have already been described. *Secondary stage*: Nonspecific localized or generalized maculopapular rash, which often involves the palms and soles. Irregular zones of hair loss give the head a moth-eaten appearance. **Condylomata lata** and mucosal ulcers have already been described. Enlargement of spleen and lymph nodes may occur. *Tertiary stage*: Signs of aortic valvular insufficiency or aneurysm of the thoracic aorta, ataxia, paresis, dementia. Formation of **gummata** (rubbery fibrotic masses) in skin, bones, and liver.

Diagnostic Tests: Examination of material from a chancre or mucocutaneous ulcer by darkfield microscopy or fluorescent antibody testing confirms presence of *Treponema pallidum*. Serologic tests (**VDRL**, **RPR**) react to treponemal antigens, but may be falsely positive in autoimmune disorders. More specific tests for treponemal antibody (**fluorescent treponemal antibody absorption test**, **FTA-ABS**) yield reliable confirmation of the presence or absence of *T. pallidum* infection.

Course: The usual history of the disease has already been outlined. About 75% of persons with syphilis proceed to the latent stage and have no late manifestations. Treatment at any time before the late stage ordinarily yields complete cure. Without treatment, the late stage culminates in cardiovascular or neurologic death.

Treatment: A single intramuscular dose of benzathine penicillin G is usually curative. Alternative treatments are oral erythromycin or tetracycline.

Gonorrhea

Infection of the genital tract by the gonococcus.

Cause: *Neisseria gonorrhoeae* (gonococcus), a gram-negative diplococcus that is transmitted almost exclusively by sexual contact. It attacks genitourinary mucous membranes, producing a purulent inflammation that may spread to adjacent organs or the peritoneum, and may progress to scarring. Infection of the pharynx or rectum can be acquired through oral or anal sex.

History: Men: After an incubation period of 3-5 days, severe pain on urination and a thick green urethral discharge. Women: Similar symptoms sometimes occur, along with vaginal or vulvar inflammation. Often, however, there are no symptoms unless **pelvic inflammatory disease (PID)** (spread of infection to the uterus and uterine tubes) occurs. PID causes pelvic pain and fever, with variable other symptoms.

Physical Examination: In men, evident purulent urethral discharge, with inflammation of the meatus. In women, acute disease may be manifested by urethritis, cervicitis, vaginitis, inflammation of **Bartholin glands** (secretory glands lateral to the vaginal vestibule), or proctitis. If PID ensues, fever, abdominal tenderness, extreme tenderness on manipulation of cervix.

Diagnostic Tests: Stained smear of pus or secretions shows gram-negative diplococci inside WBCs. Culture on appropriate medium grows gonococci. Oral and anal specimens are positive when infection is in those areas.

Course: Acute urethral infection may resolve spontaneously, but in men it often spreads to the epididymis or prostate, or progresses to a stage of scarring, with resultant infertility. In women, spread to the vagina, cervix, uterus, tubes, and rectum often occurs. Tubal infection (**salpingitis**, PID) with scarring causes infertility and a heightened risk of ectopic pregnancy. In either sex, infection occasionally involves the skin, conjunctivae, joints, tendon sheaths, cardiac valves, or meninges.

Spread of infection from mother to newborn can cause conjunctivitis with ensuing blindness.

Treatment: Antibiotic treatment with a single dose of intramuscular ceftriaxone or oral ciprofloxacin is usually curative. It is standard practice to administer treatment for **chlamydial infection** at the same time since the infections so often occur together.

Chlamydial Infection
Urogenital infection with *Chlamydia trachomatis*.

Cause: Sexually transmitted infection of genital mucous membranes and related tissues with *Chlamydia trachomatis*, an intracellular organism similar to gram-negative bacteria. Genital chlamydial infection (urethritis and cervicitis) is the commonest bacterial STD. Screening tests are positive in 10% of asymptomatic, sexually active women.

History: Men: Urethral itching or burning, dysuria, thin serous discharge, 1-4 weeks after exposure. Anorectal pain and bleeding with rectal infection, common in gay men. Women: Dysuria and pollakiuria due to **acute urethral syndrome**; **dyspareunia** (pain with intercourse), vaginal bleeding, and vaginal discharge due to cervicitis; abdominal pain and fever due to **pelvic inflammatory disease**. Most women with chlamydial infection are asymptomatic.

Physical Examination: May be unremarkable. Thin, watery urethral discharge may be noted in males. In women, cervical inflammation with discharge indicates mucopurulent cervicitis. With development of PID, fever, abdominal pain, and cervical tenderness become evident.

Diagnostic Tests: A urethral or cervical smear may show organisms with direct fluorescence antibody examination, enzyme-linked immunosorbent assay, or DNA probe.

Course: Spontaneous resolution often occurs, but in many patients chlamydial infection has long-term consequences. In men, infection can spread to the epididymis, produce urethral stricture with resulting urinary obstruction or infertility, or trigger an autoimmune disorder called **Reiter syndrome** (arthritis, conjunctivitis, mucocutaneous lesions). In about one-fifth of infected women, infection spreads to the uterus and tubes (salpingitis, PID). Complications of PID include **tubo-ovarian abscess**, **Fitz-Hugh–Curtis syndrome** (localized peritonitis in the region of the liver), and **tubal scarring** with infertility or sterility and heightened risk of **ectopic pregnancy**. A child born to an infected mother is at risk of chlamydial conjunctivitis, with the danger of blindness.

Treatment: Oral antibiotic therapy with tetracycline, erythromycin, or a single dose of azithromycin is ordinarily curative. Treatment is often instituted on suspicion (urethritis or cervicitis with negative cultures of urine and discharge) because of the high probability of chlamydial infection in such cases. Persons treated for gonorrhea are also routinely treated for chlamydial infection as well.

Topics for Study or Discussion

1. List five causes of urinary obstruction and five conditions that predispose to urinary tract infection.

2. Mention four sites of pain in urinary tract disease and indicate the probable origin of each type of pain.

3. Define or explain: anuria, chancre, IVP, microscopic hematuria, overflow incontinence, pollakiuria, Reiter syndrome, urolithiasis.

4. Distinguish between pollakiuria and polyuria, and for each symptom mention three possible causes.

5. List three important similarities and three important differences between chlamydial urethritis and gonorrhea.

Chapter 13

Disorders of the Female Reproductive System

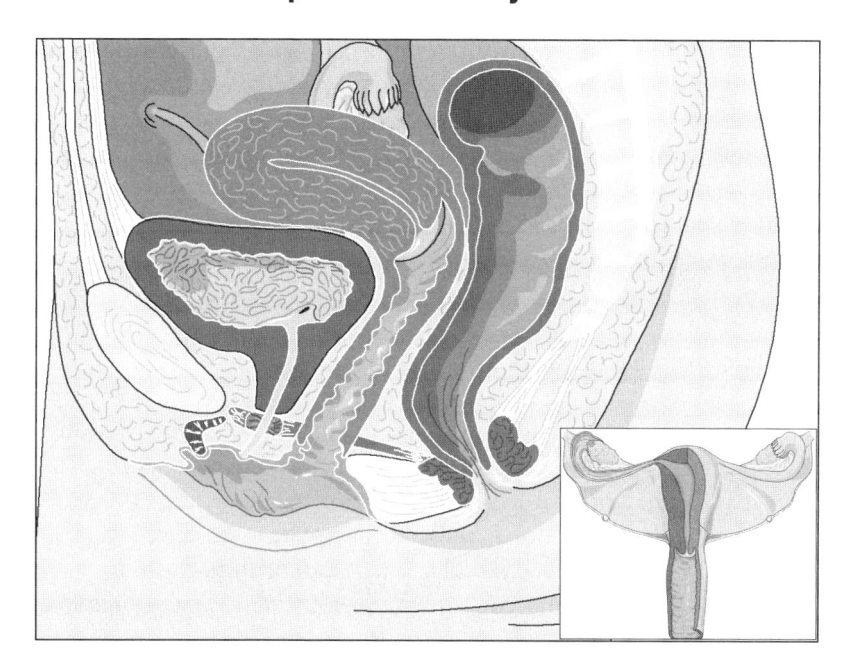

Learning Objectives

Upon completion of this chapter, the student should

- know the basic anatomy and physiology of the female reproductive system, including the breast;

- know about diagnostic methods used in assessing disorders of this system;

- have general information about common disorders affecting the system.

Anatomy and Physiology of the Female Reproductive System

The **female reproductive system** is concerned exclusively with **procreation**; unlike that of the male, it does not share structures with the urinary tract to any significant extent. The system consists of the **internal genitalia** (the ovaries, uterus, and vagina) and the **external genitalia** (the vulva, consisting of labia majora, labia minora, clitoris, and vaginal vestibule). The **uterus** is divided into the **cervix** (the lowermost portion, protruding into the vaginal vault) and the **body** (the remainder of the uterus, which lies in the pelvic cavity between bladder and rectum). The system also includes the **breasts**, which provide nourishment to the newborn child.

Gynecologic Symptoms and Signs

Gynecology is the branch of medicine that is concerned with diseases peculiar to women, chiefly diseases of the reproductive system. The following are the principal indications of gynecologic disease.

Pain, local or generalized; constant, intermittent, or related to menstruation. Various types of gynecologic pain can be distinguished:

dysmenorrhea: pain occurring with menstruation, typically felt low in the pelvis and in the low back, and often severe. The lay term for dysmenorrhea is "[menstrual] cramps."

dyspareunia: pain in the vulva, vagina, or pelvis with sexual intercourse.

dysuria: pain in the urethra or vulva with urination.

ovulatory pain: sharp pain, usually on one side of the pelvis, occurring midway between menstrual cycles (hence the common German term **mittelschmerz** 'middle pain') and due to peritoneal irritation by a small volume of blood escaping from the ovary at the time of ovulation.

Menstrual abnormalities:
    amenorrhea: absence of menstruation.
        primary amenorrhea: failure of menses to start at puberty (by age 14-16).
        secondary amenorrhea: cessation of menses that have been normal in the past.

Disorders of the Female Reproductive System • 215

anovulation: failure of ovulation to occur at the expected times.

dysfunctional uterine bleeding: irregular, unpredictable menstrual flow (too frequent or too infrequent, too heavy or too light), or amenorrhea, occurring in the absence of pregnancy, infection, or neoplasm.

hypermenorrhea: abnormally high volume of menstrual discharge.

hypomenorrhea: abnormally low volume of menstrual discharge.

menometrorrhagia: excessive menstrual bleeding occurring both during menses and at irregular intervals.

menorrhagia: regularly occurring menstrual flow that is excessive in volume and lasts longer than a normal menstrual period.

metrorrhagia: menstrual bleeding occurring at irregular but frequent intervals.

oligomenorrhea: infrequent or scanty menstrual bleeding.

polymenorrhea: menstrual bleeding that occurs with abnormal frequency.

Abnormal vaginal discharge: any discharge from the vagina that is abnormal in color, odor, or volume. Normal vaginal mucus discharge, originating from cervical glands, is nearly colorless, nearly odorless, and not heavy enough to stain underclothing except perhaps around the time of ovulation and just before onset of menses.

Vulvar burning, rawness, stinging, or itching.

A lump, swelling, or ulcer of the external genitalia, perineum, perianal region, pubes, or groin.

Breast symptoms: pain, local or generalized swelling, palpable lump, discharge or bleeding from nipple.

Diagnostic Procedures in Gynecology

History: age at **menarche**, menstrual history, sexual history, obstetric history, pelvic pain, bleeding, discharge, or other symptoms of gynecologic disease, general medical and surgical history.

Physical examination: general medical examination with attention to the abdomen and pelvis and to the breast.

A standard **pelvic examination** consists of the following elements:

Inspection and palpation of the external genitalia and perineum, with particular attention to the urethral orifice and adjacent **Skene glands**, the vaginal vestibule and adjacent **Bartholin glands**, the integrity of the pelvic floor, and any redness, swelling, ulceration, scarring, or other abnormal lesions.

Examination of the vaginal vault and the uterine cervix with the help of a vaginal **speculum**, which has adjustable anterior and posterior leaves that distend the vagina. Acetic acid or Lugol solution may be applied to the cervix to highlight zones of abnormal (possibly malignant) tissue.

Palpation of pelvic organs: cervix and body of uterus, **adnexa** (organs adjacent to the uterus—ovaries and tubes), bladder, pelvic walls and floor, rectum. **Bimanual examination** is performed with one or two fingers in the vagina and the palm of the other hand on the lower abdomen. **Rectovaginal examination** is performed with the index finger of one hand in the vagina and the middle finger of the same hand in the rectum.

A standard **breast examination** consists of the following elements:

Inspection of the breasts with the subject in the upright position, first with arms at sides, then with arms raised, and finally with hands pressed against hips to render underlying muscles taut.

Palpation of each breast in both the upright and supine positions, with attention to the axillae and assessment of nipples for inflammation, bleeding, or discharge.

Examination of cervical mucus for spinnbarkeit: When the **estrogen level** is high but the **progesterone** level is low (the conditions existing just before and just after **ovulation**), a specimen of cervical mucus can be drawn out into strings or strands several centimeters in length. This property is called **spinnbarkeit** (German, 'ability to be drawn out into a string'). When both estrogen and progesterone are present in large amounts, cervical mucus loses this property, and attempts to draw it out into a string fail. The physiology of the menstrual cycle is discussed fully below.

Basal body temperature: Daily determination of oral temperature on arising is useful in confirming and dating ovulation. Daily graphing of basal body temperature will show a rise of 0.75-1.0°F (0.2-0.5°C) approximately one day after ovulation.

Colposcopy: Examination of the cervix with an illuminated low-power microscope, which facilitates identification of suspicious cervical lesions requiring biopsy.

Pap (Papanicolaou) smear: Removal of superficial cells from the vagina and cervix for cytologic examination, to judge hormonal effect and to identify abnormal cell changes due to inflammation, infection, **dysplasia** (cell abnormalities heralding eventual development of malignancy), or actual malignancy. Specimens are taken from three areas: 1) the vaginal vault, with a flat wooden spatula; 2) the **squamocolumnar junction** (transition line between the squamous epithelium of the vagina and the columnar epithelium of the endocervical canal), with a specially shaped wooden spatula (**Ayre spatula**); 3) the **endocervical canal,** with a bristle brush to ensure sampling of columnar epithelial cells. Interpretation of the Pap smear, usually reported according to the **Bethesda system**, includes assessment of the adequacy of the specimen (presence of columnar cells from the endocervical canal); detection of hormonal effect (estrogen, progesterone); identification of inflammatory or degenerative changes in cells; and identification of dysplastic or malignant changes in cells. Often infections (candida, trichomonas, herpes simplex, human papillomavirus) can also be reliably detected.

Smear and culture: Microbiologic study of secretions or other materials from the cervix, vagina, urethra, rectum, or from superficial lesions, to identify causes of infection.

Urine studies: Culture, colony count, and sensitivity to identify urinary tract infection.

Imaging: Plain x-ray studies, pelvic ultrasound, CT, MRI.

Pregnancy testing, usually by identification and measurement of the beta fraction of human chorionic gonadotropin (beta hCG) in serum.

Determination of blood levels of various hormones: estrogens, TSH (thyroid stimulating hormone), T_4 (thyroxine), FSH (follicle-stimulating hormone), LH (luteinizing hormone), prolactin.

Biopsy: Removal of tissue from the cervix, the endometrium, or another part of the reproductive system for histologic examination to identify infection, neoplasm, or other abnormality. Cervical biopsy is colposcopically directed, and may involve removal of plugs of tissue with a punch-type instrument or removal of a cone of tissue including the entire squamocolumnar junction.

Dilatation and curettage (D&C): Scraping of the endometrium, after stretching of the cervix with graded dilators, to obtain specimen material for the diagnosis of endometrial disease. This procedure, performed under anesthesia (general, spinal, or intravenous), is also used therapeutically for various endometrial disorders.

Culdoscopy: Endoscopic inspection of the **cul-de-sac (pouch of Douglas)**, the lowermost part of the peritoneal cavity, which lies between the uterus and the rectum. The instrument is introduced vaginally under anesthesia.

Laparoscopy: Inspection of pelvic viscera through a **laparoscope**, a tubular instrument with illumination and magnification, inserted through a small incision in the abdominal wall. Minor surgical procedures can be performed through the instrument.

Menstrual Disorders

Menstruation is the normal monthly discharge of blood and tissue from the uterus that results when ovulation is not followed by conception (see box). **Menarche**, the first onset of menstruation, occurs at puberty, between the ages of 11 and 15. **Menopause**, the final cessation of menstruation, occurs ordinarily during the late 40s or early 50s. The normal **menstrual cycle** (interval from the first day of one menstrual period to the first day of the next menstrual period) is 21-35 days; the average is about 28 days. The normal **menstrual period** (time of menstrual flow) is 3-7 days; the average is 5 days. In lay and even professional parlance, the terms *menstruation, menses, menstrual flow*, and *menstrual period* are often used of any vaginal bleeding, even when it is evident that the bleeding in question is not normal menstrual flow. Similarly, the terms *cycle* and *period* are often applied to vaginal bleeding that is wholly irregular ("anovulatory cycle," "irregular periods").

The normal menstrual cycle depends on an intricate and interrelated series of chemical and biologic events. At puberty the hypothalamus secretes a neurohormone, **gonadotropin-releasing hormone (GnRH)**, which stimulates the pituitary to release its gonadotropic hormones, **follicle-stimulating hormone (FSH)** and **luteinizing hormone (LH)**.

FSH causes the ovary to begin producing estrogen, which is responsible for the development of secondary sexual characteristics (pubic and axillary hair, nipple and breast development, broadening of hips, feminine distribution of body fat). FSH also stimulates the monthly development or maturation of an **ovarian (graafian) follicle**, one of hundreds of immature microscopic units, each of which contains an **ovum** or female sex cell (**gamete**).

> The English words *menses, menstrual,* and *menstruation,* and the Greek words *dysmenorrhea, menopause,* and many related terms, are all derived from the same Indo-European root meaning 'moon' and, by extension, 'month'. From earliest antiquity, women noticed that their menstrual cycles (interval from beginning of one menstrual period to the beginning of the next one) were normally the same number of days as the cycles of the moon (from one full moon to the next). Naturally the superstition followed that the two are related as cause and effect.
>
> *Mensis,* the Latin word for 'month', is widely used in medicine (always in the plural) to refer to menstruation. Note that *menses* can have either of two meanings: 'a single menstrual period' ("Menses began on April 14"), or 'menstruation in general' ("Menses began at age 12").
>
> *Men,* the cognate Greek word for 'month', appears in medical terms as the combining form *men(o)-: menarche, menorrhagia, polymenorrhea.* The same Greek word appears in *meniscus* (Greek *meniskos,* 'little moon', hence 'crescent moon') referring to the semilunar shape of the fibrocartilaginous menisci of the knee joint.
>
> The notion of a connection between lunar cycles and menstrual cycles is deeply entrenched and ineradicable. Numerous women relate their menses to the calendar month ("My period always starts on the seventh"). In March, primary care physicians see many women who think their periods are late because February, having only 28 days, has foiled expectations based erroneously on the day of the month.

Under the influence of **estrogen**, the **endometrium** (lining of the uterus) undergoes changes concurrently with ripening of the follicle, to prepare it for implantation of the fertilized ovum should conception occur. This **proliferative phase** of endometrial development lasts 10-15 days, from the end of the last menstrual period to the time of ovulation.

Ovulation is the release of a mature ovum from its **ovarian follicle** into the pelvic cavity, from which it ordinarily passes into the uterine tube on the same side as the ovary from which it emerged, and so to the uterus. If sexual intercourse takes place around the time of ovulation, spermatozoa advancing through the female genital tract typically encounter the ovum during its passage through the uterine tube, and fertilization takes place in the tube. The fertilized ovum then migrates into the uterine cavity and implants on the endometrium.

At ovulation, the pituitary release of LH greatly increases. This hormone stimulates the follicle from which the ovum was released to evolve into a **corpus luteum** (Latin, 'yellow body'), a small but powerful secretory organ that produces the hormone **progesterone**. The function of progesterone is to make further preparations for the development of the fetus should **fertilization** occur. The most striking early effect is a more lush development of the endometrium (secretory phase), with marked thickening, and formation of microscopic coiled glandular structures.

If **conception** and **implantation** of a fertilized ovum do not occur, then the corpus luteum degenerates and ceases to produce progesterone. The endometrium, deprived of its stimulation, becomes ischemic and sloughs, with resultant menstrual flow. Menses predictably begin 14 days after ovulation if fertilization has not occurred.

If a fertilized ovum is implanted on the secretory endometrium, it forms a **placenta** (a disc of tissue from which the **umbilical cord** passes to the fetus; it serves for the interchange of oxygen, nutrients, and wastes between maternal and fetal circulation). The placenta produces progesterone and gradually takes over this function from the corpus luteum (which may, however, persist through at least the first half of pregnancy). The placenta also produces **human chorionic gonadotropin (hCG)**, the basis of virtually all current pregnancy tests.

The menstrual cycle is delicately regulated by various feedback mechanisms. For example, falling levels of either FSH or LH stimulate hypothalamic production of GnRH, and rising levels suppress GnRH.

Dysfunctional Uterine Bleeding

Unusually heavy or light bleeding from the uterus, typically unpredictable, or amenorrhea, in the absence of pregnancy or any demonstrable abnormality (neoplasm, infection) of the uterus.

Causes: Most cases are due to **anovulation** (failure to ovulate). This is a common occurrence and can result from physical or emotional stress, marked weight loss (as in anorexia nervosa or stringent dieting), strenuous exercise (running, gymnastics), excess or deficiency of thyroid hormone, polycystic ovary disease, recent discontinuance of oral contraceptives, lactation, and other causes. About one-third of patients with amenorrhea have elevated levels of **prolactin**; in rare cases, this is due to overproduction of prolactin by a pituitary tumor.

History: Unusually heavy or light bleeding, typically irregular; often, amenorrhea lasting for 3 or more cycles. Symptoms of underlying disease may also be present.

Disorders of the Female Reproductive System • 221

Physical Examination: Generally unremarkable. May show obesity or emaciation, stigmata of thyroid or ovarian disease (goiter, exophthalmos, hirsutism), or other evidence of an underlying disorder. Cysts may be palpable in the ovaries. Presence of normal breast development and axillary and pubic hair confirms normal estrogen effect. A palpable, nontender uterus of normal size and shape rules out congenital absence of the uterus (in primary amenorrhea) and helps to exclude uterine tumors or infection.

Diagnostic Tests: A pregnancy test is always done to rule out normal or **ectopic pregnancy** or recent miscarriage or abortion. Determination of blood levels of estrogen, LH, FSH, T_4, TSH, and prolactin is standard. In amenorrhea in which pregnancy has been ruled out, oral administration of a progesterone (medroxyprogesterone acetate) for 5 days is normally followed within 10 days by a discharge of blood from the uterus if the endometrium is healthy and the estrogen level adequate. Absence of a response suggests a severe uterine disorder (endometrial scarring) or estrogen deficiency due to pituitary or ovarian disease. Pelvic ultrasound may help to confirm the presence or absence of uterine or ovarian disease. Laparoscopy may be needed for definitive diagnosis. CT or MRI of the head may be performed if a pituitary tumor is suspected.

Course: Depends on the underlying condition. Extremely heavy bleeding can lead to shock or anemia.

Treatment: Depends on the underlying condition. For many patients, a course of oral contraceptive provides cyclical hormone levels sufficient to induce what seem like normal menstrual cycles and flow. Clomiphene may be given to an anovulatory woman who wants to conceive. **Hyperprolactinemia** (abnormal elevation of prolactin) in the absence of a pituitary neoplasm is treated with bromocriptine. Thyroid, ovarian, or pituitary disease, or abnormalities of pelvic anatomy and physiology, may require other specific treatment.

Dysmenorrhea and Premenstrual Syndrome (PMS)

Dysmenorrhea

Pelvic pain occurring with menstruation.

Causes: *Primary*: "Normal" menstrual cramps, occurring in 50-75% of all women, and due to uterine vasoconstriction and spasm resulting from withdrawal of progesterone effect. *Secondary*: Endometriosis, PID, use of an **IUD (intrauterine contraceptive device)**, tumor of the uterus, cervical stenosis (due, for example, to scarring after induced abortion).

History: Cramping pain felt low in the pelvis, often radiating to the back or inner thighs, often accompanied by nausea, diarrhea, headache, or prostration. Pain begins usually on the first day of the menstrual period and lasts 1-2 days. In secondary dysmenorrhea, symptoms are more variable.

Physical Examination: Generally unremarkable in primary dysmenorrhea. Endometriosis, salpingitis, or uterine neoplasm may be detected as a cause of secondary dysmenorrhea.

Diagnostic Tests: In secondary dysmenorrhea, pelvic ultrasound or MRI may identify the underlying cause. Diagnostic D&C may disclose a cause within the uterine cavity. Laparoscopy identifies endometriosis or PID.

Course: Primary dysmenorrhea tends to diminish in severity after age 25, and particularly after childbirth. Without treatment, secondary dysmenorrhea may continue throughout the reproductive years.

Treatment: Nonsteroidal anti-inflammatory drugs (ibuprofen, naproxen, mefenamic acid) usually provide good symptomatic relief. Oral contraceptives may be prescribed for more sustained control. Endometriosis is treated with drugs or surgery.

Endometriosis

Growth of endometrial tissue outside of the uterus, particularly in the ovaries and on the pelvic walls.

Cause: Unknown. The problem affects about 2% of American women. Implants of endometrial tissue can occur in a wide variety of locations, including any peritoneal surface, the rectal mucosa, and the ovaries (causing **endometrial** or **"chocolate" cysts**, so-called because of their color).

History: Severe dysmenorrhea, often beginning days before the onset of menstruation and continuing for a week or more. Pain is constant and may be diffuse, with rectal pain and dyspareunia. Many patients are **infertile** (unable to conceive). Rectal bleeding may occur from implants in the rectum.

Physical Examination: Tender nodules of endometrial tissue may be palpated in the pelvis, particularly the **cul-de-sac** (lowermost part of pelvic cavity, between uterus and rectum), the ovaries, or the rectum.

Diagnostic Tests: Ultrasound, MRI, or barium enema may identify endometrial implants. Often laparoscopy is required to arrive at a definitive diagnosis. At laparoscopy, endometrial implants often appear as hemorrhagic cysts or **"powder burn" lesions** on peritoneal surfaces.

Course: Pain (including dyspareunia) and infertility tend to persist throughout the reproductive years. Medical or surgical treatment may diminish pain, but most treatment methods may further impair fertility.

Treatment: Analgesics and various hormone analogues (leuprolide, nafarelin, oral contraceptives) or hormone inhibitors (danazol) may help. Focal endometriosis may be ablated laparoscopically with a laser. For severe or generalized disease, hysterectomy (removal of uterus), oophorectomy (removal of ovaries), or both may be indicated.

Premenstrual Syndrome (PMS, Premenstrual Tension, Late Luteal Phase Dysphoria)

A group of distressing physical and psychologic symptoms experienced in varying degrees and proportions by many women during the week preceding onset of menstruation: swelling of breasts, ankles, and about waist, breast soreness, weight gain, irritability, drowsiness, depression, changes in appetite and libido. The cause is unknown, but hormonal and possibly psychological or psychosocial factors are thought to play a part. Treatment is largely supportive: counseling and a regular program of exercise; restriction of sodium, caffeine, alcohol, and sugar; drug therapy with danazol, tranquilizers, or hormones.

Pelvic Neoplasms

Uterine Myoma (Fibromyoma, Fibroid)

A common benign neoplasm of uterine muscle.

Cause: Unknown.

History: There may be no symptoms. Abdominal or pelvic pain or pressure, heavy vaginal bleeding, dysmenorrhea, urinary frequency, infertility.

Physical Examination: Pelvic examination shows one or more discrete, firm masses in the uterine wall. With heavy bleeding there may be tachycardia, pallor, or even shock.

Diagnostic Tests: With heavy bleeding the hemoglobin level may be low. Ultrasound or MRI studies can clearly delineate the nature of the problem.

Course: Uterine myomas tend to grow larger and more numerous with time. With significant bleeding there is a risk of chronic anemia or sudden onset of shock. Myomas in the pregnant uterus can lead to fetal loss, premature or difficult labor, or severe postpartum hemorrhage.

Treatment: Small or solitary myomas can be removed surgically (**myomectomy**). If tumors are large or numerous, **hysterectomy** (removal of the uterus) may be indicated. Before surgery, leuprolide or nafarelin is administered to reduce the size and vascularity of tumors.

Pelvic Inflammatory Disease (PID), Salpingitis, Endometritis

Acute or chronic bacterial infection of the uterus and tubes.

Causes: Sexually transmitted infection with *Neisseria gonorrhoeae* or *Chlamydia trachomatis* ascending from the lower genital tract; infection with other organisms (streptococci, *Haemophilus influenzae*) may be bloodborne. Risk factors include **nulliparity** (never having borne a viable child), nonwhite race, smoking, and sexual contact with many partners.

History: Pelvic pain, chills, fever, menstrual irregularities, purulent vaginal discharge, dyspareunia. Acute symptoms are more likely to occur during menses. With **Fitz-Hugh–Curtis syndrome**, right upper quadrant pain.

Physical Examination: Fever, abdominal tenderness; marked tenderness on manipulation of cervix and palpation of adnexa. Right upper quadrant tenderness in **Fitz-Hugh–Curtis syndrome**.

Diagnostic Tests: The white blood cell count is variably elevated. Smear and culture of material obtained from the cervix or cul-de-sac by culdoscopy may identify the infecting organism. Pelvic ultrasound and laparoscopy are used to refine the diagnosis.

Course: In about 25% of patients, the condition becomes recurrent or chronic even after treatment, with pelvic pain, infertility, and increased risk of ectopic pregnancy. Complications of PID include **tubo-ovarian** abscess with danger of rupture into the peritoneal cavity, and Fitz-Hugh–Curtis syndrome, a localized peritonitis in the right upper quadrant.

Treatment: Hospitalization, intravenous antibiotics (cefoxitin, clindamycin). For milder disease, outpatient treatment with oral antibiotics may suffice. Surgical drainage of abscesses; for severe disease, hysterectomy with bilateral salpingo-oophorectomy.

Carcinoma of the Cervix

A slowly growing, invasive carcinoma of the uterine cervix, predominantly of squamous-cell origin.

Causes: Squamous cell carcinoma of the cervix develops as a consequence of **cervical dysplasia** (**cervical intraepithelial neoplasia, CIN**), which in turn is caused in a majority of cases by cervical infection with **human papillomavirus** (genital wart virus), particularly types 16, 18, and 31. The progression from CIN to invasive carcinoma typically takes 5-10 years. Peak incidence of cervical carcinoma occurs in the late 30s. Risk factors for cervical carcinoma are smoking, prolonged use of oral contraceptives, sexual contact with many partners, HIV infection.

History: Irregular vaginal bleeding or spotting, particularly after intercourse; abnormal vaginal discharge; bowel or bladder pain or dysfunction.

Physical Examination: Cervical ulceration. With advanced disease, evidence of pelvic invasion or metastasis; a **fistula** (abnormal passage or communication) between the vagina and the bladder or rectum may occur.

Diagnostic Tests: CIN can be detected early by routine Pap smear, and calls for follow-up in the form of colposcopy, cervical biopsy, and possibly surgical or laser excision of a cone of cervical tissue including the entire squamocolumnar junction. These provide precise information about the type and stage of disease.

Course: Severe bleeding may occur from ulceration and erosion of the cervix and surrounding tissues. Extension can lead to bilateral ureteral obstruction, with resultant kidney failure, or to rectovaginal or vesicovaginal fistula. The 5-year survival rate with treatment is about 60%.

Treatment: Early removal of localized disease by conization or, preferably, hysterectomy. In advanced disease, radiation is an alternative to radical surgery.

Endometrial Carcinoma
Adenocarcinoma of the uterine lining.
Causes: Unknown. Most patients are over 50. The risk is increased in childless women, those with obesity, diabetes mellitus, or polycystic ovary disease, and those who have taken postmenopausal estrogen replacement therapy without progesterone, or have been treated for breast cancer with tamoxifen.
History: Abnormal vaginal bleeding, particularly postmenopausal bleeding; pelvic pressure or pain.
Physical Examination: Often unremarkable. There may be uterine enlargement or pelvic tenderness.
Diagnostic Tests: Endometrial biopsy or, occasionally, Pap smear will show malignant cells. Ultrasound examination helps to assess the nature and extent of the problem.
Course: Extension and metastasis occur eventually. With prompt treatment, the 5-year survival rate is about 80%.
Treatment: Removal of uterus, tubes, and ovaries (**bilateral salpingo-oophorectomy**), with supplemental radiation. Progesterone may be given to palliate metastatic disease.

Vaginitis, Vulvovaginitis
Inflammation of the vagina and vulva, generally due to infection and manifested by vaginal discharge and vulvar itching or pain. Most cases are due to one of three organisms:
Candida albicans, a yeastlike fungus, frequently causes vulvar pruritus and a thick white curdy discharge. Infection is more common in diabetes mellitus and pregnancy and in women taking oral contraceptives or broad-spectrum antibiotics. Examination shows intense erythema of the vulva and curdy white material in the vaginal vault. A wet preparation of this material in potassium hydroxide examined microscopically identifies the causative organism. Culture may also be performed. Treatment is with topical antifungal medicines (miconazole, terconazole, clotrimazole) in vaginal suppositories, creams, or ointments, or with oral fluconazole in a single dose. Recurrences are common.
Trichomonas vaginalis is a sexually transmitted protozoan parasite that causes vulvar itching and vaginal discharge. Vaginal examination shows erythema, particularly of the cervix (**"strawberry cervix"**), and a watery, frothy, malodorous, yellowish-brown discharge. Wet preparation

of vaginal discharge shows motile protozoa. Treatment is with oral metronidazole for the patient and all sexual partners. (Symptoms in men are usually absent; dysuria and urethral discharge may occur.)

Gardnerella vaginalis is at least one of the organisms involved in **bacterial vaginosis**, a mixed vaginal infection that causes a thin grayish discharge with a foul fishy odor but not much vulvar irritation or itching. Microscopic examination of discharge material shows **clue cells** (epithelial cells heavily studded with bacteria). Treatment is with oral or vaginal metronidazole or clindamycin.

Disorders of the Breast

The **breasts** consist of glandular elements (dormant except during pregnancy and lactation) and their duct system (discharging at the nipple), interpersed with variable amounts of fat.

Fibrocystic Disease (or Condition) of the Breast (Cystic Mastitis, Mammary Dysplasia)

Formation of benign but painful cysts in the breasts.

Cause: Probably inappropriate response of breast tissue to ovarian hormones. The condition affects as many as one-third of all women between the ages of 25 and 50. The theory that caffeine (from coffee, tea, and chocolate) exacerbates symptoms remains unproven.

History: One or more lumps in the breast, typically painful and tender, and more so just before the onset of menses. Lumps are frequently multiple and may change markedly in size within a period of 2-3 days. Lumps typically disappear eventually, but meanwhile others often develop.

Physical Examination: One or more fluctuant, usually tender masses in one or both breasts. Occasionally nipple discharge is noted.

Diagnostic Tests: Needle aspiration of a cyst usually leads to its disappearance. Biopsy material obtained by fine-needle aspiration or other method from a solid or cystic mass helps to rule out malignant change. Biopsy may show **hyperplasia** of epithelial tissues, associated with an increased risk of malignant tumor of the breast. Mammography and ultrasound examinations may help to distinguish cysts from solid tumors.

Course: Fibrocystic disease tends to persist, with remissions and exacerbations, until menopause, and then to resolve completely and permanently. Forms of fibrocystic disease associated with proliferation of epithelial elements carry a slightly higher risk of progression to carcinoma of the breast.

Treatment: Analgesics, education, close observation for persisting or dominant lump, which may prove to be a solid tumor requiring further observation. For severe disease, danazol and, rarely, mastectomy may be advised.

Fibroadenoma of the Breast

A benign solid tumor of the breast, occurring typically in younger women. The mass is not usually tender and may be discovered accidentally. It is firm, discrete, spherical, and about 1-5 cm in diameter. Occasionally more than one tumor may be found. Aspiration does not yield fluid and does not collapse the lesion. The principal concern is in distinguishing fibroadenoma from adenocarcinoma, and in the small risk of progression of this lesion to **cystosarcoma phyllodes**, a rapidly growing tumor that is not histologically malignant but tends to recur after excision. Treatment of fibroadenoma is simple excision under local anesthesia.

Carcinoma of the breast is discussed in Chapter 5.

Topics for Study or Discussion

1. Mention two effects of GnRH (gonadotropin releasing hormone) and two effects of FSH (follicle stimulating hormone).

2. Briefly describe how a Pap (Papanicolaou) test is done and what it shows.

3. Define or explain: anovulation, CIN, clue cell, dyspareunia, menarche, mittelschmerz, spinnbarkeit, *Trichomonas vaginalis*.

4. Compare and contrast breast and cervical carcinoma as to incidence, mortality rate, risk factors, and measures for early detection.

5. Name five conditions that can cause amenorrhea and five conditions that can cause heavy uterine bleeding.

Chapter 14

Disorders of the Metabolism, Nutrition, and Endocrine Function

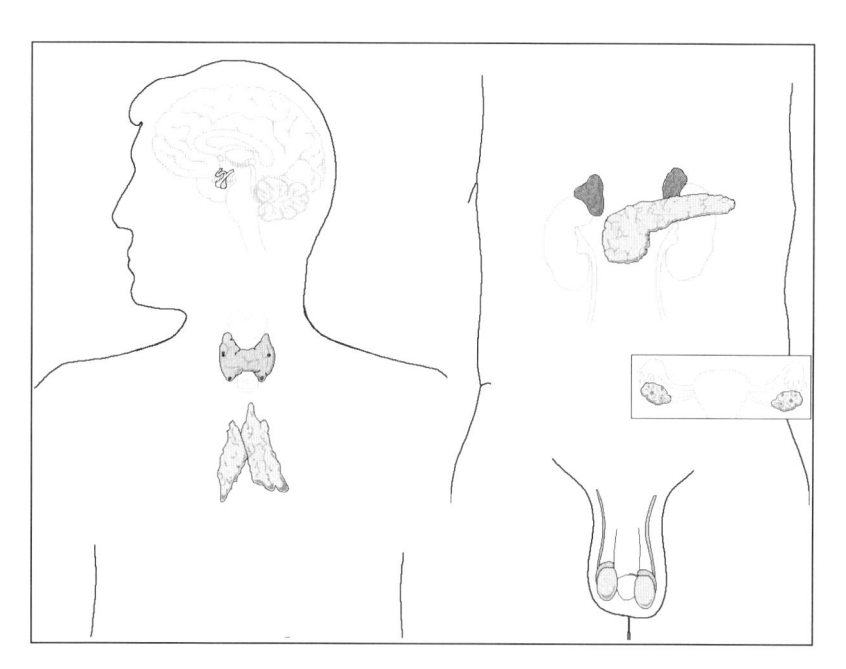

Learning Objectives

Upon completion of this chapter, the student should

- have basic information about the physiology of metabolism and nutrition;

- know the functions of the principal endocrine glands;

- know signs, symptoms, and treatments of common metabolic disorders.

Metabolism and Nutrition

Metabolism is a general term for the sum of all the chemical and electrical processes that occur in the living body. A principal part of metabolism is the **oxidation** of foods so as to release energy in tiny amounts that are usable at the cellular level. Most metabolic processes are at least partially under the control of hormones.

A **hormone** is a chemical messenger or mediator produced by a cell, tissue, or gland. Hormones are released into the circulation, and perform their functions at sites remote from their origins. Some hormones stimulate cellular functions, while others inhibit them. A **tropic hormone** stimulates the cells of a remote gland to produce its secretion, and a **releasing hormone** (**relin**) promotes release of a specific hormone into the circulation.

Many of the important hormones are produced by **endocrine** ("internal secretion") **glands** (also called ductless glands because their secretions pass directly into the circulation)—**pituitary, thyroid, adrenal**, and others. Some of these endocrine glands (for example, the **pancreas** and the **gonads**), perform nonhormonal functions as well.

Nutrition refers to the intake and use of foods by the body. Each of the three main types of food (**protein, fat, carbohydrate**) has its own function in human nutrition.

A normal adult requires one gram of protein per kilogram of body weight per day to supply sufficient materials for maintenance and repair of tissues and organs and for production of intracellular enzymes, hormones, and other substances. **Proteins** are built up of long strands of **amino acids**, which are relatively simple nitrogen-containing organic compounds. Only 20 different amino acids have been found in all the complex proteins of the human organism. About half of these can be synthesized in the body; the rest, called **essential amino acids**, must be obtained from the diet.

Carbohydrate (consumed in the form of **starches** and **sweets**) is the most important source of energy in most diets. Carbohydrate foods are chemically degraded in the digestive system to simple sugars, especially **glucose**, a 6-carbon sugar that is the most plentiful in the blood and the principal fuel of cellular energy metabolism.

Fats (lipids) are oily or greasy substances built up of **fatty acids** (long, straight-chain organic acids). Fats in the diet come mainly from animal foods, but the term fat is often extended to include oils of plant origin.

All three basic types of food can be and are burned in the body as fuel. The amount of energy that a foodstuff can supply can be determined by burning the food outside the body in a **calorimeter** (a small furnace equipped with a sensitive means of measuring heat production). The energy released by food is measured in calories per gram (cal/g). The large calorie or kilocalorie (kcal, 1000 calories) is a more convenient unit of measure in nutrition; in modern parlance, **kilocalories** are usually called simply **calories**.

Whereas proteins and carbohydrates both supply about 4 calories (kcal) per gram, fats supply about 9. The active adult requires 2500-4000 kcal/day to meet the energy demands of basic life processes (1200-1800 kcal) plus those imposed by physical exertion. In the average middle-class American diet, 50% of calories come from carbohydrate, 35% from fat, and 15% from protein.

By convention, the subject of nutrition also includes materials usually not thought of as foods: water, minerals, and vitamins. **Water** is the most abundant substance in the body and the principal constituent of blood. **Intracellular fluid** accounts for about 40% of total body weight, **interstitial fluid** (in tissue spaces, outside of cells) another 15%, and **plasma** (the fluid part of blood) about 5%. The water content of plasma, and indirectly that of the intracellular and interstitial compartments, is regulated within narrow limits by a complex system of checks and balances involving the sensation of thirst, perspiration, gastrointestinal fluid losses, renal excretion and reabsorption of water and electrolytes, and other chemical processes.

Essential dietary **minerals** include iron (needed for the production of red blood cells and as a catalyst in many metabolic processes), calcium (a principal constituent of bones and teeth), sodium, potassium, zinc, magnesium, and many more.

Vitamins are organic compounds, normally present in many foods, that the human body needs in trace amounts, usually to serve as boosters or catalysts in essential metabolic processes.

Disorders of nutrition are relatively common, and have many causes, among them overeating, alcoholism, stringent dieting, anorexia nervosa, malabsorption due to inherited abnormalities or to gastrointestinal disease or surgery, and any severe chronic disease including metastatic carcinoma. Specific vitamin deficiencies occur but are rare in our culture. Most nutritional deficiencies are complex and occur as part of a more general pattern of illness. The most common nutritional disorder, except among the extremely poor, is not undernutrition but **exogenous obesity**: **overweight** due to consumption of calories, mostly from fat and carbohydrate, in excess of metabolic requirements. As little as 15-20 pounds of overweight is associated with heightened **mortality** due to cardiovascular disease, metabolic disease, and even malignant disease.

Disorders of Endocrine Function

Diseases of the pituitary, thyroid, adrenal, and parathyroid glands, and diabetes mellitus, are discussed in this section.

Diseases of the Pituitary Gland

The **pituitary gland** or **hypophysis**, situated on the undersurface of the brain, consists of two distinct masses of endocrine tissue. The anterior pituitary (**adenohypophysis**) produces hormones that regulate the development and function of other endocrine glands: **thyroid stimulating hormone (TSH)**, **adrenocorticotropic hormone (ACTH)** which stimulates the adrenal cortex, and the gonadotropins: **follicle-stimulating hormone (FSH)** and **luteinizing hormone (LH)**, which stimulate gonadal functions. The anterior pituitary is also the source of **growth hormone** (**somatotropin**, which regulates the natural growth process) and **prolactin** (required for lactation after pregnancy).

The posterior pituitary (**neurohypophysis**) is in direct continuity with the part of the brain called the **hypothalamus**. It produces two hormones: **oxytocin**, which stimulates uterine contractions in labor; and **vasopressin (antidiuretic hormone, ADH)**, which helps to control water balance by promoting reabsorption of water by the kidneys.

Hypopituitarism

Deficiency of pituitary hormones, with resultant structural and functional disturbances.

Causes: Benign or malignant neoplasms of the pituitary gland or surrounding tissues, cerebral vascular disease, infection, trauma, shock, autoimmune disease.

History: Weakness, fatigue, weight loss, diminished **libido**, amenorrhea.

Physical Examination: Wasting, loss of axillary and pubic hair, hypotension. Visual field defects may be noted if a causative tumor affects the optic chiasm.

Diagnostic Tests: The levels of pituitary hormones (ACTH, TSH) in the serum are diminished, as well as the levels of hormones produced by organs stimulated by these hormones (T_4, cortisol). Fasting blood sugar and sodium are depressed, lipids increased.

Course: Any stressing illness can precipitate shock, vascular collapse, and death.

Treatment: Surgical excision of a tumor, if present. Endocrine replacement therapy as needed (cortisol, thyroid hormone, gonadal hormones).

Acromegaly, Gigantism

Overgrowth of body structures in adulthood (**acromegaly**) or in childhood (**gigantism**) due to excessive **somatotropin** (growth hormone).

Cause: Benign pituitary adenoma producing abnormal amounts of somatotropin. May occur as part of multiple endocrine adenomatosis.

History: Excessive long-bone growth (when onset is before puberty); excessive growth of hands, feet, jaw. Weakness, amenorrhea, headache, hoarseness, sleep apnea, sweating.

Physical Examination: Coarse facial features, hypertension, visual field defects, cardiomegaly.

Diagnostic Tests: Serum level of growth hormone is elevated, and is not suppressed by administration of oral glucose. The blood sugar is elevated. X-ray of the skull may show an enlarged **sella turcica** (the saddle-shaped bony depression in which the pituitary rests). MRI may show a pituitary tumor.

Course: Premature cardiovascular disease. Other complications include pituitary failure, hypertension, diabetes mellitus, cardiac enlargement and failure, carpal tunnel syndrome, and visual field defects.

Treatment: Surgical excision of the tumor is usually successful. Radiation may also be used. Bromocriptine is administered to reduce the level of growth hormone. Octreotide, a synthetic analog of **somatostatin** (a hormone that inhibits production and release of growth hormone) is also effective.

Diabetes Insipidus

A disorder in which deficiency of antidiuretic hormone (ADH, vasopressin) leads to excessive output of urine containing no sugar.

Cause: Failure of the posterior lobe of the pituitary to produce ADH because of trauma, infection, neoplasm, or inherited pituitary disease.

History: **Polyuria** (increased urine output), **polydipsia** (excessive thirst).

Physical Examination: There may be signs of dehydration. The pulse may be rapid and the blood pressure low.

Diagnostic Tests: The serum sodium is elevated. The urine contains no sugar. Administration of vasopressin corrects polyuria.

Course: Complications include dehydration and hypernatremia (depletion of serum sodium).

Treatment: Desmopressin administered intranasally or intramuscularly controls polyuria and polydipsia.

Diseases of the Thyroid Gland

The **thyroid gland**, whose name means "shield-shaped," is situated in the front of the neck overlying the junction of the **larynx** and **trachea**. The thyroid gland produces two iodine-containing hormones, **thyroxine** (T_4) and **triiodothyronine** (T_3), which circulate in the blood bound to a plasma protein (**thyroid binding globulin, TBG**). These hormones influence general metabolism, chiefly by regulating gene transcription of body proteins (including growth hormone).

The term **goiter** refers to a palpable and often visible enlargement of the thyroid gland. Goiter can occur with elevated, normal, or decreased levels of thyroid hormone, depending on its cause.

Hypothyroidism

A syndrome resulting from deficiency of circulating thyroid hormone. When the disorder appears at birth or in early infancy it is called **cretinism**; hypothyroidism occurring after early childhood is called **myxedema**.

Causes: Congenital absence or hypoplasia of the thyroid gland; intrinsic thyroid disease (**Hashimoto thyroiditis**), deficiency of dietary iodine, goitrogenic foods or medicines, deficiency of pituitary thyroid stimulating hormone.

History: Weakness, lethargy, myalgia, constipation, depression, intolerance to cold, polymenorrhea, weight gain, hoarseness.

Physical Examination: Dry, sallow skin, brittle hair and nails, thinning of scalp hair and outer thirds of eyebrows, puffy face, sluggish speech, bradycardia, nonpitting edema. Goiter when disease is due to iodine deficiency, antithyroid agents, or thyroiditis.

Diagnostic Tests: The T_4 and other measures of thyroid hormone are depressed, the TSH level elevated (except when disease is due to pituitary TSH deficiency). There may be reduction of red blood cells, blood sugar, and sodium, and elevation of cholesterol. Antibody to thyroid may be found in Hashimoto thyroiditis.

Course: With treatment the prognosis is excellent. Complications of untreated disease include coronary artery disease, congestive heart failure, heightened susceptibility to infection, psychosis, and coma.

Treatment: Deficiency of thyroid hormone can be corrected by administration of levothyroxine. Maintenance treatment must be continued indefinitely unless a treatable cause of hypothyroidism can be found and eliminated.

Hyperthyroidism (Thyrotoxicosis)

A syndrome resulting from excessive thyroid hormone in the circulation.

Causes: The principal cause is autoimmune disease of the thyroid gland, with production of thyroid-stimulating immunoglobulin by the immune system. This condition (**Graves disease**) is 8 times commoner in women and usually comes on between ages 20 and 40. Graves disease may be accompanied by other autoimmune disorders (pernicious anemia, myasthenia gravis, diabetes mellitus). Less common causes of hyperthyroidism are acute thyroiditis and inappropriate administration of thyroid hormone.

History: Restlessness, nervousness, fatigue, intolerance to heat, sweating, palpitations, weight loss, frequent bowel movements, menstrual irregularities, enlargement of thyroid gland (goiter). In Graves disease, bulging of eyes, conjunctival drying or irritation.

Physical Examination: Tachycardia, warmth and moistness of skin, resting tremor of hands, hyperactive deep tendon reflexes, loosening of nails. In Graves disease, diffuse or nodular enlargement of thyroid, sometimes with arterial **bruit** (a vascular hum synchronous with heartbeat, heard with a stethoscope); **exophthalmos** (undue prominence of eyes due to edema of orbital contents), staring gaze, lid lag (slowness of upper eyelids to move with eye movements).

Diagnostic Tests: The levels of T_3 and T_4 are elevated, and TSH is depressed. The radioactive iodine uptake is increased. Thyroid-stimulating immunoglobulin is present in the serum. Antinuclear antibody may also be present. There may be mild anemia and hypercalcemia.

Course: Complications include atrial fibrillation, paralysis, and hypercalcemia.

Treatment: End-organ effects of thyroid hormone (tachycardia, tremor, restlessness) can be reduced by beta-blocker treatment. Glandular hyperactivity can be reduced by antithyroid medicines (propylthiouracil, methimazole), radioactive iodine, or thyroidectomy.

Thyroiditis

Thyroiditis is a general term for inflammation of the thyroid gland. Several types are recognized, differing in their causes, symptoms, and effects on thyroid function. Two of the more common types are discussed below.

Hashimoto Disease
(Chronic Lymphocytic Thyroiditis)

A relatively common disorder, often asymptomatic. It occurs more frequently in women, and tends to run in families.

Cause: Development of antibodies to one's own thyroid tissue.

History: Gradual painless enlargement of the thyroid gland, with symptoms of mild hypothyroidism. Often there are no symptoms at all.

Physical Examination: The thyroid gland is enlarged, symmetric, firm, and nontender.

Diagnostic Tests: The erythrocyte sedimentation rate is elevated. Testing of serum may disclose presence of autoantibodies to thyroid tissue. Thyroid function tests give variable results.

Course: Tendency to resolve spontaneously, but may lead to progressive decline of thyroid function.

Treatment: Thyroid hormone supplementation and long-term observation for progression of hypothyroidism.

DeQuervain Disease (Subacute Thyroiditis, Granulomatous Thyroiditis, Giant Cell Thyroiditis)

Cause: Probably viral infection of the thyroid gland.

History: Acute, painful enlargement of the thyroid gland, with dysphagia. There may also be malaise and symptoms of thyrotoxicosis.

Physical Examination: The thyroid gland is enlarged and tender. Signs of hyperthyroidism may be present.

Diagnostic Tests: The sedimentation rate is markedly elevated and the radioactive iodine uptake is reduced. Antibody to thyroid tissue may be present in the serum.

Course: Self-limited.

Treatment: Aspirin. If hypothyroidism is present, thyroid hormone supplementation is given. Propranolol is used to control transitory thyrotoxicosis.

Disorders of the Parathyroid Glands

The four **parathyroid glands** are so called because they lie on or in the capsule of the thyroid gland. These glands produce **parathyroid hormone (PTH)**, which regulates the serum calcium level within narrow limits. Calcium control is important for proper maintenance of bones and teeth; more critically, the level of calcium in the serum and in tissue fluids exerts a potent influence on nerve and muscle function. Parathyroid hormone maintains the level of calcium in serum by moving calcium ions out of the bones, reducing the renal clearance of calcium, and increasing the rate of intestinal absorption of calcium. **Calcitonin**, a hormone produced by the thyroid gland, is also involved in regulation of serum calcium.

Hypoparathyroidism

Causes: The most common cause is accidental removal of the parathyroid glands during thyroidectomy. Rarely the parathyroid glands may be damaged by trauma, infection, neoplasm, or chemical poisons, or by autoantibodies, which may be formed in the polyglandular autoimmune syndrome, discussed later in the chapter.

History: With acute onset, tetany, tingling of face, hands, and feet, muscle cramps, carpopedal spasm (painful cramps of wrists and ankles), laryngospasm with respiratory obstruction, seizures. With more chronic onset, mental retardation, abnormalities of bones and teeth, cataract, parkinsonlike disorder due to calcification of basal ganglia.

Physical Examination: The skin may be dry and coarse. Deep tendon reflexes are hyperactive, and the **Chvostek sign** (twitching of face after percussion over facial nerve in front of ear) and **Trousseau sign** (spastic contraction of the hand after application of a constricting cuff to the arm) are positive.

Diagnostic Tests: The serum calcium is low and the serum phosphorus is high. Excretion of phosphorus in the urine is reduced. The level of parathyroid hormone in the serum is low.

Treatment: Calcium replacement, intravenously in acute tetany, and vitamin D. Treatment must be continued indefinitely.

Hyperparathyroidism

Causes: Hyperplasia, adenoma, or carcinoma of a parathyroid gland. Adenoma may occur as part of **multiple endocrine adenomatosis**, discussed later in this chapter.

History: Bone pain; weakness, fatigue, polyuria, polydipsia, urolithiasis.

Physical Examination: Unremarkable.

Diagnostic Tests: The serum calcium is elevated, the phosphorus depressed. Urinary calcium and phosphorus are both elevated. X-ray may show osseous or dental abnormalities, or cysts or pathologic calcification of the kidneys.

Course: Complications include peptic ulcer, pancreatitis, renal damage.

Treatment: Surgical removal of neoplasm. Reduction of serum calcium by administration of furosemide or other agents.

Diseases of the Adrenal Glands

The **adrenal glands** are two crescent-shaped caps of endocrine tissue, one situated on top of each kidney. Each adrenal gland consists of two essentially different bodies of endocrine tissue: the **outer cortex**, and the **inner medulla**.

The adrenal cortex produces three classes of hormones, two of which play crucial roles in the control of sugar, protein, and mineral metabolism. The **glucocorticoids** (principally **cortisol**) increase glucose production by the liver, affect protein and fat metabolism, help to regulate blood pressure, mediate many of the responses of the body to stress, and tend to suppress immune and inflammatory responses. The **mineralocorticoids** (principally **aldosterone**) regulate electrolyte and water balance by promoting renal retention of sodium ions of potassium, hydrogen, and ammonium ions. **Adrenal androgens** play a minor role in reproductive physiology in both men and women. They are chiefly of interest as a cause of hirsutism and virilization in certain adrenal diseases.

The **adrenal medulla** is part of the **sympathetic nervous system** (see Chapter 18). Cells of the adrenal medulla are stimulated directly by sympathetic nerve endings to produce **epinephrine**, **norepinephrine**, and **dopamine**, which (although not essential to life) play a critical part in the body's response to severe stress. These hormones affect many tissues, increasing the rate and force of cardiac contractions, relaxing the smooth muscle of the bronchi, constricting some blood vessels and dilating others, stimulating liver and muscle tissue to produce and release glucose, and controlling fat breakdown and insulin production.

Adrenal Insufficiency (Addison Disease)

An acute or chronic deficiency of **cortisol** and related hormones from the adrenal cortex.

Causes: Degeneration of the adrenal cortices, usually as an autoimmune phenomenon sometimes involving other endocrine glands as well. Other diseases (infection, malignant tumors) may account for destruction of the adrenal glands in rare cases. Deficiency of pituitary ACTH also causes some adrenal insufficiency, but not the full-blown clinical picture of Addison disease. **Adrenal crisis** may be precipitated by severe physical stress (surgery) or systemic disease (meningococcemia) or by sudden withdrawal of steroid therapy.

History: Weakness, easy fatigability, anorexia, nausea, vomiting, diarrhea, abdominal pain, amenorrhea, emotional lability. In **addisonian crisis**, fever, confusion, collapse, coma.

Physical Examination: Weight loss, wasting, hypotension, sparseness of axillary hair; increased pigmentation of skin, especially over pressure points, skin creases, and nipples. In crisis, severe hypotension and evidence of dehydration.

Diagnostic Tests: The eosinophil count is elevated. The serum sodium is low, the potassium and BUN (blood urea nitrogen) elevated.

Serum cortisol is abnormally low and does not rise in response to administration of ACTH. Chest x-ray shows a small, vertical heart.

Course: Without treatment, steady progression is likely. Addisonian crisis can be rapidly fatal. Fluid and electrolyte depletion, wasting, cardiovascular collapse.

Treatment: The basic treatment is replacement of missing corticosteroids. Supportive treatment and elimination of any identifiable underlying or precipitating cause are important. In crisis, intravenous fluid and electrolyte replacement may be lifesaving.

Cushing Syndrome (Hyperadrenocorticism)

A syndrome due to prolonged elevation of adrenal cortical hormones in the circulation.

Causes: The most frequent cause of **Cushing syndrome** today is medicinal administration of adrenocortical hormones. The condition can also result from production of excessive adrenocortical hormones by a neoplasm of the adrenal cortex, from medicinal administration of ACTH, or from production of ACTH-like substances by other neoplasms (such as bronchogenic carcinoma). When excessive adrenal cortical activity results from an elevated level of adrenocorticotropic hormone (ACTH) from a tumor (basophil adenoma) of the pituitary, the condition is called **Cushing disease**.

History: Increasing obesity, stretch marks especially on trunk and thighs, acne, easy bruising, impaired wound healing, weakness, thirst, headache, amenorrhea or impotence, increased body hair, personality change.

Physical Examination: Truncal obesity, moon face, buffalo hump (soft tissue prominence over upper back), protuberant abdomen with purple **striae** (stretch marks), hirsutism, acne, hypertension.

Diagnostic Tests: Blood glucose is elevated and potassium is low. The serum level of cortisol is high and does not fall after administration of dexamethasone, a synthetic corticosteroid. Urinary excretion of cortisol is also increased. In Cushing disease and other disorders due to excessive ACTH, the blood level of ACTH is elevated. Otherwise the ACTH level is subnormal, its production by the pituitary having been suppressed by high circulating levels of corticosteroid. An adrenal tumor may be shown by abdominal CT scan. Tumor of the pituitary is identified by cranial MRI.

Course: Depends on the origin of the problem. Untreated Cushing syndrome can be complicated by osteoporosis, nephrolithiasis, psychosis, heightened susceptibility to infection, and consequences of hypertension and diabetes mellitus; it is generally fatal within a few years.

Treatment: Discontinuance of corticosteroid treatment, or reduction of dose. Surgical removal of a causative pituitary or adrenal neoplasm. Ketoconazole or metyrapone can be used to suppress cortisol levels when surgery is not feasible.

Congenital Adrenal Hyperplasia

A genetically determined deficiency of the enzymes normally involved in the formation of cortisol. The resulting deficiency of cortisol leads to overproduction of ACTH by the pituitary, which in turn stimulates excessive androgen production by the adrenal glands. Signs of abnormality due to excessive androgen levels are evident at birth or shortly after: **virilization** of female children, **precocious** genital development of males. Signs of adrenal insufficiency include electrolyte and water imbalances, which may be evident within the first few days of life. Laboratory studies show elevation of androgen (dehydroepiandrosterone) in serum and urine. Serum ACTH levels are increased and cortisol levels are diminished. Treatment is lifelong replacement of missing adrenal cortical secretion with dexamethasone or prednisone.

Disorders of Pancreatic Endocrine Function

The digestive function of the pancreas is discussed in Chapter 11. As mentioned earlier, the **pancreas** is an **endocrine** gland as well as an exocrine one (one that produces a secretion released through a duct). The endocrine function of the pancreas is performed by the **islets of Langerhans**, tiny aggregations of endocrine cells interspersed among the exocrine secretory elements.

The **B** or **beta cells** of the islets of Langerhans produce insulin, which increases glucose utilization and exerts other complex influences on the metabolism of carbohydrates, proteins, and fats. The **A** or **alpha cells** produce **glucagon**, an inhibitor of glucose activity, and the **D** or **delta cells** produce somatostatin, which inhibits secretion of growth hormone by the anterior pituitary.

Diabetes Mellitus

A disorder of metabolism in which body cells are unable to use glucose as fuel because of a deficiency of insulin. Two major types of diabetes are recognized.

Insulin-Dependent Diabetes Mellitus (IDDM)

Cause: A lack of insulin in the circulation due to failure of pancreatic B cells to respond to normal stimuli to insulin production. This type of diabetes shows a familial tendency. Failure of insulin production may be due to toxic, infectious, or autoimmune damage to B cells in genetically predisposed persons.

History: **Polyuria** (increased output of urine), **polydipsia** (excessive thirst), **polyphagia** (excessive appetite), weakness, and weight loss, coming on gradually or suddenly, usually in a person under 40 years of age. With fulminant onset, IDDM may present as **ketoacidosis** with dyspnea, drowsiness, collapse, and coma.

Physical Examination: Unremarkable in uncomplicated diabetes. In ketoacidosis: tachypnea, tachycardia, hypotension, flushing, fruity breath, and stupor or coma. Symptoms of cardiovascular, neurologic, or ocular complications may be evident in long-established or neglected disease.

Diagnostic Tests: Fasting blood sugar is over 140 mg/dL and 2-hour postprandial blood sugar is over 200 mg/dL. Sugar is present in the urine. Serum cholesterol is often elevated. In ketoacidosis, ketones are found in the serum and the urine, and there is chemical evidence of metabolic acidosis (low blood pH, low blood HCO_3). Glycosylated hemoglobin (HbA_{1c}) reflects blood sugar levels over the preceding few weeks and is used to monitor control. Laboratory studies may also show evidence of systemic complications (infection, renal disease).

Course: IDDM is a lifelong derangement of carbohydrate metabolism. In most patients, careful attention to diet and general health and proper use of insulin permit good control of blood sugar and fair protection against complications. Diabetes predisposes to numerous other conditions, including hypercholesterolemia, atherosclerosis, ocular cataracts and retinopathy, renal disease, infections of the urinary tract, skin, and other tissues, neuropathy, and microvascular disease in the extremities.

Treatment: IDDM is by definition a disease that must be treated with insulin as a condition of the patient's survival. The mainstay of treatment, however, is diet, with limitation of total calories and restriction of carbohydrate and cholesterol. Increased fiber helps to stabilize carbohydrate metabolism, and artificial sweeteners are substituted for sugar. Injections of insulin are given one to four times a day, the dose being adjusted to the patient's needs as shown by home testing of urine or, preferably, blood. A variety of insulin products are available with different patterns of absorption and peak activity. The proper management of diabetes requires scrupulous attention to general health, care of the skin and the feet, and vigorous treatment of complications. Diabetic ketoacidosis is treated with intravenous fluids, insulin, and general supportive measures.

Non-Insulin-Dependent Diabetes Mellitus (NIDDM, Nonketotic Diabetes Mellitus)

Cause: A relative deficiency of circulating insulin accompanied by insensitivity or resistance of tissues, particularly liver and muscle, to insulin effect. There is a genetic predisposition to this form of diabetes, but the mechanism of transmission is unknown. NIDDM accounts for 90% of all cases of diabetes mellitus. Most patients are over 40 and obese.

History: The condition may remain asymptomatic for months or years. Polyuria, polydipsia, and sometimes weakness or fatigue occur as in insulin-dependent disease, but weight loss and ketoacidosis do not occur.

Physical Examination: Unremarkable except for obesity, unless complications have developed. Hypertension is often present.

Diagnostic Tests: Fasting blood sugar over 140 mg/dL; 2-hour postprandial blood sugar over 180 mg/dL. There is sugar in the urine. Ketones are not found in serum. The cholesterol is often elevated. With advanced disease there may be chemical or electrocardiographic evidence of complications.

Course: Mild non-insulin-dependent diabetes mellitus may cause few symptoms, particularly with treatment. Complications are the same as those for insulin-dependent diabetes mellitus, with the exception of ketoacidosis. Complications typically do not develop as rapidly or become as severe as in IDDM.

Treatment: Dietary restriction of carbohydrate alone may suffice to control blood sugar levels and abolish symptoms of polyuria and fatigue. Cholesterol restriction is also advised. When diet does not control hyperglycemia, oral drugs (sulfonylureas, biguanides) are prescribed. In rare instances, optimal control depends on the use of insulin. Care of general health and avoidance of skin injury and infection are important in the management of all forms of diabetes.

Multiple Endocrine Neoplasia

At least three genetically determined disorders have been identified in which benign or malignant neoplasms occur in two or more endocrine glands, particularly the parathyroid glands and pancreatic islets. Pancreatic tumors may produce insulin, gastrin, VIP (vasoactive intestinal polypeptide), or other hormonelike substances.

Polyglandular Deficiency Syndrome

Any of several familially determined autoimmune disorders in which deficiencies in the hormonal products of two or more endocrine glands result from autoantibodies directed against the glands.

Topics for Study or Discussion

1. Give three examples of diseases caused by endocrine deficiency, three examples of diseases caused by excessive hormone production, and three examples of endocrine disorders present (but not necessarily evident) at birth.

2. List five general types of substances that are essential in the human diet.

3. Define or explain: Addison disease, carbohydrate, glucose, goiter, hormone, insulin, metabolism, thyrotoxicosis, thyroxine, vasopressin.

4. The pituitary gland is called the master gland because it controls other glands. List four endocrine glands whose function is regulated by the pituitary, and four types of endocrine disorder that can result from pituitary disease.

5. Mention some examples of feedback control between two hormones or the glands that produce them.

Chapter 15

Disorders of Blood Cells, Blood-Forming Tissues, and Blood Coagulation

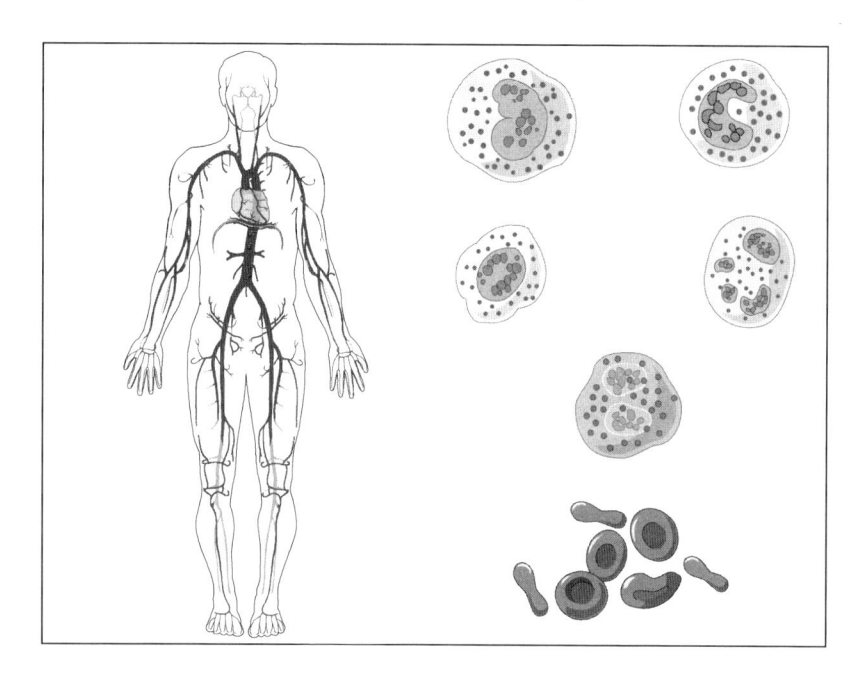

Learning Objectives

Upon completion of this chapter, the student should

- know the basic anatomy and physiology of the blood cells and lymphatic system;

- have a general knowledge of diagnostic procedures and treatments used in diseases of hemolymphatic disorders;

- understand signs, symptoms, and treatment of common diseases affecting this system.

Anatomy and Physiology

The **blood** is an opaque, viscous fluid that can be classed as a tissue because of its complex structure and cellular components. Nearly half of the volume of the blood is made up of formed or cellular elements: **red blood cells**, **white blood cells**, and **platelets**. These are suspended in a fluid medium called **plasma**, whose chief component is water. Plasma carries **electrolytes**, **proteins**, **nutrients**, **wastes**, and **dissolved gases**. Among the proteins is **fibrinogen**, which under certain conditions is converted to **fibrin**, the insoluble material that is responsible for blood clotting. Plasma from which the fibrin has been removed is called **serum**.

Red blood cells (RBCs, **erythrocytes**) contain **hemoglobin**, a complex iron-containing protein that transports oxygen from the lungs to tissues and carbon dioxide from tissues to the lungs. On microscopic examination, red blood cells appear as flat, round, faintly pink discs with both faces concave. When seen on edge they thus have a dumbbell appearance.

Red blood cells are formed in **bone marrow** and released into the circulation as needed to maintain the normal red blood count. The process of red cell production is called **erythropoiesis**. It depends on adequate supplies of iron, protein, certain vitamins (especially folic acid and vitamin B_{12}), and a hormone produced in the kidney (erythropoietin). After about three months, a red blood cell disintegrates and is removed from the circulation in the spleen; the iron is recycled.

Mature red blood cells have no nuclei. The presence of many nucleated red blood cells in the circulation indicates increased production and release of red blood cells. The presence of **reticulocytes** (red blood cells containing fragments of nuclear material that can be detected by staining) has the same significance.

White blood cells (WBCs, **leukocytes**) differ from red blood cells in being somewhat larger and far less numerous, having nuclei, and lacking a reddish tinge. In addition, white blood cells are subdivided into several distinct categories on the basis of origin, form, and function.

White blood cells that arise and mature in bone marrow are called **myeloid cells**. They fall into two major groups: **granulocytes** (so called because they have stainable **granules** in their cytoplasm) and **monocytes** (so called because each has a solitary, non-lobed nucleus). Monocytes are **phagocytes** (cells that engulf and destroy dead tissue, bacteria, and other foreign material). Similar cells called **histiocytes** appear in various tissues and organs of the body (spleen, liver).

Granulocytes are also called **polymorphonuclear leukocytes** because their nuclei are characteristically divided into two to five lobes. These are further classified on the basis of the appearance of their granules after staining by a standard method (Wright or Giemsa stain) as **eosinophils**, with coarse reddish-orange granules; **basophils**, with dark blue to black granules; and **neutrophils**, with fainter granules that take up equal amounts of blue (basic) and red (acidic) stains.

Eosinophils are phagocytes and function in allergic and other immune responses. Basophils contain histamine, heparin, and other active biochemical agents, which they release as appropriate. Neutrophils, the most numerous polymorphonuclear leukocytes and in fact the most numerous white blood cells, function primarily as phagocytes. Their numbers in the circulation rise soon after any injury or inflammatory process occurs, and they are transported by the blood to the site of trouble. Here they leave the circulation and enter the tissues to surround, engulf, and destroy devitalized tissue or invading microorganisms. Less mature neutrophils, whose nuclei are not divided into lobes, are called **band cells** or simply **bands**.

The only white blood cells not produced in the bone marrow are **lymphocytes**. These arise from precursor cells in the marrow but develop to maturity in lymphoid tissue (spleen, thymus gland, tonsils, lymph nodes). Their classification and functions are discussed in Chapter 4.

Platelets are not cells and have no nuclei. They are small round or oval bodies formed in bone marrow by cells called **megakaryocytes**. They function in blood coagulation. **Coagulation** is a complex process, in which, by various possible reaction chains, soluble fibrinogen is converted to insoluble fibrin. An intact coagulation mechanism depends on sufficient numbers of normally functioning platelets and on the presence in the plasma of adequate levels of a number of proteins, any of which can be congenitally deficient.

Diagnostic Procedures in Hematologic Disease

Complete Blood Count (CBC): Enumeration and classification of formed elements in the blood, generally with electronic instruments

248 • Human Diseases

rather than by visual inspection. The components of the complete blood count are as follows.

Red blood cell count (RBC): Enumeration of red blood cells in a standard volume of blood (reported as cells/mm^3 or /L).

Hemoglobin (Hb, Hgb): Measurement of concentration of hemoglobin in whole blood (reported in g/dL or mmol/L).

Hematocrit (Hct): Proportion of mass of cellular elements in blood to total blood volume, after centrifugation, reported as a decimal (if cell mass is 44% of total blood volume, the hematocrit is reported as 0.44); reflects chiefly red blood cell volume.

White blood cell count (WBC): Enumeration of white blood cells in a standard volume of blood (reported as cells/mm^3 or /L). A count of 7000/mm^3 would be reported in SI units as 7 x 10^9/L.

Platelet count (Plt): Enumeration of platelets in a standard volume of blood (reported as platelets/mm^3 or /L).

From the first three values (RBC, Hb, Hct), three **red cell indices** are calculated as follows:

Mean corpuscular hemoglobin (MCH): Hgb/RBC; average weight of hemoglobin per red blood cell (reported as pg/cell).

Mean corpuscular hemoglobin concentration (MCHC): Hgb/Hct; average concentration of hemoglobin in red blood cells (reported as g/dL or g/L).

Mean corpuscular volume (MCV): Hct/RBC; average size of red blood cells (reported in μm^3 or fL)

Stained smear of peripheral blood: This examination allows a detailed inspection of all formed elements, with an estimate of their size, shape, staining properties, maturity, and other structural features, and identification of abnormal cells or immature forms not normally found in peripheral blood.

Differential count of white blood cells: Determination of the relative proportions of the six principal white blood cells (mature neutrophils, band neutrophils, eosinophils, basophils, lymphocytes, and monocytes). This examination can be performed either by visually inspecting a stained smear of blood and counting 100 cells, or by sophisticated electronic equipment. Proportions are reported as percents (lymphocytes 30%) but may also be given as integers without units (lymphocytes 30). Multiplying the relative count of a particular cell type by the total number of white blood cells in the specimen yields the absolute count of that cell type. If lymphocytes make up 30% of all white blood cells, and the total white blood cell count is 7000/mm³ (7 x 10⁹/L), then the absolute lymphocyte count is 2100 x 10⁶/L.

Bone marrow biopsy: An examination of bone marrow removed by aspiration from the sternum or iliac crest. The marrow may be smeared and stained like whole blood, or it may be compacted, embedded in wax, and sectioned before staining like a specimen of solid tissue.

Erythrocyte sedimentation rate (ESR) (sed rate): Determination of the rate at which erythrocytes settle in a specimen of anticoagulated blood standing in a glass column of standard dimensions. Principally an index of inflammation, which accelerates sedimentation of cells by leading to production of acute phase reactants (serum proteins generated as part of the inflammatory process).

Reticulocyte count: Enumeration of reticulocytes (immature red blood cells) as an estimate of red blood cell production.

Serum iron, serum iron-binding capacity, serum ferritin: These are all measures of the iron available for erythropoiesis. Ferritin is the plasma protein that carries iron in bound form.

Osmotic fragility test: Determination of the osmotic concentration of a solution of saline that will cause hemolysis of red blood cells; altered in conditions affecting the chemical or physical structure of cells.

Hemoglobin electrophoresis: Analysis of the various hemoglobins, normal and abnormal, found in the patient's blood.

Sickling test: Application of chemicals that cause sickling of red blood cells from persons with sickle cell anemia or sickle cell trait.

Carboxyhemoglobin: A measure of the percent of hemoglobin that has formed carboxyhemoglobin with inhaled carbon monoxide.

Assays of serum B_{12} and folate: To determine adequacy of these vitamins for RBC production.

Serum indirect-reacting bilirubin: A measure of the formation of bilirubin by breakdown of RBCs.

Clotting time: The time in which a specimen of blood clots under standard conditions.

Prothrombin time: A measure of prothrombin activity; the standard test to monitor therapy with the oral anticoagulant warfarin.

Activated partial thromboplastin time: A specialized coagulation test to identify deficient clotting factors; the standard test to monitor therapy with the intravenous or intramuscular anticoagulant heparin.

Coagulation factor assay: Chemical or immunologic tests to measure concentrations of various coagulation factors in the blood.

Disorders of Red Blood Cells

Anemia

A reduction in the number of red blood cells in the circulation, due to deficient production, destruction within the body (**hemolysis**), or hemorrhage.

Iron Deficiency Anemia

Anemia due to deficient iron stores; the most common type of anemia.

Cause: Depletion of iron stores usually results from chronic or recurring blood loss (gastrointestinal hemorrhage, menstruation, repeated blood donation). It can also occur in certain metabolic states (pregnancy, chronic infection) and, rarely, because of inadequate iron intake (vegetarians, dieters).

History: Fatigue, poor exercise tolerance, palpitations, shortness of breath. Dysphagia occurs in **Plummer-Vinson syndrome** (due to formation of esophageal webs). **Pica** (eating non-food materials such as clay).

Physical Examination: Pallor, tachycardia, smooth tongue, brittle nails, cheilosis (chapping and fissuring of lips).

Diagnostic Tests: The red blood cell count is abnormally low. With advanced disease, cells become **microcytic** (smaller than normal; MCV reduced) and **hypochromic** (containing less hemoglobin than normal; MCH reduced). Abnormal cells, including **target cells** (cells so thin that the central positions of opposite sides touch, causing a bull's-eye appearance), may occur. The serum iron and serum ferritin are abnormally low. Administration of iron produces a prompt improvement in the red blood cell count, with elevated reticulocyte count. Diagnostic evaluation may include an aggressive search for a site of blood loss.

Treatment: Oral iron replacement continued for several months restores the red blood cell studies and serum iron and ferritin to normal.

Pernicious Anemia

A chronic anemia due to deficiency of vitamin B_{12} absorption.

Cause: Pernicious anemia is an inherited autoimmune disorder that typically does not cause symptoms until after the age of 35. The biochemical cause is lack of secretion of intrinsic factor by glands in the gastric mucosa, with resultant failure to absorb vitamin B_{12}. All patients have **gastric achlorhydria** (lack of hydrochloric acid in gastric juice). Neurologic symptoms (ataxia, confusion, dementia) eventually occur.

History: Gradual onset of weakness, paresthesia in the fingers and toes, dysequilibrium, anorexia, sore tongue, and diarrhea.

Physical Examination: Pallor, icterus. The tongue appears red and smooth. Ataxic gait, diminished sense of vibration and position in extremities; later, loss of perception of light touch and pinprick.

Diagnostic Tests: The red blood cell count is low. Red blood cells are large (**macrocytosis**; increased MCV) and variable in size (**anisocytosis**). The reticulocyte count is low. Polymorphonuclear leukocytes have multilobulated nuclei. Bone marrow smear shows large precursors of red blood cells with abnormal morphology. The serum indirect bilirubin is elevated. The serum vitamin B_{12} is abnormally low. The **Schilling test** (administration of radioactively tagged B_{12} orally before and after administration of intrinsic factor) shows an increase in the urinary excretion of B_{12}. Endoscopy shows atrophic gastritis, and chemical studies indicate achlorhydria.

Course: This is an irreversible condition requiring lifelong treatment, without which neurologic damage may become irreversible. There is a heightened risk of gastric carcinoma in persons with achlorhydria.

Treatment: Administration of vitamin B_{12}, usually by injection, regularly throughout life (once a month after a loading period with more frequent doses).

Hemolytic Anemia

Anemia due to abnormal destruction of red blood cells.

Hereditary Hemolytic Anemia

Hereditary **hemolytic anemias** are due to genetically induced abnormalities in the structure of the red blood cell (**spherocytosis, elliptocytosis**, sickle cell disease) or sensitivity to certain biochemical challenges (glucose-6-phosphate dehydrogenase deficiency).

Sickle Cell Anemia

A congenital abnormality of red blood cells causing hemolytic anemia and other adverse effects.

Cause: An autosomal recessive gene, present in 8% of African-Americans, results in formation of variable amounts of an abnormal hemoglobin (**hemoglobin S**). Persons with the homozygous form (abnormal gene inherited from both parents) have significant numbers of abnormal red blood cells, which are subject to **sickling** (assumption of a sickle-shaped distortion), with a tendency to hemolysis and formation of arterial obstructions in the presence of reduced arterial oxygen, acidosis, or other biochemical alterations in blood. Persons with the heterozygous form are said to have **sickle cell trait**; they rarely or never have symptoms.

History: Weakness, poor exercise tolerance, jaundice, ulcers of the shins, susceptibility to infections, hemolytic crises (acute episodes of bone pain in extremities and back).

Physical Examination: Jaundice, hepatomegaly, splenomegaly, cardiomegaly.

Diagnostic Tests: The red blood count is abnormally low and the bilirubin is elevated. The blood smear shows reticulocytes, nucleated red blood cells, target cells, and sickled cells. Laboratory screening for sickling is positive, and hemoglobin electrophoresis shows the presence of hemoglobin S. Persons with sickle cell trait have smaller amounts of hemoglobin S on electrophoresis, and their blood counts and smears are normal. Prenatal diagnosis can be made by studying fetal DNA.

Course: Complications include ischemic necrosis of bone, osteomyelitis due to *Staphylococcus* or *Salmonella*, splenic and renal infarction, increased risk of infection, retinopathy with visual loss, formation of bilirubin gallstones.

Treatment: Largely supportive, with avoidance of precipitating factors. For hemolytic crisis, oxygen inhalation and blood transfusion.

Glucose-6-Phosphate Dehydrogenase (G-6-PD) Deficiency

An inherited deficiency of the enzyme glucose-6-phosphate dehydrogenase, which causes episodes of hemolytic anemia in response to infection or on exposure to certain drugs or foods.

Cause: Absence of glucose-6-phosphate dehydrogenase from red blood cells. An X-linked recessive disorder seen primarily in males of African, Mediterranean, or Asian ancestry. Occurs in 10-15% of African-American men.

History: Jaundice at birth. In later life, susceptibility to episodes of hemolysis (manifested by weakness, jaundice, and dark urine) during infections or after eating fava beans or taking certain drugs (quinidine, quinine, nitrofurantoin, sulfonamides, phenazopyridine, and others).

Physical Examination: During hemolytic episodes: pallor, jaundice, possibly evidence of congestive heart failure. At other times, no physical findings.

Diagnostic Tests: During hemolytic episodes: anemia, reticulocytosis, abnormally shaped red blood cells on smear. Elevation of indirect bilirubin. At other times: no hematologic abnormalities, but deficiency of G-6-PD in red blood cells.

Course: Hemolytic episodes occur during infections or after consumption of certain drugs and foods, and sometimes spontaneously. They are rarely severe or life-threatening.

Treatment: Avoidance of drugs known to induce hemolysis, and fava beans. Prompt treatment of severe or systemic infection. Life expectancy is significantly reduced.

Acquired Hemolytic Anemia

Causes: Acquired hemolytic anemias result from formation of antibody to one's own red blood cells in certain systemic diseases (lupus erythematosus, leukemia, lymphoma), in response to certain drugs (methyldopa, quinidine), or for unknown reasons (50%).

History: Gradual or abrupt onset of fatigue and dyspnea due to anemia. There may be a family history of hemolytic anemia.

Physical Examination: Pallor, jaundice, splenomegaly.

Diagnostic Tests: The red blood cell count is low, the reticulocyte count elevated. Indirect bilirubin is elevated in serum. The **direct Coombs test** is positive, indicating sensitization of the patient's red blood cells. The **indirect Coombs test** may also be positive, indicating presence of anti-RBC antibody in serum.

Treatment: If anemia is severe, blood transfusion may be indicated. Corticosteroid treatment may block hemolysis. In severe or refractory cases, splenectomy, immunosuppressive agents, and immune globulin are often beneficial.

Erythroblastosis Fetalis
(Hemolytic Disease of the Newborn)

Hemolytic anemia affecting a newborn, due to destruction of fetal red blood cells by antibodies formed by the mother's immune system.

Cause: The child's red blood cells contain some antigen not found in the mother's red blood cells. If fetal and maternal blood become mixed (as in trauma, amniocentesis, or chorionic villus biopsy), the maternal immune system may form antibody to this antigen, which then enters the fetal circulation and causes hemolysis. Mixing of blood during delivery stimulates maternal antibody that cannot affect the child just born, but will affect any future fetuses having the same red cell antigen.

The usual cause of severe erythroblastosis is presence of the D antigen of the Rh system in the red blood cells of a fetus borne by an **Rh-negative** mother. Milder degrees of hemolysis occur with other red blood cell incompatibilities, including those in the **ABO system**. The mother is unaffected in hemolytic disease of the newborn. The incidence of the disorder has been much reduced by the administration to Rh-negative mothers of **high-titer Rho (D)** immune globulin during each pregnancy and immediately after delivery.

History: Jaundice becoming evident within hours of birth. Pallor, generalized swelling, lethargy, poor feeding, spasms.

Physical Examination: Jaundice, pallor (often masked by jaundice), anasarca (generalized edema), pleural effusion, ascites (fluid in the abdominal cavity), enlargement of liver and spleen, cardiac murmurs, lethargy, spasticity, hyperactive reflexes, cardiac or pulmonary failure.

Diagnostic Tests: The red blood cell count is low and the unconjugated (indirect-reacting) bilirubin is high. Blood glucose may be depressed. Increased numbers of nucleated red blood cells and reticulocytes are found in the circulation. The direct Coombs test shows the red blood cells of the newborn to be coated with hemolytic antibody. The indirect Coombs test on the mother's blood confirms that she has formed antibody to fetal red cell antigen.

Course: Very mild cases may resolve spontaneously, but even with treatment a child showing profound jaundice and lethargy in the first 24 hours may die. Stillbirths are not uncommon. Anemia may correct itself over a few days once further exposure to maternal antibody ceases. However, severe anemia may lead to cardiac failure or death. A more severe threat is marked elevation of bilirubin, which is toxic in the newborn to the basal ganglia of the brain. Deposition of unconjugated bilirubin in the nerve tissue of the basal ganglia, called **kernicterus**, produces spasticity and unless quickly treated and reversed may lead to a parkinson-like movement disorder and often mental retardation and deafness.

Treatment: Exchange transfusion (replacement of fetal blood, a little at a time, with donor blood lacking harmful antigen) may be needed if anemia is profound or hyperbilirubinemia very high. Respiratory and cardiac function may require support.

Aplastic Anemia

Failure of marrow production of red blood cells (also white blood cells and platelets).

Cause: Damage to bone marrow by chemicals (benzene), drugs (chloramphenicol), radiation, neoplastic infiltration, or autoantibodies.

History: Gradual onset of weakness, fatigue, dyspnea, headache.

Physical Examination: Pallor, purpura or petechiae, tachycardia, oral or pharyngeal infection or ulceration.

Diagnostic Tests: The red blood cell, white blood cell, and platelet counts are abnormally low. Marrow smear shows hypoplastic or acellular marrow.

Treatment: Blood transfusion to correct anemia. Oxygen and control of hemorrhage as needed. Antibiotics for infection. Corticosteroids, immunosuppressive agents, colony stimulating factors. Marrow transplantation if possible.

Polycythemia Vera

A myeloproliferative disorder in which the red blood cell count is abnormally high.

Cause: A clonal stem cell disorder leading to increase in all cellular elements of bone marrow and peripheral blood, most conspicuously erythrocytes but to a lesser degree granulocytic leukocytes and platelets. Onset is usually between 50 and 60 years of age.

History: Headaches, dizziness, tinnitus, visual blurring, fullness in the epigastrium, redness of skin, pruritus (worse after a hot bath).

Physical Examination: Reddish-purple skin and mucous membranes. Hypertension, splenomegaly, hepatomegaly.

Diagnostic Tests: Red blood cell count, hemoglobin, and hematocrit are increased, as well as white blood cell and platelet counts. Serum iron and ferritin are reduced. Marrow biopsy shows increased cellularity.

Course: Average survival time is 10-12 years. Arterial and venous thromboses, hemorrhage, and infection are common complications. As the disease progresses, the marrow cells become replaced by fibrous tissue, and zones of **extramedullary hematopoiesis** (formation of red blood cells elsewhere than in the marrow) develop in the spleen and liver. Secondary gout may develop as a result of rapid DNA turnover with excessive uric acid production. Many cases evolve into a terminal acute leukemia-like blast stage.

Treatment: Phlebotomy to reduced blood volume and red blood cell count. Radioactive phosphorus, busulfan, chlorambucil, hydroxyurea.

Diseases of White Blood Cells

Leukemia

Any of several disorders characterized by increased white blood count and the appearance of immature and abnormal white blood cells in the circulation. **Leukemias** result from genetic abnormality of **stem cells** in the bone marrow, due either to mutation of cells or to chromosomal aberrations occurring before conception. As a consequence, the body produces increased amounts of one or more types of blood cells (erythrocytes, granulocytes, monocytes, lymphocytes, platelets), which are abnormal in structure and function. Leukemias vary broadly in clinical features and course. Three common types are discussed here.

Acute Lymphocytic Leukemia (Acute Lymphoblastic Leukemia, ALL)

A rapidly progressive hematologic malignancy of children.

Cause: Mutation of lymphocyte precursor cells, possibly due to drugs, radiation, or genetic predisposition or chromosomal aberration. Onset is in childhood, usually before age 5.

History: Pallor, weakness, irritability, repeated infections, bleeding tendency, bone pain, headache, stiff neck, vomiting, cranial nerve palsies and other neurologic abnormalities.

Physical Examination: Pallor, lethargy, neurologic findings, evidence of opportunistic infections, hemorrhagic phenomena.

Diagnostic Tests: The white blood cell count may be low, elevated, or normal. Anemia and thrombocytopenia are often present. Serum levels of uric acid and creatinine may be elevated. Bone marrow examination shows replacement of normal elements by infiltrations of **blast cells**. Cerebrospinal fluid shows **lymphoblasts** (extremely immature lymphocytes) in central nervous system involvement. Imaging studies including radionuclide bone scans may show abnormalities due to infiltration of organs or tissues by malignant lymphoblastic cells.

Course: The disease is ordinarily fatal in less than six months. With vigorous treatment, many patients achieve long-term survival and apparent cure. Anemia, thrombocytopenia, susceptibility to infection, invasion of the central nervous system (50%), and infiltration and damage of the liver and other organs often prove lethal.

Treatment: Chemotherapy with vincristine, daunorubicin, or asparaginase, combined with corticosteroid. For central nervous system involvement, cranial irradiation and injection of methotrexate intrathecally (into the subarachnoid space). Control of anemia (transfusions if necessary), bleeding, and infection; personal and family counseling.

Chronic Myelogenous Leukemia (CML)

A malignancy of the marrow characterized by markedly elevated levels of circulating white blood cells formed there, with immature and abnormal cells.

Cause: The **Philadelphia chromosome**, the first oncogene to be associated with a specific malignancy; this is a reciprocal translocation of strands of genes between chromosomes 9 and 22. It results in malignant proliferation of myelogenous (marrow-produced) white blood cells (granulocytes and monocytes), which, however, retain their functions for years, until the disease reaches its terminal stage. Onset generally occurs in middle life (30s, 40s, and 50s).

History: Weakness, fatigue, fever, night sweats, bone pain.

Physical Examination: Low fever, enlargement of the spleen, tenderness over the sternum due to hyperactive marrow.

Laboratory Tests: Marked elevation of the white blood cell count (100,000-500,000/μL), with modest increases in immature forms. Other cells in the circulation are generally normal in number and form. The uric acid may be elevated. Marrow smear shows increased cellularity and increased immature white blood cells. Chromosomal studies identify the Philadelphia chromosome.

Course: Usual survival is less than 5 years. However, long-term survival, and apparent cure, occur in half of patients who undergo successful bone marrow transplantation. The disease typically ends in a phase of greatly accelerated production of wholly immature and undifferentiated **stem cells (blastic crisis)**, in which marrow dysfunction can lead to marked anemia, bleeding disorders, and toxemia.

Treatment: Largely supportive and palliative. Chemical suppressants of marrow activity (hydroxyurea, interferon alfa) lower white blood counts and mitigate symptoms. In the blast stage, chemotherapy protocols including vincristine, daunorubicin, and prednisone provide brief remission. Allogeneic bone marrow transplant (from a sibling or unrelated donor matched with respect to critical antigens, particularly HLA) is apparently curative in about one-half of patients, and is more effective in younger patients.

Chronic Lymphocytic Leukemia

A malignancy of B lymphocytes.

Cause: Malignant change in a B-cell precursor, with formation of a clone of abnormal, immunologically incompetent cells. This results in infiltration of bone marrow and other tissues with abnormal **lymphocytes** and failure of immune response. Most cases occur in the middle-aged and elderly.

History: Gradual onset of weakness and fatigue, often with enlarged lymph nodes. In some asymptomatic patients the condition is discovered incidentally on routine blood testing.

Physical Examination: Enlargement of lymph nodes, liver, spleen, or all of these. Pallor or jaundice may be present.

Diagnostic Tests: Relative and absolute lymphocytosis (increase in the percentage of lymphocytes among white blood cells, and in their total number). The lymphocytes are small but normal in appearance. Bone marrow may show infiltrations of lymphocytes. Red blood cell or platelet count may be reduced. There may be a deficiency of IgG in serum.

Course: Typically chronic, with mild or absent symptoms. Most patients survive 5-10 years after diagnosis. Possible complications include autoimmune hemolytic anemia, thrombocytopenia, and lymphoma (development of a malignant solid neoplasm of lymphoid tissue).

Treatment: Largely supportive and palliative. Chlorambucil, fludarabine, and adrenal corticosteroids may be used in severe or terminal disease. Splenectomy may be needed to control hemolytic anemia.

Lymphoma

A malignant tumor consisting of lymphocytes. Several types are recognized.

Hodgkin Disease
Cause: Unknown. Genetic influences and viral infection have been implicated, but without conclusive proof.
History: Painless enlargement of one or more lymph nodes, fever, sweats, pruritus, abdominal pain (aggravated by alcohol).
Physical Examination: Enlargement of lymph nodes, possibly spleen; fever.
Diagnostic Tests: Lymph node biopsy shows **Reed-Sternberg** cells (characteristic large cells with two nuclei).
Prognosis: The overall survival rate is about 50%; with early diagnosis and treatment, about 80%.
Treatment: Radiation, chemotherapy.

Non-Hodgkin Lymphoma
A variegated group of lymphocyte malignancies. Oncogenes have been identified for some types.
History: Painless enlargement of lymph nodes, fever, sweats, weight loss, abdominal pain.
Physical Examination: Enlargement of lymph nodes, spleen.
Diagnostic Tests: The peripheral blood may be normal. Lymph node biopsy shows characteristic malignant changes, and bone marrow biopsy shows infiltration of abnormal lymphoid aggregates. The serum LDH is elevated. Chest x-ray and CT scan of the abdomen and pelvis may show hilar and abdominal or pelvic lymphadenopathy.
Treatment: Radiation, chemotherapy, bone marrow transplantation.

Multiple Myeloma
A malignant tumor of plasma cells.
History: Bone pain, usually in the back or ribs. Onset is usually in later life.

Physical Examination: Pallor, bone tenderness, neurologic abnormalities.
Diagnostic Tests: The red blood cell count is low, the erythrocyte sedimentation rate elevated. The serum calcium level is elevated. Serum protein electrophoresis shows abnormal proteins, and **Bence Jones protein** appears in urine. Marrow biopsy shows infiltration of abnormal plasma cells. X-rays show lytic lesions in ribs, spine, other bones.
Complications: Renal failure, amyloidosis, cardiomegaly, neurologic impairment.
Prognosis: Average survival is about 3 years.
Treatment: Radiation, chemotherapy, marrow transplant.

Coagulation Disorders

Numerous disorders of blood coagulation have been identified, some acquired but the majority inherited. They fall into three categories: **disorders of platelets**, **abnormalities of platelet function**, and **disorders of clotting factors**. A major distinction among coagulation disorders is between platelet disorders and deficiencies of one or more plasma coagulation proteins.

Thrombocytopenia
Deficiency of platelets in the circulation, which can result from diminished production, accelerated destruction, or sequestration in the spleen.

Idiopathic Thrombocytopenic Purpura (ITP, Immune Thrombocytic Purpura)
An acquired hemorrhagic disorder due to autoimmune destruction of platelets.
Cause: Antiplatelet antibody formed in response to acute viral infection (acute ITP) or other factors (chronic ITP). **Acute ITP** occurs chiefly in children between 2 and 6 who are recovering from a viral illness such as varicella or infectious mononucleosis. **Chronic ITP** is a disease of adults affecting more women than men by a ratio of 4:1.
History: *Acute*: Sudden onset of easy bruising, nosebleeds, blood in urine or stool. *Chronic*: Insidious onset of bruising, heavy menstrual

flow, and spontaneous bleeding from mucosal surfaces (epistaxis, hematemesis, hematochezia or melena, hematuria).

Physical Findings: Petechiae, purpura, ecchymoses; frank or occult blood in sputum, urine, stool. Blood blisters in the mouth.

Diagnostic Tests: Marked lowering of the platelet count in peripheral blood. Prolonged bleeding time and abnormal clot retraction. Bone marrow shows normal to hyperactive platelet production. Serologic studies show antibody bound to platelets.

Course: In acute ITP, spontaneous return of platelet count to normal usually occurs within six months. In chronic disease the course tends to be protracted. Severe hemorrhage and anemia due to chronic blood loss are unusual, but can occur. The most dangerous kind of hemorrhage is intracranial.

Treatment: Acute ITP requires mainly support, observation, and treatment of severe complications. In chronic ITP, splenectomy and therapy with corticosteroids or other immunosuppressive agents are usually required.

Glanzmann Disease (Thrombasthenia)

An inherited coagulation disorder (autosomal recessive) in which platelets occur in normal numbers, but do not function normally because of deficiency or absence of platelet membrane glycoprotein. The condition is more common in persons of Semitic or Indian origin. Symptoms are the same as for thrombocytopenia: bruising, epistaxis, menorrhagia, and other spontaneous mucosal bleeding. Laboratory studies show normal numbers of platelets in the circulation, but tests of platelet function (clot retraction, observation for adhesion and aggregation) yield abnormal results. Treatment is with platelet transfusions and oral iron supplementation. Allogeneic bone marrow transplant is sometimes successful.

Hemophilia

A hereditary clotting disorder leading to spontaneous hemorrhages.

Cause: Very low levels of coagulation **factor VIII** (antihemophilic globulin, AHG), due to an X-linked recessive genetic defect. Males are affected almost exclusively, but genetic transmission is by female carriers. Approximately one male in 10,000 is affected.

History: Abnormal bleeding in response to mild trauma, or even spontaneously: hemarthrosis (bleeding into joints), gastrointestinal bleeding, and excessive bleeding after surgery or dental extractions or from open wounds occur most commonly. Aspirin aggravates the bleeding tendency.

Physical Examination: Pallor and tachycardia (after recent hemorrhage). Evidence of local hemorrhage into joints or muscles or subcutaneously, or from skin wounds or surgical sites.

Diagnostic Tests: Anemia and reticulocytosis after hemorrhage. The **partial thromboplastin time** (**PTT**) is prolonged, but other standard tests for coagulation defects (platelet count, prothrombin time, fibrinogen level) yield normal results. The plasma level of factor VIII is low, typically less than 5% of normal.

Course: With careful avoidance of trauma and aspirin, and infusions of factor VIII as needed, most patients can lead essentially normal lives. Recurrent **hemarthroses** may lead to permanent damage to joints. Administration of blood products can result in transmission of infections such as AIDS and hepatitis B and C. Some patients form antibody to factor VIII and so fail to derive benefit from infusions of it.

Treatment: Modification of lifestyle so as to reduce the danger of trauma. Avoidance of aspirin. Treatment of severe bleeding and suspicion of bleeding (as in closed head injury) with infusions of factor VIII concentrate. Aminocaproic acid may be used when the response to factor VIII is inadequate. Preoperative administration of desmopressin acetate, which temporarily boosts factor VIII levels.

Topics for Study or Discussion

1. List three hematologic disorders that are genetically induced, three that are acquired, and three that are invariably fatal.

2. Which formed elements of the blood have no nuclei?

3. Define or explain: Bence Jones protein, hemolysis, lymphoblast, Philadelphia chromosome, reticulocyte, thrombocytopenia.

4. Which hematologic disorders are treated with splenectomy? Why? Which disorders are sometimes helped by bone marrow transplants?

5. During the 1980s, the mortality of hemophilia among children drastically increased. Why? How was this trend reversed?

Chapter 16

Musculoskeletal Disorders

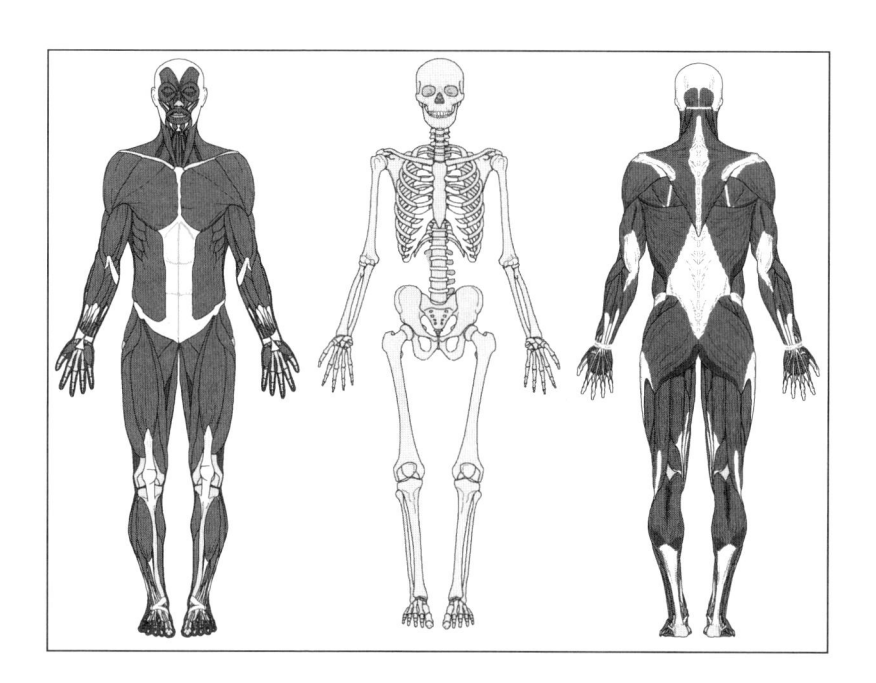

Learning Objectives

Upon completion of this chapter, the student should

• have basic information about the structure and function of the musculoskeletal system;

• know common signs, symptoms, and diagnostic measures pertaining to disorders of this system;

• have a general understanding of the cause, diagnosis, and treatment of common musculoskeletal disorders.

Anatomy and Physiology of the Musculoskeletal System

The **musculoskeletal system** comprises those structures that lend support and mobility to the body and that enable us to perform voluntary actions: bones, cartilage, muscles, and associated connective tissue structures (tendons, ligaments).

Bone is a type of tissue in which a framework or matrix of organic (protein) fibers is reinforced by deposits of calcium and phosphorus salts, which provide strength and rigidity. Bone is not inert material. It has a rich blood supply, it can heal after severe injury, and its calcium content is in equilibrium with the calcium level of the blood. Most bones are covered by a dense sheet of connective tissue called **periosteum**. Each of the long bones of the extremities is divided into a **diaphysis** (shaft), an **epiphysis** (enlarged, knobby end) and a **metaphysis** (between the diaphysis and the epiphysis). **Long bones**, and some others, are hollow and contain bone marrow in their cavities. **Bone marrow** is the site of production of red blood cells, monocytes, and platelets.

Cartilage is a noncalcified connective tissue similar to bone. In most joints, the contacting surfaces of the bones are covered by protective layers of cartilage. Some weightbearing joints (intervertebral joints, knees) contain thick cushions of tougher cartilage (**fibrocartilage**). Cartilage also provides semirigid support for the nose, the external ear, the larynx, and the trachea and bronchi.

Muscle is a unique type of tissue that has the property of contracting (shortening) under appropriate stimulation, usually neural. The respiratory, digestive, and urinary tracts contain **smooth muscle**, which is **innervated** by (receives its nerve supply from) the autonomic nervous system (discussed in Chapter 18) and is not subject to voluntary control. The muscle of the heart is also not subject to voluntary control.

The anatomic description of each **voluntary muscle** includes mention of its shape and position, its origin (bone or other structure that serves to anchor it), insertion (bone or other structure that is moved or stabilized by the muscle), action, blood supply, and innervation. Each muscle is supplied by a nerve containing **motor fibers** (to transmit impulses from the brain and spinal cord) and **sensory fibers** (for **proprioception**, that is, perception of position and movement). Each motor nerve is attached to its muscle at a motor end-plate, where nerve impulses trigger contraction of muscle fibers.

While some muscles are attached directly to the periosteum of the bones that serve as their origin and insertion, most muscles are modified at one or both ends and equipped with **connective tissue** bands that serve for attachment to muscle. A narrow, cordlike band is called a **tendon**; a broad, sheetlike connection is called an **aponeurosis**. Some tendons (for example, those at the wrist and ankle) pass through tubular sheaths that act somewhat like pulleys to control direction of pull and reduce local friction. The subcutaneous tissue overlying some bony prominences (shoulder, heel) contains one or more **bursas** (purselike cushions containing a little fluid to protect underlying surfaces and reduce friction).

A **joint** is the site at which two bones **articulate** (connect, generally in an arrangement whereby one or both can move with respect to the other). As mentioned above, the ends of bones forming a joint are usually protected by **articular cartilage** and sometimes by heavier fibrocartilage cushions (intervertebral discs, menisci of knees). The entire joint is surrounded by a capsule of **synovial membrane**, a delicate, highly vascular connective tissue that secretes a lubricating fluid in small amounts. A **ligament** is a band of inelastic connective tissue extending across the joint from one bone to the other to limit both the direction and the extent of motion at the joint. Most joints have several ligaments (the knee has twelve).

Musculoskeletal Disorders

The musculoskeletal system is subject to numerous hereditary, developmental, traumatic, inflammatory, and degenerative disorders. The cardinal symptoms of most of these are pain, tenderness, stiffness, muscle weakness, other disabilities related to impairment of structure or function, or any combination of these. Diagnosis is based chiefly on the history and physical examination, although x-ray and other imaging techniques and (in selected cases) blood and other laboratory studies, including electromyography, may be required. Treatment relies heavily on analgesics, muscle relaxants, rest, and physical therapy.

A few of the more common musculoskeletal disorders are discussed below. Musculoskeletal injuries are dealt with in Chapter 6. However, many of the conditions described below are due, at least sometimes, to trauma, often of the chronic, repetitive type.

Hereditary and Developmental Disorders

Muscular Dystrophy

This term includes a number of inherited disorders of voluntary muscle tissue having various clinical features. Some begin in infancy and others in middle age; some cause death within a few years and others progress slowly and have little impact on lifestyle or life expectancy. Progressive muscular weakness and wasting of muscle tissue are features of most types of **muscular dystrophy**. In some types, enlargement of affected muscles (**pseudohypertrophy**) occurs. Some are associated with mental retardation or other defects. Diagnosis is made by history (including family history), physical examination, electromyography, muscle biopsy, and detection of elevated serum creatine kinase. Prenatal diagnosis is possible. Treatment is purely supportive, and consists of physical therapy and regular exercise.

Scoliosis

Lateral curvature of the spine in the erect position, due to malalignment of vertebrae. Two types are recognized. **Structural scoliosis** affects the vertebrae primarily. It may be caused by bone, nerve, or muscle disease, but in 90% of cases the cause is unknown. In most of these cases a genetic cause is likely. This type of scoliosis is both commoner and more severe in women. Onset is around the age of puberty. **Nonstructural scoliosis** occurs as a result of abnormality or disease other than in the affected vertebrae. Many cases are due to significant discrepancy in leg length, which brings about a compensatory curve in the upper spine to keep the head and shoulders level.

In both types of scoliosis, there is usually some rotational deformity of the spine in addition to lateral curvature. Generally there are no symptoms at first, and detection is made on routine physical examination, chest x-ray, or school screening. Direct inspection of the back often fails to disclose mild scoliosis, especially in overweight patients. When a person with scoliosis bends forward from the waist, one side of the thorax appears more prominent than the other because of the rotatory component of the deformity. X-ray examination and measurement of the curvature is needed for precise diagnosis.

A curvature of more than 20° is considered significant, particularly because it is likely to progress. When significant scoliosis is detected before the mid-teens, vigorous efforts are made to correct it before spinal growth ceases. Correction is by bracing or casting. In severe or neglected cases, surgical fusion of the spine may be indicated. Untreated scoliosis may lead to severe deformity and disability, even compromise of cardiac and pulmonary function.

Osgood-Schlatter Disease

During fetal development, long bones are formed by deposition of calcium in a cartilage matrix. Until long bone growth is complete, in the mid to late teens, growth centers at the epiphyses remain soft to allow for continuing longitudinal growth. Undue stress on some of these growth centers, due to physical and especially athletic activity, may cause local inflammation and pain. **Osgood-Schlatter disease** affects the **tibial tubercle**, where the tendon running down from the patella inserts on the front of the upper end of the tibia. The condition is commoner in boys and is usually bilateral. Symptoms are pain at the site, particularly after exertion, and limping. A firm tender mass can be felt. Spontaneous resolution occurs within a few months to two years. Treatment is with rest, analgesics, and occasionally splinting.

Legg-Calvé-Perthes Disease

Avascular necrosis (death of tissue due to loss of blood supply) of the head of the femur, occurring in children near the middle or end of the first decade of life. Symptoms are hip pain and limping. Imaging studies including radionuclide scan can show altered physical and chemical properties of the affected part of the femur. Spontaneous healing occurs after two or three years, but may leave the child with a badly deformed femoral head and serious hip joint malfunction. Treatment is by splinting or casting to keep the hip in abduction during weightbearing, and occasionally surgery.

Disorders of Muscles, Tendons, Ligaments, and Bursas

Tendinitis (Tenosynovitis)

Inflammation of a tendon or, more precisely, of a **tendon sheath**. The cause is usually repetitive or extreme strain on the tendon, as in an occupational or athletic setting. The symptoms are pain on active or passive movement of the part, localized tenderness over the tendon, and sometimes swelling and **crepitus** (rubbing or grating sound) with movement. Disability may be severe but spontaneous resolution usually occurs if the inciting activity can be stopped. Treatment is with analgesics and anti-inflammatory agents, wrapping or splinting, and local heat. Injection of adrenal corticosteroid into the site of inflammation often yields prompt if temporary relief, but repeated injections may lead to complications, including rupture of the tendon.

Bursitis

Inflammation of a **bursa**, usually due to local trauma, often repetitive (kneeling on concrete, working overhead). Inflammation can also result from local infection or as an extension from an inflamed joint. Onset is typically sudden; initial symptoms are sharply localized pain and tenderness and often pronounced swelling, with fluctuancy due to accumulation of inflammatory fluid within the affected bursa. The diagnosis is usually evident from the history and physical examination. If infection is suspected, the bursa must be aspirated and the fluid examined by smear and culture for pathogenic microorganisms. Treatment options include rest, immobilization if necessary, local heat, nonsteroidal anti-inflammatory drugs, local corticosteroid injections, and antibiotics for infection if present. Common sites of bursitis are subdeltoid (near the point of the shoulder), olecranon (near the point of the elbow), prepatellar (overlying the patella; housemaid's knee), popliteal (**Baker cyst**; fluctuant swelling of the bursa behind the knee joint, which communicates with the joint space, as a result of local trauma or disease), and calcaneal (near the point of the heel).

Fibromyalgia Syndrome

A syndrome of chronic musculoskeletal pain accompanied by weakness, fatigue, and sleep disorders.

Cause: Unknown. The condition occurs almost exclusively in adult women with onset before age 50. Depression and viral infection have been proposed as underlying causes in some cases. The disorder sometimes occurs in hypothyroidism.

History: Chronic widespread aching and stiffness, typically bilaterally symmetrical and involving particularly the neck, shoulders, back, and hips, which is aggravated by use of affected muscles. Usually there are associated fatigue, a sense of weakness or inability to perform certain movements, paresthesia, difficulty sleeping, and headaches.

Physical Examination: Trigger points: sharply localized and extremely tender points, particularly in the neck and back, and often bilaterally symmetric. Some of these points may correspond to sites of pain and others may be painless until palpated. Otherwise examination is normal. There is no fever or local swelling or redness, and joints are not involved.

Diagnostic Tests: Complete blood count, erythrocyte sedimentation rate, and imaging studies yield uniformly normal results.

Course: The condition tends to be chronic, with moderate to severe disability, but symptoms can usually be mitigated by treatment. Symptoms do not progress, and objective signs of disease never develop.

Treatment: Education, exercise, physical therapy. Psychoactive medicines such as amitriptyline and chlorpromazine occasionally help.

Disorders of Cartilage

Herniated Disc (Herniated Nucleus Pulposus, HNP; Slipped Disc)

Extrusion of the soft center of an **intervertebral disc**, with symptoms due to pressure on adjacent spinal nerves.

Cause: *Predisposing cause*: Degeneration of the intervertebral disc due to aging or other pathologic process. *Precipitating cause*: Lifting or straining that puts unusual force on the disc.

History: Pain in the back or extremities, often of sudden onset and associated with lifting or straining. The pain may radiate along the course of an extremity like an electric shock, and may be associated with paresthesia and hypesthesia. Movement or coughing may aggravate pain. Bowel or bladder function may be affected.

Physical Examination: There may be tenderness at the site of herniation. Neurologic examination may show impairment of deep tendon reflexes due to compression of dorsal nerve roots (afferent component of reflex arc; see Chapter 18).

Diagnostic Tests: CT and myelography may show bulging or displacement of a disc. MRI is a more sensitive technique for showing herniation.

Course: Prolonged disability may occur if the condition is left untreated, although milder cases may often be asymptomatic.

Treatment: Bed rest, analgesics, and muscle relaxants usually provide symptomatic relief. With radiologic evidence of severe or progressive disease or significant neurologic impairment, **laminectomy** (cutting through the posterior arch of one or more vertebrae) and removal of herniated disc material are indicated.

Torn Meniscus

The **menisci** are crescent- or C-shaped pads of fibrocartilage within the knee joint, one medial and one lateral, that cushion shocks between the femur and the tibia. Injury to a meniscus is common and usually results from twisting the knee joint with the foot planted, often in an athletic setting. The patient hears a pop and feels sudden severe pain. Swelling develops soon, and the knee may lock or buckle with weight-bearing. Meniscal tears do not heal. The medial meniscus is torn ten times as often as the lateral meniscus. A piece broken off a meniscus remains in the joint as a **loose body**, and may impair mobility.

Examination shows effusion of fluid into the joint space, crepitus, and a positive **McMurray test**: extension of the knee from full flexion with the leg and foot externally rotated causes an audible or palpable snap in medial meniscus tear; extension with the leg and foot internally rotated causes a snap in lateral meniscus tear. Treatment is with ice, elevation, a bulky compression dressing, and crutches, with attention to maintaining mobility and muscle strength and tone in the quadriceps muscle (the large, four-headed muscle on the front of the thigh that extends the knee joint). Mild tears may eventually become asymptomatic. For persistent symptoms, arthroscopic (but occasionally open) surgery is required, with removal of loose fragments and reshaping of remaining cartilage.

Chondromalacia Patellae

Degeneration of the cartilage layer on the back of the patella (kneecap), with resulting pain in the knee. The cause is unknown, but most cases arise in active teenagers or young adults. Often a history of trauma is obtained. Any disturbance in the normal alignment of the knee and the patella can cause chronic trauma to the back of the patella, with resultant degenerative changes (roughening, fraying, even complete loss of cartilage). The principal symptom is pain with walking, especially on stairs, and with squatting. Physical examination shows tenderness on manipulation of the patella and sometimes swelling and crepitus. X-rays are negative. Some cases resolve spontaneously with rest and anti-inflammatory medicines. **Quadriceps exercises** (repeatedly bringing the knee into full extension, with tensing of the muscles of the front of the thigh) often help to correct muscle imbalances. Shaving the roughened posterior surface of the patella arthroscopically may relieve pain. If tracking of the patella in its groove on the anterior femur is grossly deviant, surgical transplantation of the patellar tendon may be needed.

Disorders of Bone

Osteoporosis

A disorder in which the density of bone is inadequate for its normal supporting function.

Causes: The most important cause is postmenopausal deficiency of estrogen. Other causes include genetic disorders (Marfan syndrome, osteogenesis imperfecta), endocrine disorders (diabetes mellitus, Cushing disease, thyrotoxicosis, hyperparathyroidism), rheumatoid arthritis, and prolonged immobilization.

History: Backache, reduction of stature, **kyphosis** (forward hunching of the upper spine), pathologic fractures.

Physical Examination: Unremarkable except for features noted above.

Diagnostic Tests: X-ray examination shows demineralization of bone and may also show compression fractures of vertebrae. Bone density can be more accurately assessed by CT scan or other methods.

Treatment: Administration of calcium along with vitamin D, calcitonin (oral or nasal), biphosphonates, or other agents to promote remineralization of bone. Estrogen is given to postmenopausal women; men with reduced androgen levels are treated with testosterone. Physical therapy, increased mobility.

Paget Disease

A degenerative disorder of bone occurring most commonly in middle-aged and elderly persons.

Cause: An abnormal process of bone breakdown and erratic repair, of unknown cause, resulting in softening and swelling of bone. The disease shows a familial tendency. Viral infection has been implicated in some cases.

History: There may be no symptoms, but most patients experience bone pain, hunching of the back (kyphosis), bowing of the shins, pathologic fractures, and (with cranial involvement) increasing hat size, cranial nerve palsies, and deafness.

Physical Examination: Warmth over affected bones and typical deformities.

Diagnostic Tests: Serum alkaline phosphatase and often serum calcium are elevated. X-rays and bone scans localize lesions and permit accurate assessment of severity.

Course: Progressive deformity. Abnormal bone occasionally undergoes malignant change.

Treatment: Calcitonin (oral or nasal), biphosphonates, or pamidronate.

Osteomyelitis

Bacterial infection of bone.

Cause: Infection with staphylococci, streptococci, or other organisms. Bacteria may be introduced directly into bone tissue (gunshot wound, surgery, compound fracture) or migrate there from adjacent soft-tissue infection (sinusitis, deep abscess) or a remote source (systemic infections such as typhoid or tuberculosis, bacteremia in IV drug abusers). Osteomyelitis due to salmonella frequently occurs as a complication of sickle cell disease and other inherited hemoglobin abnormalities.

History: Gradual or sudden onset of bone pain, fever, and chills.

Physical Examination: Fever, tenderness of site of infection. In severe infection there may be signs of toxemia.

Diagnostic Tests: The erythrocyte sedimentation rate is elevated. Causative organisms can be cultured from material aspirated from infected bone or from the blood. Serologic studies can identify infection due to salmonella. X-ray or, preferably, CT and MRI studies show local swelling, decalcification, and eventually erosive destruction of bone.

Course: Without prompt treatment, infection may become chronic. Bone destruction can lead to severe deformity and disability.

Treatment: Rest, immobilization, analgesics. Antibiotics based on culture findings. Surgical drainage of the infection site. Severe or advanced disease may require radical surgical excision of infected bone (**saucerization**). Physical therapy as needed.

Disorders of Joints

Arthritis

Inflammation of one or more joints. Arthritis is not just one disease, but a group of many (perhaps over 200) that have joint inflammation as their common feature. Rheumatoid arthritis is discussed in Chapter 4. Two other types are described below.

Degenerative Joint Disease (DJD; Osteoarthritis)

A joint disorder characterized by degeneration of articular cartilage.

Cause: Unknown. Familial factors may be operative. Cartilage protecting articular surfaces of bones degenerates, allowing bony surfaces to touch and erode each other. Hypertrophy of bone at the affected site adds to symptoms. Onset of symptoms is typically in early middle-age. Trauma, overweight, and the presence of other orthopedic disorders in the area of the affected joint may precipitate or accelerate symptoms.

History: Gradual onset of pain and stiffness in joints, particularly the intervertebral joints, hips, and knees; pain is aggravated by activity and relieved by rest.

Physical Examination: Stiffness, crepitus, and occasional swelling of affected joints. **Heberden nodes** (small firm nodules at the distal interphalangeal joints of the fingers) may be present.

Diagnostic Tests: X-rays show narrowing of joint spaces due to destruction and wearing away of cartilage; increased density (**eburnation**) of articular ends of bone due to mutual compaction after loss of protective cartilage; and hypertrophy of bone near the joint, with formation of **osteophytes** (outgrowths of bone from the surface) variously described as beaking, lipping, and **bridging** (forming a bridge from one bone to the other).

Course: Progressive pain and stiffening of joints, with eventual deformity and disability, may occur.

Treatment: Rest, physical therapy, prescribed exercise programs, correction of underlying causes if possible, weight reduction in overweight patients, mild analgesics (acetaminophen). Surgical replacement of the hip or knee joint reduces pain and improves mobility.

Gout

A systemic disease with joint symptoms due to deposition of **urate crystals**.

Causes: Elevation of serum uric acid due to overproduction, impaired excretion, or both. Some forms of gout are hereditary. Signs and symptoms of gout can be precipitated by certain drugs (thiazide diuretics, nicotinic acid, low-dose aspirin), malignancies of blood-forming tissues and other disorders characterized by rapid breakdown of cellular nucleic acid, renal disease, hypothyroidism, and lead poisoning (saturnine gout; see box). Nearly all patients are men over 40.

History: Recurrent acute episodes of severe pain, tenderness, and swelling, usually affecting a single joint, often occurring at night, and separated by symptom-free intervals. The first metatarsophalangeal joint is most often affected. After the acute episode, itching and scaling of the skin overlying the affected joint. Eventual development of nodules in soft tissues.

Physical Examination: Redness, swelling, and exquisite tenderness of the affected joint. **Tophi** (nodular deposits of urate crystals with local inflammation) may appear in cartilage (the outer ear), in tissues around joints (subcutaneous tissue, tendons), or at other sites.

Diagnostic Tests: The serum uric acid level is generally elevated, as well as the erythrocyte sedimentation rate. Microscopic examination of material aspirated from affected joints or tophi shows urate crystals. In chronic disease, x-rays may show tophi in bone as punched out (**radiolucent**) areas.

Course: Without treatment an acute attack can last for days or weeks. Chronic disease may lead to joint destruction, deformity, and disability. Uric acid kidney stones are a common complication. With advanced disease, renal failure may occur.

Treatment: An acute attack of gout is promptly aborted by colchicine, nonsteroidal anti-inflammatory agents, or corticosteroid. Rest and immobilization may also be important in shortening the attack. Options for prophylactic treatment between attacks include drugs that inhibit uric acid production (allopurinol) or increase its excretion (probenecid). Colchicine can also be used. Abstinence from certain foods

> The metal **lead** has been known and used from antiquity. Medieval alchemists considered it one of the "elements" according to their primitive systems. They gave symbolic names to these elements based on the names of the heavenly bodies as then known. Thus, gold was symbolized by the sun, silver by the moon, quicksilver by the planet Mercury (which is still the usual English name of the element), and lead by Saturn. Compounds or effects of lead were therefore labeled "saturnine," a usage that continues to this day in the somewhat uncommonly heard term "saturnine gout," meaning a kind of gout induced by lead poisoning. What is another meaning of saturnine? Where does it come from?

(liver, sweetbreads, anchovies) and alcohol is usually recommended, but the impact of dietary restrictions is minimal in a patient taking adequate doses of prophylactic medicine.

Topics for Study or Discussion

1. Name three musculoskeletal disorders that can be inherited, three that can result from repetitive trauma, and three that can lead to chronic disease and disability.

2. Consult a reference book and list five types of arthritis not discussed in this book.

3. Define or explain: aponeurosis, bursa, crepitus, epiphysis, fibromyalgia, kyphosis, laminectomy, meniscus, tophus.

4. Name some musculoskeletal disorders that show a decided preference for persons of one gender. What does this difference in incidence suggest to you?

5. Orthopedists treat sprains, fractures, scoliosis, Legg-Calvé-Perthes disease, and tendinitis. Rheumatologists treat rheumatoid arthritis, fibromyalgia, and lupus erythematosus. How would you distinguish their fields of interest and expertise? In which practice would you expect to find a preponderance of women patients?

Chapter 17

Diseases of the Eye

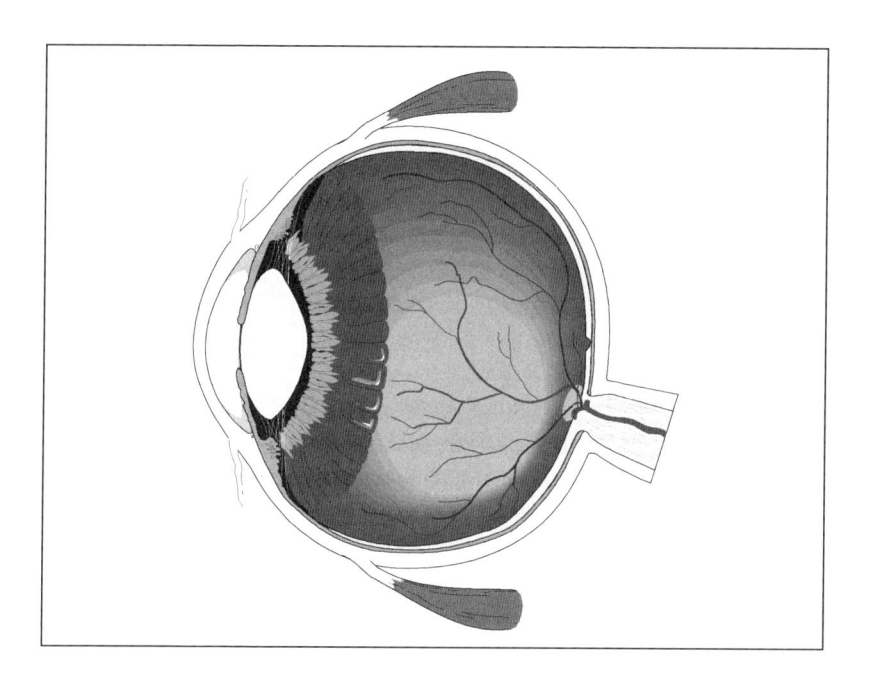

Learning Objectives

Upon completion of this chapter, the student should

- know the basic anatomy and physiology of the eye;

- have a general knowledge of diagnostic procedures and methods of treatment used in ocular diseases;

- understand signs, symptoms, and treatments of common diseases affecting the eye.

Anatomy and Physiology of the Eye

Each **eye** is a roughly spherical structure protected on all sides except the front by the bones and soft tissues of the orbit. Blood vessels and nerves enter at the back of the eye. The **eyeball** (bulb, globe) consists of three concentric layers: the outer **sclera**, a tough coat of connective tissue; the pigment layer or **uveal tract**, a delicate, spongy, vascular membrane of pigmented cells; and the innermost layer, the light-sensitive **retina**.

Anteriorly the sclera is modified to form the transparent **cornea**, through which light rays enter the eye. The uveal tract consists of three parts: the **iris**, which regulates the amount of light entering the eye; the **ciliary body**, which adjusts the focus of the eye; and the **choroid**, which underlies the retina. The retina is a layer of specialized nerve cells that are stimulated by light rays within the visible range. Nerve fibers of these cells unite to form the **optic nerve**.

The **ocular fundus** is the rear wall of the eye as viewed through the pupil with an **ophthalmoscope** (discussed below). The fundus consists of the retina and its arteries and veins and the **disc** (optic nerve head). The disc appears as a round, ivory-colored plaque raised somewhat from the surrounding retina and having a shallow central depression, the **cup**. The disc lies on the nasal side of the fundus, not at its center. The central portion of the retina, concerned with central vision and hence the most sensitive, appears as a faint yellow spot, the **macula lutea**. The retinal vessels (branching arteries, each closely accompanied by a vein) emerge from the center of the disc.

The optic nerve passes back through an aperture in the orbit and crosses the optic nerve of the opposite eye, with which it exchanges some fibers. Behind the crossing, the newly assorted bundles of fibers, called the **optic tracts**, carry visual impulses into the brain.

On their way to the retina, light rays pass through both the cornea and the **lens**, a transparent structure suspended just behind the cornea. The shape of the lens can be altered by the pull of muscles originating in the ciliary body, and this alteration adjusts the focal distance of the eye. The iris, the colored part of the eye, lies between the cornea and the lens, and controls the amount of light entering the eye by changing the diameter of the **pupil**, the black-appearing round aperture in the middle of the iris.

Diseases of the Eye • 279

The part of the eye lying anterior to the lens contains a watery fluid, the **aqueous humor**, which is produced by the ciliary body and drains into small veins in the anterior chamber at the "drainage angle" (the slight angle between cornea and sclera). The space occupied by the aqueous humor is divided into the **anterior chamber** (between cornea and iris) and the **posterior chamber** (between iris and lens). Behind the lens, the cavity of the eye is filled with a somewhat denser fluid, the **vitreous humor**. Both humors are refractive media, participating in the transmission and refraction of light rays.

The **eyelids** are folds of skin, supplied with oil and sebaceous glands and lash follicles, that shut out light and provide a watertight seal over the eyes. The medial or nasal junction or angle between upper and lower lids is called the **inner canthus**; the lateral or temporal angle is called the **outer canthus**. The visible part of the sclera is covered by a delicate vascular membrane, the **conjunctiva** (**bulbar conjunctiva**), which is continuous with the lining of the inner surfaces of the eyelids (**palpebral conjunctiva**). The conjunctiva does not extend over the cornea.

A **lacrimal gland** is situated near the front of each **orbit**, above and lateral to the eyeball. This gland produces **tears**, which moisten, lubricate, and cleanse the eyeball.

Tears flow downward and medially to drain by way of the lacrimal **puncta** (minute openings at the inner canthus) and nasolacrimal ducts into the nose.

Each eye is equipped with six **extraocular muscles**, which produce eye movement and control the direction of gaze. Three **cranial nerves** (III, oculomotor; IV, trochlear; and VI, abducens) supply these six muscles. In addition, the oculomotor nerve sends motor branches to the upper eyelid, the ciliary body (focus), and the iris (light/dark adaptation). Coordination of the movements and position of the two eyes and fusion of their images into a single three-dimensional one takes place in the brain.

Symptoms and Signs of Ocular Disease

Argyll Robertson pupil: a pupil that constricts when the subject focuses on a near object, but not when the eye is stimulated with light; due to central nervous system disease, most often syphilis.

Blepharospasm: spasm of the eyelids, usually due to local irritation, **photophobia**, or both.

Chemosis: marked watery edema and bulging of the conjunctiva.

Coloboma (iridis): a congenital defect in the iris, in which a wedge-shaped segment is absent, giving a keyhole appearance to the pupil; similar defects are created by certain types of ocular surgery.

Cupping of the disc: As noted above, the normal optic nerve head has a slight central depression (**physiologic cupping**). Increase in the depth of the cup occurs with increased intraocular pressure (**glaucoma**) or atrophy of the optic nerve.

Diplopia: double vision; seeing two overlapping two-dimensional images instead of one three-dimensional image; may result from injury or disease of one or both eyes or from failure of fusion of images in the cerebral cortex, due to alcohol, drugs, fever, infection, neoplasm, or trauma.

Ectropion: eversion (turning outward) and drooping of the lower eyelid, exposing the conjunctival surface and allowing overflow of tears.

Entropion: inward turning of the margin of the lower eyelid, often so that the lower lashes touch the eyeball.

Epiphora: chronic overflow of tears from the lower eyelid onto the cheek; may be due to blockage of the nasolacrimal duct or to deformity of the lower lid (ectropion).

Exophthalmos: abnormal bulging of the eye between the lids; may be due to local disease (orbital cellulitis or neoplasm) or (when bilateral) to systemic disease (Graves disease).

Hyphema: presence of blood in the anterior chamber.

Hypopyon: presence of pus in the anterior chamber.

Itching of the eye or eyelid.

Lacrimation (tearing): increased flow of tears.

Miosis: sustained constriction of the pupil, which may be due to ocular or nervous system disease or to the effect of drugs (pilocarpine, morphine).

Mydriasis: sustained dilatation of the pupil, which may be due to ocular or nervous system disease or to the effect of drugs (atropine, cyclopentolate).

Nyctalopia: marked reduction of visual acuity at night (that is, under conditions of near-darkness).

Nystagmus: a rhythmic back-and-forth movement of the eyes usually due to congenital abnormality or central nervous system disease.

Ocular discharge: a serous, mucous, or purulent material formed on conjunctival surfaces, often gluing the eyelids together and producing crusting of the eyelashes; usually due to infection or allergy.

Pain in the eye, which may be a superficial irritation or scratchy feeling on the cornea or sclera (as from an abrasion or ulcer) or a deep, throbbing pain within the eyeball (as in acute glaucoma).

Papilledema: swelling of the optic disc, as observed with an ophthalmoscope; usually due to increased intracranial pressure ("choked disc") (hemorrhage, neoplasm, disturbance of cerebrospinal fluid circulation) or intrinsic eye disease (optic neuritis). (When disc edema is due to inflammation, the term **papillitis** is preferred to papilledema.) The disc appears edematous and perhaps injected, and the retinal vessels as they emerge from the swollen disc appear to be kinked ("stepping" of vessels). **Papilledema** is roughly quantified as the difference in focal distance between the disc and the surrounding retina, as determined by ophthalmoscopic examination and measured in diopters.

Photophobia: aversion to bright light, which causes a sense of pain in the eye, usually because of irritability or spasm of the iris.

Ptosis: drooping of an upper eyelid that cannot be fully corrected by voluntary effort.

Redness of the eye, due either to local inflammation and hyperemia of the conjunctiva or to hemorrhage in the sclera.

Scotoma (visual field defect): a blind spot; a gap in the visual field of one or both eyes in which objects cannot be seen. A scotoma that appears identical in each eye is always due to a disease or condition of the central nervous system (for example, migraine headache). A scotoma may appear as a black hole or may show flashes or swirls of white or colored light.

Strabismus: a general term for any condition in which the direction of gaze is different in the two eyes, as noted by an observer.

Trichiasis: a growing inward of some eyelash hairs, with resultant irritation of the eye.

Visual impairment, ranging from slight indistinctness of distant objects to complete blindness. Visual impairment may be of gradual or sudden onset, unilateral or bilateral, static or progressive, reversible or permanent.

Xerophthalmia: abnormal dryness of the eye, usually due to decreased flow of tears.

Diagnostic Procedures in Ophthalmology

Inspection of the eye and adjacent structures with adequate illumination and often with magnification. For a thorough examination, the eyelids must be retracted and the patient must move each eyeball through a full range of positions.

Fluorescein dye may be applied to the cornea and conjunctiva, and the surface of the eye examined with a cobalt blue light, to detect injuries, ulcerations, or foreign bodies.

Slit lamp examination. A slit lamp is a low-power microscope with built-in illumination projected through a narrow slit. This instrument enables the physician to view a magnified cross-sectional image of the anterior structures of the eye: cornea, anterior chamber, iris, and lens. Significant abnormal findings on slit lamp examination include **flare and cells** (diminished clarity of the aqueous humor due to protein leakage from the iris; swirls of inflammatory cells in the anterior chamber due to inflammation) and **keratic precipitates** (KPs) (whitish deposits of inflammatory cells on the posterior surface of the cornea).

Funduscopic examination: Inspection of the **fundus** (the rear of the interior of the eye, consisting of the retina, its blood vessels, and the optic nerve head). The examination is performed with an **ophthalmoscope**, an instrument with a light source and a set of changeable lenses to enable the examiner to focus on the fundus regardless of refractive errors in the subject's lens. Possible findings with the ophthalmoscope include swelling or cupping of the disk, vascular and other abnormalities associated with retinopathy (discussed later in this chapter), and retinal detachment.

Vision testing: Usually performed with standard charts containing letters or words of various sizes. For assessment of distant vision, the **Snellen chart** is placed 20 feet from the subject, and visual acuity is recorded as the smallest line of type in which the subject can read more than half the letters correctly. Each line is designated by the distance at which a person with normal vision can read it. Thus, 20/20 vision is normal, while 20/80 vision means that the subject must be as close as 20 feet to read a type size that a normal person can read at 80 feet. For near vision testing, lines or paragraphs are printed in various sizes of type on a card that can be held in the hand. Testing may involve finding the smallest print that the subject can read at a standard distance, or finding the range of distances through which the subject can read a particular size of type. The eyes are tested both separately and together. For children and illiterates, charts with pictures or symbols are used.

Visual field testing: Use of a black felt sheet or screen mounted on a wall to map areas of impaired or absent vision. An **Amsler grid** consists of a network of lines, usually white on black, around a central point at which the subject is instructed to gaze while the examiner moves a small object through various parts of the visual field to detect defects.

Perimetry: A means of assessing peripheral vision by testing the subject's ability to discern moving objects or flashing lights at the extreme periphery of the visual fields.

Tests for color-blindness: Usually these are printed figures made up of variously sized dots in various colors and shades. Persons with normal color vision perceive numbers against a background of differently colored dots. Colorblind persons see only a scattering of dots.

Refraction: Determination of near and distant vision more precisely than is possible with vision charts. The instrument used enables the examiner to try a large number of lenses of standard magnification so as to determine the refractive error of each eye and hence the strength of the corrective lens that must be prescribed to correct the error. The instrument is also used in detecting and measuring astigmatism (described later in this chapter).

Tonometry: Determination of the pressure of the aqueous humor, to detect glaucoma. Tonometers of various types are used.

Orbital imaging: X-rays or MRI of the skull with emphasis on the orbit(s) to identify orbital or intraocular foreign body.

Retinal arteriography: Imaging of the retinal arteries with fluorescein injected into an arm vein.

Electroretinography: Instrumental determination of changes in electrical potential of the retina in response to light stimuli; identifies visual abnormalities due to retinal disease.

Ophthalmology is the branch of medicine that is devoted to the prevention, diagnosis, and treatment of eye diseases. This is an exceedingly complex field, which can only be touched on in a book of this scope. The rest of the chapter is devoted to discussions of some of the commoner eye diseases. Numerous terms are defined above and below; however, there is no glossary at the end of the chapter. If you encounter unfamiliar words, look them up in the index.

Inflammatory Diseases of the Eye

Conjunctivitis
Inflammation of the conjunctiva.

Causes: Infection, allergy, injury (including injuries due to chemicals, heat, or other radiant energy), or other process affecting the anterior part of the eye. Infection may be due to viruses (particularly certain adenovirus types) or bacteria (including chlamydia and gonococcus). Transmission is generally by hand contact. Neonatal conjunctivitis is acquired from an infected birth canal.

History: Soreness, itching, or irritation of one or both eyes, with redness of the conjunctiva; inability to tolerate contact lenses. Depending on cause and severity, lacrimation or mucopurulent discharge that crusts the lashes and glues the eyelids together, swelling of the eyelids, blurring of vision, or photophobia may also occur.

Physical Examination: Patchy or diffuse injection of the conjunctiva, sometimes with coarsely granular appearance ("cobblestoning," typical of some allergic conjunctivitis). Lid edema, blepharospasm, lacrimation, ocular discharge, photophobia, chemosis (typically allergic), and sometimes blepharitis, keratitis, or enlargement of preauricular lymph nodes (nodes in front of the ear). Slit lamp examination precisely locates areas of inflammation.

Diagnostic Tests: Microscopic examination of conjunctival scrapings can identify infection due to chlamydia. Culture is necessary to confirm gonococcal conjunctivitis.

Course: Most conjunctivitis is benign and self-limited. Untreated gonococcal conjunctivitis can spread to the cornea, causing perforation and blindness. Chlamydial conjunctivitis is of two kinds. *Chlamydia trachomatis* types A-C cause **trachoma**, a severe conjunctivitis with keratitis, often leading to lid deformity and blindness. Types D-K cause a milder infection, **inclusion conjunctivitis**, which typically resolves without sequelae. Seasonal or perennial allergic conjunctivitis is typically recurrent or chronic during times of exposure to allergens.

Treatment: Allergic conjunctivitis is treated with topical vasoconstrictors, mast cell stabilizers (cromolyn, lodoxamide), and corticosteroids. Systemic antihistamines and steroids may be required. Bacterial infection is treated with topical sulfonamide or antibiotic drops. Both forms of chlamydial conjunctivitis respond to systemic tetracycline, doxycycline, or erythromycin. Gonococcal conjunctivitis is treated with systemic ceftriaxone.

Hordeolum (Stye)

An acute staphylococcal abscess, typically small, that forms near the margin of an upper or lower eyelid. Treatment is with warm compresses and topical sulfonamide or antibiotic. Incision and drainage may be necessary.

Chalazion

A chronic, nontender fibrotic nodule in an eyelid, resulting from nonresolution of a stye that has developed in a conjunctival gland. The lesion may grow large and become cosmetically objectionable. Treatment is incision and curettage.

Keratitis

Inflammation of the cornea.

Causes: Keratitis may result from injury (chemical, abrasion, erosion, puncture, contact lens wear), infection (bacterial, viral, fungal, or protozoan), or systemic disease. Bacteria causing keratitis include pneumococcus, staphylococcus, *Pseudomonas*, and *Moraxella*. Syphilitic and tuberculous keratitis (due to systemic infection) also occur. Viral keratitis may be due to herpes simplex virus or varicella-zoster virus. Keratitis in contact lens wearers may be due to the protozoan parasite *Acanthamoeba*.

History: Pain in the eye, aggravated by opening and closing the lid; lacrimation, photophobia, visual blurring. There may be a history of corneal trauma (fingernail scratch, cigarette ash, airborne foreign body) or of systemic infection (tuberculosis, syphilis).

Physical Examination: Conjunctival injection, particularly near to the corneal rim. Photophobia, lacrimation, watery or purulent discharge. Staining of the cornea followed by examination with cobalt blue light shows ulceration or other epithelial defects.

Diagnostic Tests: Microscopic examination or culture of scrapings from the cornea may indicate a causative organism.

Course: Certain infections (herpes simplex virus, *Acanthamoeba*) cause progressive and severe damage if untreated, with visual loss due to corneal scarring. Thinning and bulging (descemetocele) of an inflamed zone of cornea may also occur. Corneal infection can extend to the sclera, iris, or optic nerve.

Treatment: Specific antimicrobial treatment, if available, is mandatory. Topical antibiotics usually suffice in bacterial keratitis. Viral infections are treated with topical idoxuridine or trifluridine and systemic acyclovir. Topical steroids are used in selected cases.

Uveitis

Uveitis is inflammation of any part of the **uveal tract**. Inflammation of the iris is called **iritis**; of the ciliary body, **cyclitis**; and of the choroid, **choroiditis**. Uveitis may occur as a feature of various granulomatous diseases (syphilis, tuberculosis, toxoplasmosis, sarcoidosis) or may appear in various systemic inflammatory diseases (ulcerative colitis, Crohn disease, psoriasis, ankylosing spondylitis, Reiter syndrome, Behçet syndrome). **Anterior uveitis** (iritis, cyclitis, iridocyclitis) causes unilateral ocular pain, visual blurring, and photophobia.

Examination of the eye shows constriction of the pupil and a flush of redness around the rim of the cornea. Photophobia may be evident. Slit lamp examination shows cells and flare of the aqueous humor, keratic precipitates (KP) of the posterior corneal epithelium, and sometimes hypopyon or distortion of the pupil by adhesions (**synechiae**; singular synechia). (Anterior synechiae form between the iris and the posterior surface of the cornea; posterior synechiae between the iris and the anterior surface of the lens.) **Posterior uveitis** (choroiditis) causes gradual loss of vision in one eye, with minimal discomfort. Examination shows cells in the vitreous, and may indicate inflammatory changes in the retina.

The erythrocyte sedimentation rate is elevated. Laboratory studies and chest x-ray may indicate other manifestations of an underlying process and make possible a precise diagnosis. Treatment is with corticosteroids topically or systemically. Mydriatics are given to dilate the pupil and reduce the risk of posterior synechiae. Underlying infection requires specific treatment.

Glaucoma

An ocular condition in which the pressure of the aqueous humor is abnormally high. Two types are recognized.

Open Angle Glaucoma

The most common type of glaucoma, consisting of a persistent elevation of intraocular pressure.

Cause: Unknown; apparently related to decreased reabsorption of aqueous humor from the anterior chamber of the eye. However, the drainage angle is not demonstrably narrowed, hence the name (contrast the next condition). Both eyes are about equally affected, and the condition runs in families.

History: Gradual loss of peripheral vision. Appearance of halos around lights, especially at night, when intraocular tension is very high.

Physical Examination: Increased cupping of the optic disc (increased **cup:disc ratio**).

Diagnostic Tests: Intraocular tension, as determined by **tonometry**, is elevated (normal 10-21 mmHg). Visual fields are diminished.

Course: Optic atrophy, with partial to complete loss of vision within 15-20 years if untreated.

Treatment: Long-term treatment with miotics: beta-adrenergic blocking agents (timolol, levobunolol, metipranolol), epinephrine, pilocarpine). Laser trabeculectomy surgery may be undertaken in refractory cases to improve drainage.

Narrow Angle Glaucoma

Acute onset of unilateral ocular pain and visual loss due to sudden obstruction of the outflow of aqueous humor.

Cause: *Predisposing*: A narrow anterior chamber angle (more common in the elderly, in persons with hypermetropia, and in Asians). *Precipitating*: Prolonged dilatation of the pupil, such as occurs in a darkened theater or after administration of certain drugs (anticholinergic medicines orally, mydriatic drops for eye examination).

History: Sudden onset of pain in one eye, with blurring of vision, halos around lights; often nausea, vomiting, and abdominal pain.

Physical Examination: Redness of the eye, steamy cornea, dilated nonreactive pupil.

Diagnostic Tests: Tonometry shows markedly elevated intraocular pressure.

Course: Severe and permanent visual loss occurs if acute glaucoma is not promptly treated.

Treatment: IV acetazoleamide and mannitol are administered to reduce intraocular pressure. Laser **iridectomy** (destruction of a wedge of iris) permits drainage of the anterior chamber. The unaffected eye is usually operated on prophylactically as well.

Cataract

An ocular lens that has become cloudy or opaque because of intrinsic physical or chemical change.

Causes: Largely unknown. Infantile cataracts occur after maternal rubella or when the child has galactosemia. Cataract can occur in various systemic diseases (diabetes mellitus, hypoparathyroidism) or as a complication of other ocular disease (uveitis, glaucoma) or injury (penetrating injury of the lens, ionizing radiation). The most common type is **senile cataract**, occurring as part of aging, with onset after age 50. The risk is increased by cigarette smoking.

History: Gradual painless loss of vision, not improved by glasses, and seeing rings or halos around lights at night.

Physical Examination: Inspection confirms the presence of partial or complete opacity of one or both lenses. A fully developed cataract, with severe impairment of vision, is called "**ripe**." Slit lamp examination gives more precise information about the type, extent, and location of lenticular opacity.

Course: Without treatment the entire lens eventually becomes opaque and vision is lost. Surgery restores vision at any stage by removing the lens.

Treatment: Surgical removal of the opaque lens by a variety of techniques, leaving the posterior capsule of the lens intact. Surgical extraction is now less frequently used than fragmentation with ultrasound (**phacoemulsification**). A synthetic lens is usually implanted at the time of cataract extraction.

Disorders of the Retina

Retinopathy

A general term for degenerative disorders of the retina, usually accompanied by loss of vision and often due to systemic disease. Two types will be discussed here.

Hypertensive Retinopathy

Degenerative retinal changes due to impairment of blood supply to the retina and choroid in persons with very high, or chronic, hypertension, with variable degrees of visual loss. Chronic hypertension accelerates the development of arteriosclerosis, and many of the physical findings are due to vascular changes. The **Keith-Wagener-Barker** classification is often used to grade funduscopic observations:

Grade I—focal or diffuse narrowing of retinal arterioles, with reduction of the arteriole-venule ratio (**AV ratio**; normally 4:5) to 3:4 or 1:2; narrowed arterioles may be described as having a **copper-wire** or **silver-wire** appearance.

Grade II—further narrowing of arterioles, with reduction of the AV ratio to 1:2 or 1:3; crossing phenomena or **AV nicking** (tapering of a venule where an arteriole crosses it).

Grade III—all of the above, with **"flame"** (flame-shaped) hemorrhages and **cotton wool spots** (exudates); these are fluffy opaque zones of degenerative change following microscopic infarction and hemorrhage in the retina.

Grade IV—all of the above, with papilledema.

Close observation of the changes of hypertensive retinopathy is of value in judging hypertensive vascular damage elsewhere in the body. There is no treatment.

Diabetic Retinopathy

Degenerative vascular changes in the retina occurring in diabetes mellitus, particularly in poorly controlled diabetes; the principal cause of legal blindness before age 65.

Two forms are recognized. In **proliferative retinopathy** there is formation of new blood vessels (**neovascularization**) in the retina, with visual loss and a risk of vitreous hemorrhage and retinal tears. The condition is detected by fluorescein angiography and treated by laser photocoagulation (occasionally, surgery).

In **nonproliferative retinopathy**, changes are limited to venous dilatation, **microaneurysms** (appearing as tiny red spots adjacent to vessels), retinal hemorrhages and **hard** (sharp-bordered) **exudates**, and retinal edema. Waning, partially resolved retinal edema leaves folds or tucks in the retina, which appear as whitish streaks, often arranged in fanlike configurations. A complete encirclement of the macula by radially disposed streaks constitutes a macular "star figure." Visual impairment correlates poorly with extent of disease. Laser coagulation is the usual treatment. Maintaining good control of diabetes reduces the risk of severe retinopathy.

Macular Degeneration

Age-related loss of central vision due to atrophic or exudative changes in the macula lutea of the retina. Onset is usually after age 50 and the condition typically progresses to complete loss of central vision (legal blindness), with preservation of peripheral vision and the ability to walk and recognize familiar faces and objects. Medical and surgical treatment are ineffectual.

Retinitis Pigmentosa

An inherited degenerative disorder of the retina, causing progressive visual loss beginning usually in childhood. Ophthalmoscopic examination shows edema of the disc and scattered spiderlike patches of pigment in the retina. There is no effective treatment.

Retinal Detachment

Separation of the retina from the choroid as a result of trauma or degenerative changes, particularly in older persons. Myopia and cataract surgery predispose to detachment. The patient experiences visual disturbances (blurring, visual field defects) and may report seeing a curtain floating in the field of the affected eye. The problem tends to be progressive and may lead to complete blindness if the macula becomes separated. Ophthalmoscopic examination shows one or more free margins of retina floating in the vitreous, and sometimes tears in the retina. Treatment is by **retinopexy**—reattachment with cryotherapy applied to the sclera opposite the site of detachment or laser coagulation applied to free retinal margins. Placement of the detached segment may be facilitated by injection of gas under slight pressure into the cavity of the vitreous humor. Occasionally open surgery is required.

Disorders of Ocular Movement

Strabismus
A disorder of ocular motility in which the two eyes do not look in exactly the same direction, and cerebral fusion of their images into a three-dimensional one cannot occur.

Heterophoria is a transient deviation of one eye from the normal position with respect to the other. It may occur as a slight congenital weakness or imbalance of ocular muscles that is symptomatic only in the presence of fatigue. Other causes include fever, alcohol, and drug use. Inward deviation of one eye is called **esophoria**, outward deviation is called **exophoria**, and normal positioning of both eyes is called **orthophoria**.

Heterotropia is a persistent deviation of one or both eyes, due to congenital ocular muscle weakness or imbalance. Inward deviation is called **esotropia**, outward deviation **exotropia**. If one eye is consistently affected, central suppression of its image eventually occurs, with resulting **amblyopia** (dulling of vision that cannot be corrected with a lens). Treatment of heterotropia must be carried out before amblyopia has developed. Treatment consists of prismatic lenses that permit images to fuse, occlusion of one eye to preserve the vision of the other, exercises to improve strength and coordination of ocular muscles, and surgery to bring the eyes into line.

Paralytic strabismus results from paralysis of one or more eye muscles due to congenital abnormality, trauma, infection, multiple sclerosis, herpes zoster, neoplasm, or hemorrhage. Surgical treatment may be helpful in selected cases.

Nystagmus is involuntary rhythmic movements of the eyes, typically bilateral, due to congenital abnormality, multiple sclerosis, or central nervous system tumor, infection, or hemorrhage, or intoxication (chronic alcoholism). Transitory nystagmus occurs after riding on a merry-go-round or in the presence of vertigo. There is no treatment for nystagmus other than removing the cause, if it can be detected.

Visual Impairment
Emmetropia: Normal vision.

Hyperopia (farsightedness): The focus of light rays passing into the eyes lies behind the retina, due to a congenitally short anteroposterior diameter of the eyeball. Treatment is with corrective lenses.

Myopia (nearsightedness): The focus of light rays passing into the eye lies in front of, rather than on, the retina, because of a congenitally long anteroposterior diameter of the eyeball. This condition, much commoner than the preceding, shows a familial tendency and when severe it predisposes to glaucoma. Treatment is with corrective lenses.

Astigmatism: The image falling on the retina is distorted because the curvature of the cornea is not the same in all axes (that is, the cornea is not spherical). Correction is with lenses having a cylindrical curvature to neutralize the effect of corneal distortion.

Presbyopia: Loss of normal accommodation with aging, due to diminished elasticity of the eyes, with inability to focus on objects or print near to the eye. Treatment is with corrective lenses for reading. Persons with myopia as well as presbyopia require bifocals or even trifocals to provide a choice of focal distances.

Topics for Study or Discussion

1. Name and describe four ocular symptoms or signs that are due to intrinsic eye disease, and four that are due to neurologic or systemic disease.

2. What is the anatomic boundary between the aqueous humor and the vitreous humor? Between the anterior chamber and the posterior chamber?

3. Define or explain: canthus, fundus, keratitis, lacrimation, ptosis, retinopathy, scotoma, slit lamp.

4. List three disorders limited to the eye that can cause blindness, and three systemic conditions that can cause blindness.

5. Name and describe three abnormalities of vision and three malfunctions of extraocular muscles.

Chapter 18

Diseases of the Nervous System

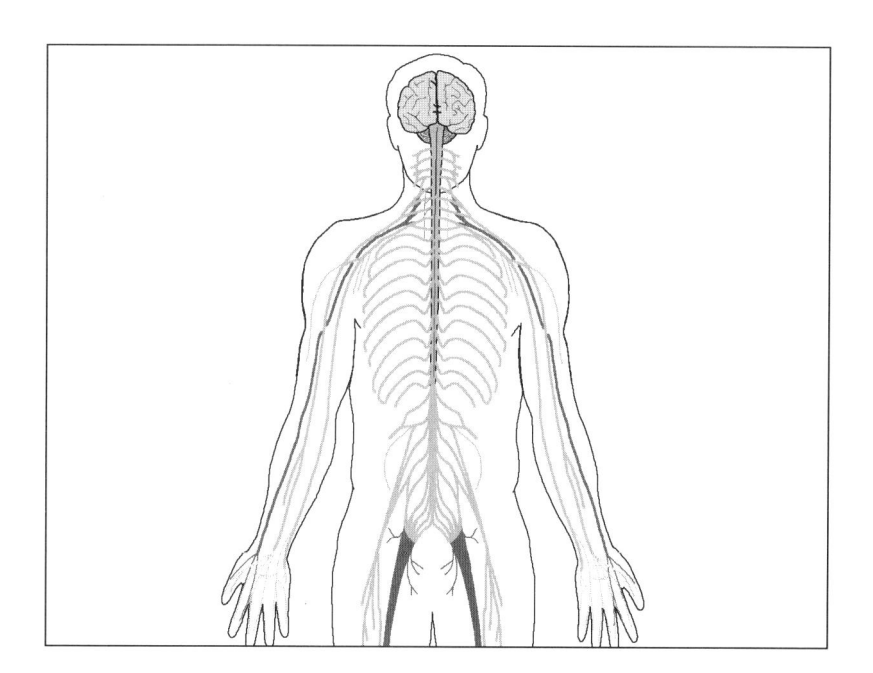

Learning Objectives

Upon completion of this chapter, the student should

- know the basic anatomy and physiology of the nervous system;

- have a general knowledge of diagnostic procedures and treatments used in neurologic disease;

- understand signs, symptoms, and treatments of common diseases affecting the nervous system.

Anatomy and Physiology of the Nervous System

The **nervous system** is an exceedingly complex arrangement of nerve cells and their fibers that extends throughout the body and receives, processes, and interprets sensory stimuli; initiates and coordinates voluntary muscular movement; regulates autonomic processes such as heartbeat, vascular constriction and dilatation, bronchiolar caliber, sweating, and gastrointestinal secretion and motility; carries out complex mental functions and operations including memory and recall of past events, recognition of persons and objects, abstract reasoning and practical problem solving, judgment, and language production and comprehension; and is the seat of mood and emotions.

All nerve tissue is made up of **nerve cells** and their processes. Although nerve cells vary widely in structure and function, all conform to a basic pattern. Each nerve cell (**neuron**) consists of a cell body containing a nucleus; one or more short treelike processes, called **dendrites**; and a single long, straight process, the **axon**. Dendrites conduct nerve impulses toward the cell body, and are therefore called **afferent processes**; axons conduct impulses away from the cell, and are therefore called **efferent processes**. The point of contact between processes of two different cells is called a synapse. Chemical substances called neurotransmitters are produced in infinitesimal quantities at nerve endings, and serve to transmit nerve impulses, either stimulating or inhibiting, across the synapse.

The axons of some nerve cells are enveloped in a thin layer of fatty white material called **myelin**. The **myelin sheath** serves as an electrical insulator. Nerve tissue consisting of many myelinated fibers is called **white matter**; tissue consisting chiefly of nerve cell bodies is called **gray matter**.

The nervous system is divided into two major sections: the **central nervous system**, consisting of the brain and spinal cord; and the **peripheral nervous system**, consisting of the peripheral motor and sensory nerves and the **autonomic nervous system**. The **brain**, which entirely fills the cranial cavity, is traditionally broken down into major parts on the basis of gross anatomic features:

The **cerebrum**, made up of two symmetric hemispheres and concerned with the higher mental processes; its surface, the **cerebral cortex**, is thrown into deep convolutions like the kernel of a walnut. The convexities (raised areas) are called **gyri**, and the grooves between them are called **sulci**. Deeper grooves (**fissures**) divide each hemisphere into four lobes: **frontal, temporal, parietal,** and **occipital.**

The **cerebellum** lies behind the cerebrum and looks like a smaller version of it, as its name implies. Its principal function is coordination of voluntary motor activity.

Four structures—diencephalon, mesencephalon or midbrain, pons, and medulla oblongata—compose, from front to back, the **ventral surface of the brain**; the last two make up the **brain stem**. The medulla continues below the skull as the **spinal cord**.

The brain and spinal cord are covered by three protective membranes called **meninges**. The outer membrane, the **dura mater**, is in contact with the bony interior of the skull and spinal column. Within the dura is the delicate **arachnoid membrane**, and within that is the **pia mater**, which lies on the surface of the brain and spinal cord.

Within the cerebrum and the diencephalon is a system of communicating hollow chambers (the two **lateral ventricles**, the **third ventricle**, and the **fourth ventricle**). **Cerebrospinal fluid** (CSF) is a watery medium that is both formed and reabsorbed within the skull, and serves primarily as a shock absorber. It surrounds the brain and spinal cord in the subarachnoid space and also fills the ventricular system and the hollow central canal of the spinal cord.

Twelve pairs of cranial nerves (traditionally represented by Roman numerals) emerge from the ventral surface of the brain and brain stem and serve important sensory and motor functions, chiefly within the head:

I. **Olfactory**: sense of smell.
II. **Optic**: vision.
III. **Oculomotor**: innervates four of the six extraocular muscles and also the ciliary body, the iris, and the upper eyelid.
IV. **Trochlear**: innervates the superior oblique muscle of the eye.
V. **Trigeminal**: sensory nerve supply to the face, nose, and mouth; motor supply to the muscles of mastication.
VI. **Abducens**: innervates lateral rectus muscle of eye.
VII. **Facial**: motor supply to the muscles of facial expression; also stimulation of tear and salivary glands; some sensory functions, including taste on the anterior two-thirds of the tongue.
VIII. **Vestibulocochlear**: hearing and equilibrium.
IX. **Glossopharyngeal**: motor and sensory branches to the ear, tongue, and throat; taste sensation from the posterior third of the tongue.

296 • Human Diseases

X. **Vagus**: sensory fibers to the ear, tongue, and throat; motor fibers to thoracic and abdominal viscera.
XI. **Accessory** (spinal accessory): motor innervation of two voluntary muscles of the neck: trapezius and sternocleidomastoid.
XII. **Hypoglossal**: motor innervation of the tongue.

The **spinal cord** is made up largely of axons of nerve cells, some with cell bodies in the brain (carrying motor impulses to various spinal segments) and others with cell bodies in the cord itself (carrying sensory impulses from spinal segments to various brain centers). Whereas the visible surface of the cerebral cortex is made up of gray matter (cell bodies), with white matter inside, in the spinal cord the white matter, consisting of ascending and descending myelinated nerve fibers, is on the outside, and the gray matter is within.

The **peripheral nervous system** comprises all nerve tissue outside the brain and spinal cord. Its two major divisions are the **spinal nerves** and the **autonomic nervous system**. Spinal nerves are those that originate in the spinal cord and pass between pairs of vertebrae to supply the body with sensation and voluntary motor power. There are 31 sets of spinal nerves, one arising from each spinal segment; these segments correspond closely to the cervical, dorsal, lumbar, and (fused) sacral vertebrae.

Each spinal segment gives off a pair of nerve roots on each side: a **dorsal (sensory) root** and a **ventral (motor) root**. Each dorsal root has a visible node or swelling (**ganglion**) containing cell bodies of sensory nerves. The dorsal and ventral roots fuse to form **segmental nerves**, which pass forward around the body and give off branches to all external surfaces and internal structures, particularly muscles of the trunk and extremities.

Each visible and named peripheral nerve is a bundle of thousands of myelinated axons of motor neurons whose cell bodies lie in the brain and spinal cord, and of dendrites of sensory nerves, whose cell bodies are located in the dorsal root ganglia. **Motor nerves** send signals to voluntary muscles throughout the body. **Sensory nerves** carry impulses from sensory structures in the skin that respond to pain, pressure, light touch, hot, and cold; from visceral sensors that respond to pressure or stretching and pain; and from proprioceptive sensors in voluntary muscles that signal the brain as to their position, tension, and movement.

The **autonomic nervous system** is a purely motor system concerned with automatic or involuntary activities or processes, such as heart rate and digestion. The bodily effects of emotion (tachycardia, sweating, pallor, sense of constriction in the chest) largely result from the actions of the autonomic nervous system.

Nerves of the sympathetic or thoracolumbar division arise from a series of ganglia lying along each side of the thoracic and lumbar segments of the spinal cord, but outside the spinal column. These communicate with the spinal cord and with one another by both myelinated and nonmyelinated fibers. The **sympathetic nervous system** is concerned with the so-called fight or flight response mediated by **epinephrine** and **norepinephrine**. Nerves of the sympathetic division are distributed to the eye, where they cause pupillary dilatation; the heart, where they increase the pulse rate; the lungs, where they cause bronchodilatation; and skin, where they constrict blood vessels, stimulate secretion of sweat, and cause erection of hairs.

The **parasympathetic** or **craniosacral** division of the autonomic nervous system provides motor innervation to cranial, thoracic, abdominal, and pelvic viscera, generally of an opposite nature to sympathetic innervation. That is, parasympathetic activity occurs chiefly during periods of rest or quiet, and is associated with cardiac rates and with such physiologic processes as gastrointestinal secretion and motility, and sexual activity.

Parasympathetic nerves arise only from the brain and from sacral segments of the spinal cord. Three cranial nerves (III, VII, and IX) send parasympathetic fibers to structures in the head (iris, ciliary body, salivary glands; a fourth (X) sends fibers to thoracic, abdominal, and pelvic viscera (heart, lungs, digestive system). Parasympathetic nerves from sacral segments of the spinal cord supply the urinary tract and reproductive system.

Signs and Symptoms of Neurologic Disease

Altered level of consciousness, varying from slight drowsiness or inattentiveness to confusion and disorientation to deep coma from which the subject cannot be aroused by any stimulus.

Syncope (fainting): sudden loss of consciousness, usually transitory, due to circulatory or neurologic abnormality, including central nervous system intoxication or injury, but frequently the result of strong emotion in the absence of organic disease.

Amnesia: loss of memory, recent, remote, or total.

Aphasia: impairment of the ability to communicate through spoken or written language, or to understand spoken or written language, or both.

Pain, sensed at or near the body surface, usually burning or stinging (**causalgia**) or like an electric shock, due to irritation or inflammation of nerves.

Hypesthesia: partial loss of sensation on one or more parts of the body surface.

Anesthesia: total loss of sensation on one or more parts of the body surface.

Paresthesia: a sense of tingling or prickling ("pins and needles") on a part of the body surface. The lay term "numbness" is applied indiscriminately to hypesthesia, anesthesia, and paresthesia.

Headache: local or generalized, intermittent or constant; can result from infection, neoplasm, or hemorrhage within the cranium, obstruction to the flow of cerebrospinal fluid, trauma, or migraine.

Dysequilibrium: loss of balance sense; tendency to fall without support.

Vertigo: a subjective sense of spinning. Dysequilibrium and vertigo sometimes occur together, and both are indiscriminately referred to as dizziness by the laity.

Muscle weakness (**paresis**) or complete loss of function (**paralysis**), local or widespread. Paralysis is divided into **flaccid** (absence of muscle tone and absence of reflexes) and **spastic** (muscles tight, with resistance to manipulation and hyperactive reflexes).

Spasm: sustained contraction, usually painful, of a voluntary muscle.

Tremors: shaking of parts of the body supplied by voluntary muscles, principally the arms, forearms, and hands, Tremors are divided into **resting** (occurring only when the affected muscles are not being used for purposeful activity) and **intention** (occurring only during voluntary movement).

Tic: a rapid involuntary muscle twitch, typically recurrent and stereotyped, affecting one or several body areas.

Chorea: rapid, jerky, purposeless involuntary movements of one or several muscle groups.

Athetosis: slow, writhing involuntary movements of the face or limbs.

Incoordination: jerkiness and awkwardness in activities requiring smooth coordination of several muscles.

Ataxia: impairment of complex movements due to loss of proprioceptive impulses from the muscles of the trunk or limbs.

Seizures: sudden, transitory impairment of central nervous system function, with or without loss of consciousness, and with or without local or generalized **tonic** and **clonic** contractions of voluntary muscles.

Many other signs and symptoms (visual and hearing impairment, vomiting, disturbance in bowel or bladder function, personality change) often prove to be due to diseases of the central nervous system. Mental disorders are discussed in the next chapter.

Diagnostic Procedures in Neurology

The basic diagnostic procedure in diseases of the nervous system is the **neurologic examination**, a standardized set of observations and tests performed with the physician's eyes, ears, and hands or with simple instruments. The neurologic examination is modified as dictated by the patient's complaints and condition at the time of examination. (A comatose patient cannot be expected to follow directions or stand and walk.) The following are the essential elements of the basic neurologic examination.

Mental Status Examination: Assessment of the subject's appearance, level of consciousness, mood, orientation, language ability, memory, reasoning capacity, and other elements of mental function. The mental status examination is fully discussed in the next chapter.

Cranial Nerve Examination: A systematic examination of the sensory and motor functions of the twelve cranial nerves.

I. **Olfactory**: Testing sense of smell. This assessment is often omitted, hence the frequent expression, "Cranial nerves II through XII are intact."

II. **Optic**: Testing the subject's vision with standard eye charts. Checking peripheral vision and visual fields by simple techniques. Examination of the ocular fundi with an ophthalmoscope.

III. **Oculomotor**: Testing ocular movements; observing for strabismus, nystagmus, and drooping of eyelids. Testing the ability of the pupil to constrict when stimulated by light and when focused on a near object.

IV. **Trochlear**: Extraocular movements already assessed.

V. **Trigeminal**: Sensitivity to light touch (wisp of cotton or fine brush) and pain (sterile needle) are tested over the skin of the face. The blink reflex to touching the cornea with cotton is also tested. The integrity of motor branches to the muscles of mastication is tested by having the subject open the mouth wide, and then clench the teeth together.

VI. **Abducens**: Extraocular muscles already assessed.

VII. **Facial**: Testing muscles of facial expression by having the subject wrinkle the forehead, close the eyes tightly, retract the lips so as to show the teeth, and purse the lips as for whistling. Taste on the front part of the tongue may be tested.

VIII. **Vestibulocochlear: Cold caloric test**: when ice-water is poured into the ear canal, a normal vestibular apparatus causes nystagmus with the quick component to the opposite side. Hearing is tested in each ear separately.

IX. **Glossopharyngeal**: With impairment of innervation to one side of the palate, the uvula deviates to the normal side, particularly during the gag reflex. Swallowing is affected by impairment of either the ninth or the tenth cranial nerve.

X. **Vagus**: The subject's ability to speak and to swallow is observed.

XI. **Accessory**: The subject's ability to push against the examiner's hand with each side of the chin indicates integrity of the nerve supply to the sternocleidomastoid and trapezius muscles.

XII. **Hypoglossal**: The examiner notes the symmetry of development of the tongue muscles at rest and the symmetry of movement when the tongue is protruded. Impairment of a hypoglossal nerve causes deviation of the tongue to the affected side.

Spinal Nerve Examination: Sensory innervation of the skin is assessed by the subject's ability to recognize **light touch** (wisp of cotton), **pain** (sterile needle), **hot and cold** (test tubes of hot and cold water) on various parts of the body surface. Examination may include tests of **stereognosis** (ability to recognize an object by handling it), vibratory sense (ability to sense the vibration of a tuning fork when the stem is placed on a bone near the surface, such as the elbow or the shin), **two-point discrimination** (ability to distinguish two points close together on the skin). **Proprioception** is tested by having the subject report whether a toe or finger is moved up or down by the examiner, and by observation of **stance** and **gait**. The **Romberg test** (having the subject stand with feet together and eyes open, then eyes closed) assesses position sense in the trunk and legs.

Motor innervation is tested by observation of muscle development, tone, and voluntary movement in the trunk and limbs, with comparison of the two sides. The examiner notes any wasting, paralysis, spasm or rigidity, or involuntary movements (tremors, tics, chorea, athetosis). Coordination is tested by having the subject perform **rapidly alternating movements** with the hands or feet. The **finger-to-nose** and **heel-to-shin** tests and **tandem walking** are other ways of judging coordination.

Reflexes: A **reflex** is a muscular contraction occurring in response to a sensory stimulus. All the nerve cells and fibers involved in a reflex are located in a spinal cord segment, and its sensory and motor roots form a so-called **reflex arc**; the brain is not involved.

Muscle stretch (deep tendon) reflexes occur in response to sudden stretching of a muscle, usually induced by tapping a tendon with a rubber-headed reflex hammer. Tendon reflexes are tested in several muscles of the upper and lower extremities, with comparison of the two sides.

Superficial (cutaneous) reflexes are muscle contractions in response to stroking the skin; those of the abdominal wall are tested as part of a complete neurologic examination.

Pathologic reflexes are present only in neurologic disorders. The **Babinski reflex** consists of dorsiflexion of the great toe and flaring of the other toes in response to stroking of the sole of the foot toward the toes. The **Chaddock reflex** is the same response to stroking of the side of the foot toward the toes. These and similar pathologic reflexes, along with spastic paralysis and rigidity, indicate an **upper motor neuron lesion**—interruption of motor tracts from the cerebral cortex to the spinal segment involved, without impairment of the reflex arc. Flaccid paralysis, absence of normal and abnormal reflexes, and muscle wasting indicate a **lower motor neuron lesion**—interruption of motor tracts from spinal cord to muscle.

Other Diagnostic Procedures: Besides physical examination, the physician may use other diagnostic procedures to gain more detailed or accurate information about nervous system integrity and function.

Lumbar Puncture: Withdrawal of a specimen of cerebrospinal fluid from the subarachnoid space by inserting a needle between two vertebrae (usually L4 and L5) at the lower end of the spinal cord. A **manometer** (graduated glass tube) is used to measure the pressure of the fluid at the beginning of the procedure (**opening pressure**) and the end (closing pressure). Specimens of fluid are examined microscopically (stained smear) for cells (neutrophils and lymphocytes) and pathogenic microorganisms; chemically for glucose, protein, and other substances; by culture for bacterial pathogens; and, if indicated, serologically for evidence of syphilis, Lyme disease, or other infections and by cytologic techniques for malignant cells. Normal CSF is water clear. **Xanthochromia** (yellowness) of the fluid suggests recent but not current hemorrhage. Frank blood in the specimen may indicate subarachnoid hemorrhage but may also be due to local injury by the needle (**traumatic tap**).

Electroencephalography (EEG): Measurement and recording of electrical activity from several sites simultaneously. **Electrodes** are attached with fine needles to standard sites on the scalp and the record is made on a strip of moving paper. Tracings are usually made after administration of a short-acting sedative (with the subject asleep, if possible). The effects of **hyperventilation** and of **photic stimulation** (exposure to a flashing light) are recorded also. The EEG is particularly useful in identifying and classifying seizure disorders.

Imaging studies include CT scan (with or without intravenous injection of contrast medium), MRI, and standard x-ray views of the skull. Angiography may be used to show cranial vasculature with injected contrast medium. In digital subtraction angiography, x-ray images of the head with and without contrast medium are processed by a computer, which deletes all shadows common to both films (skull bones, soft tissue profiles and interfaces), leaving only the vascular system visible. Myelography is visualization of the spinal canal (the tubular enclosure of the spinal cord formed collectively by the vertebrae) by x-ray with contrast medium introduced into the subarachnoid space by lumbar puncture. A brain scan is an examination based on the distribution of a radioactive isotope injected systemically in brain tissue.

Electrophysiologic studies: Measurement of electrical activity in nerves and muscles. Electromyography (EMG) involves insertion of fine needle electrodes into voluntary muscles. **Nerve conduction velocity** (NCV) is measured by timing the passage of nerve impulses between a stimulating and a recording electrode, which are a precisely measured distance apart.

Hereditary and Congenital Neurologic Disorders

Cerebral Palsy

A nonprogressive disorder of voluntary movement and posture control, first noted at or soon after birth. A somewhat vague term for congenital neurologic impairment that is not hereditary. Most cases are due to maternal infection or drug use, difficult labor, or obstetrical complications. Symptoms vary widely in extent and severity. Most patients have spastic paralysis. About half have seizures, about half are mentally retarded, and about half die by the age of 10. Treatment is principally supportive—physical therapy, orthopedic intervention, family counseling, and the use of drugs to control spasticity.

Congenital Hydrocephalus

Enlargement of the head by excessive fluid pressure within the ventricular system, evident at birth or within the first few weeks of life.

Causes: Obstruction to the normal outflow of cerebrospinal fluid from the ventricular system due to a congenital defect, often the result of maternal infection (toxoplasmosis, rubella, cytomegalovirus, syphilis).

Physical Examination: Abnormally large circumference of the head at birth, or disproportionate increase in head size during early infancy.

Diagnostic Tests: CT scan and ultrasonography confirm ventricular enlargement and may indicate the site of obstruction.

Course: Without treatment, progressive enlargement of the ventricular system can be expected, with damage to the cerebral hemispheres and other intracranial structures.

Treatment: Surgical insertion of a shunt from the obstructed ventricular system to the right atrium of the heart or to the peritoneal cavity.

Neural Tube Defects

A group of congenital abnormalities in the development of the central nervous system during the first two months of fetal life. Some of these are associated with defects in the skull or vertebral column. The cause is generally unknown. Some defects are genetically determined, and others may be induced by maternal infection (rubella). Prenatal diagnosis of neural tube defect can be made by the finding of elevated alpha-fetoprotein in amniotic fluid obtained by **amniocentesis** at or after 16 weeks of gestation.

anencephaly: absence of cerebral hemispheres. This condition is incompatible with life, and babies born with it typically die within hours.

microcephaly: abnormally small, maldeveloped cerebral hemispheres, typically associated with mental and motor retardation.

cranium bifidum with encephalocele: failure of the developing cranium to close in the midline either anteriorly or posteriorly, with protrusion of part of the brain through the defect. The prognosis is good with early surgical repair of the defect. A shunt procedure may be necessary to treat associated hydrocephalus.

porencephaly: one or more cysts or cavities in a cerebral hemisphere communicating with the ventricular system. There may be little or no neurologic impairment.

hydranencephaly: a more severe form of the preceding, with very little cerebral cortex remaining. Neurologic impairment is more severe.

spina bifida: a failure of closure of one or more vertebrae in the posterior midline, which may be associated with bulging of meninges (**meningocele**) or of spinal cord and meninges (**meningomyelocele**). Neurologic impairment depends on the site and extent of the defect. The prognosis is good with early surgery, but paralysis present at birth cannot be reversed.

Huntington Disease (Huntington Chorea)

A genetic disorder (autosomal dominant) characterized by progressive muscle rigidity and dementia accompanied by chorea and often seizures. Onset is by age 40 and may be in childhood. Death occurs in 5-15 years.

Tourette Syndrome (Gilles de la Tourette Syndrome)

A chronic, familial motor disorder, sometimes triggered by drugs, and characterized by **tics** (repetitive, irregular habit spasms involving particularly the face, sometimes partially repressible) and involuntary vocal utterances, sometimes obscene. Drug therapy with haloperidol or clonidine may help control tics. Supportive counseling with attention to speech and behavior problems is crucial.

Demyelinating and Degenerative Diseases

Multiple Sclerosis

A chronic sensory and motor disorder of variable presentation, due to loss of myelin from nerve cells in the central nervous system.

Cause: Patchy deterioration of the myelin sheaths of nerve tracts in the brain and spinal cord and in the optic nerve leads to deterioration of nerve function. The cause is unknown; genetic, infectious, and autoimmune factors have been suggested. Onset is usually between 20 and 40. The incidence is higher in women and in cooler latitudes. Disease is sometimes apparently precipitated by fatigue, emotional stress, pregnancy, or viral respiratory infection.

History: Irregular, intermittent or progressive impairment of sensory or motor function: hypesthesia, paresthesia, visual disturbances, disorders of equilibrium; muscular weakness, spasticity, or unsteadiness; tremors, nystagmus, diplopia, disturbances of swallowing or bladder function.

Physical Examination: Findings on neurologic examination are typically diffuse and highly variable: hypesthesia or anesthesia, irregularly distributed muscle weakness with spasticity and hyperactive deep tendon reflexes, Babinski reflex, impaired abdominal superficial reflexes, ataxia, uncoordinated (scanning) speech, tremors, nystagmus, temporal pallor of the optic discs followed by optic atrophy, visual field defects, emotional lability.

Diagnostic Tests: The spinal fluid may show moderate lymphocytosis and elevation of the gamma-globulin concentration above that of the serum. CSF electrophoresis may detect bands of antibody to myelin. The electroencephalogram may show nonspecific abnormalities. MRI of the brain and spinal cord shows multiple patchy lesions.

Course: Presenting symptoms often remit for months or years. Typically the disease progresses gradually, with remissions and exacerbations, and eventually produces some disability. Relapses may be triggered by excessive fatigue.

Treatment: Increased rest, particularly during periods of heightened symptoms. Adrenocortical steroids often mitigate neurologic impairment, particularly during acute relapses. Physical therapy and muscle relaxants are helpful in dealing with muscle weakness and spasm. Immunotherapy, plasmapheresis, and synthetic myelin protein are among treatments currently being evaluated. Psychotherapy or counseling may be necessary.

Guillain-Barré Syndrome

A chronic inflammation of peripheral nerves.

Cause: Formation of autoantibody to myelin, with resultant segmental demyelination of peripheral nerve fibers, usually reversible. Precipitating causes: acute infection (influenza, infectious mononucleosis, varicella-zoster), myocardial infarction, certain vaccines, surgery.

History: Symmetric muscle weakness, paresthesias, hypesthesias, and pain, coming on 1-4 weeks after the precipitating event. The cranial nerves and those of the upper and lower extremities may be involved. Loss of bladder control and respiratory paralysis may occur.

Physical Examination: Peripheral sensation is impaired and deep tendon reflexes are diminished or absent. The pulse and blood pressure may be elevated.

Diagnostic Tests: The spinal fluid contains elevated protein but normal cell counts.

Course: The case fatality rate is about 5%. About 80% of patients recover completely.

Treatment: Physical therapy; cardiac monitoring and pulse oximetry, with mechanical ventilation as needed. Plasmapheresis to remove antibody from serum.

Amyotrophic Lateral Sclerosis (Lou Gehrig Disease)

Progressive paralysis and wasting of muscles due to degeneration of motor neurons.

Cause: Unknown. There is a genetic predisposition, and men are affected more than women by a ratio of 3:1. Viral or autoimmune factors cannot be excluded. Possible precipitating factors include trauma, extreme stress or fatigue, viral respiratory infection, and myocardial infarction.

History: Onset, between the ages of 30 and 50, of weakness and wasting of voluntary muscles, particularly those in the hands and feet. **Fasciculations** (repeated twitching of small groups of voluntary muscle fibers) may precede any other symptoms. Eventually, with brain stem involvement, difficulty in speaking, eating, and even breathing. Depression commonly occurs with progressive deterioration.

Physical Examination: Muscle weakness and atrophy, visible fasciculations, evidence of cranial and spinal motor nerve malfunction without sensory impairment. Heightened deep tendon reflexes, spasticity, and rigidity indicate upper motor neuron degeneration.

Diagnostic Tests: Electromyography and muscle biopsy confirm loss of motor nerve supply to affected areas.

Course: Usually the disease is steadily progressive and death occurs in 2-5 years.

Treatment: Purely supportive; physical therapy, muscle relaxants; nasogastric tube or gastrostomy feedings, tracheotomy and respirator as needed.

Myasthenia Gravis

A chronic disorder of neuromuscular conduction.

Cause: Formation of autoantibody to the patient's own cholinergic receptors. The disease sometimes occurs in conjunction with other autoimmune disorders (rheumatoid arthritis, systemic lupus erythematosus), tumor of the thymus, or thyroid disease. It is commoner in women and onset is usually between the ages of 20 and 40. Severe infection or pregnancy may trigger the first evidence of disease.

History: The chief symptom is rapid fatiguing of muscles, particularly ocular, facial, and pharyngeal. Repeated movements lead to progressive weakening of the muscle, which recovers after an interval of rest.

Physical Examination: Patients may have ptosis, diplopia, difficulty in chewing or swallowing, but no muscle wasting, abnormalities of reflexes, or sensory impairment.

Diagnostic Tests: Anticholinesterase agents (intravenous edrophonium or intramuscular neostigmine) dramatically but briefly improve muscle strength and resistance to fatigue. Electromyography demonstrates progressive fatigue of stimulated muscles; serologic studies detect acetylcholine receptor antibody.

Treatment: Anticholinesterase drugs (neostigmine, pyridostigmine) and, if necessary, adrenal corticosteroids. When thymic tumor is present the thymus is surgically removed. Respiratory paralysis may require mechanical ventilation. Plasmapheresis to remove autoantibodies may be effective in severe exacerbations.

Parkinsonism (Parkinson Disease, Paralysis Agitans)

A chronic, progressive neurologic disorder causing muscle tremor and rigidity.

Cause: Unknown. Neurologic symptoms are due to deterioration and dopamine depletion in certain brain nuclei (corpus striatum, globus pallidus, substantia nigra). It is more common in men and onset is usually between 45 and 65. Certain toxic chemicals (carbon disulfide, carbon monoxide), drugs (chlorpromazine, haloperidol, and other neuroleptic drugs), and a history of encephalitis can induce parkinsonian symptoms.

History: Resting tremor, initially in one extremity, that is exacerbated by emotional stress and reduced during voluntary motion. Stiffness, rigidity, and **bradykinesia** (slowness of movement) commonly occur, with postural instability and gait disorders.

Physical Examination: Immobile, masklike face, with infrequent blinking. Reduced automatic movements such as swinging the arms while walking. Hyperactive deep tendon reflexes and resistance to passive movement of joints, often with **"cogwheel" rigidity**. A flexed posture, a shuffling and seemingly hurried (festinating) gait, and difficulty in standing from a sitting position are typical. Seborrhea (excessive secretion of sebum) on the scalp and face and excessive drooling are also often seen. The handwriting becomes smaller **(micrographia)**. There may be mild deterioration of mental function.

Course: Typically progressive, with death in about 10 years.

Treatment: Drug treatment is helpful in advanced disease: amantadine, anticholinergics (trihexyphenidyl, ethopropazine), levodopa and carbidopa, bromocriptine, and selegiline. Surgical removal of degenerating brain tissue may be a good choice in younger patients. Physical and speech therapy and counseling are important for most patients.

Infections of the Central Nervous System

Encephalitis

Inflammation of the brain due to viral infection.

Cause: Most cases of encephalitis are due to viruses transmitted by mosquitoes (Eastern and Western equine encephalitis, Japanese B encephalitis) or ticks. Numerous other viruses (coxsackievirus, herpes simplex virus, mumps virus, HIV) can cause encephalitis.

History: Abrupt onset of fever and headache, with muscle weakness or paralysis, restlessness, personality or behavioral changes, delirium, seizures, and lethargy perhaps progressing to coma.

Physical Examination: Fever, depressed level of consciousness, signs of meningeal irritation, evidence of focal or diffuse neurologic

damage including tremors, paralysis, hyperreactive reflexes, and pathologic reflexes.
Diagnostic Tests: Serologic studies can identify the causative virus. The CSF shows increase of pressure, protein, and cells. Abnormal findings on EEG are nonspecific.
Course: Most cases resolve without sequelae after a few weeks, but many are followed by residual paralysis, seizures, and parkinsonism.
Treatment: Largely supportive. Physical therapy; attention to nutrition and hydration. Drug therapy as needed to provide sedation, relieve fever and headache, and control convulsions. Herpes simplex encephalitis responds to acyclovir. In severe disease, adrenal corticosteroids may reduce cerebral edema and inflammation.

Brain Abscess

An abscess can be formed in the substance of the brain by pathogens migrating from infections of the ear or nose, or by bloodborne pathogens in patients with systemic infection. The usual agents are staphylococci and streptococci. Headache and drowsiness or delirium are the presenting symptoms, followed by seizures, coma, and focal neurologic abnormality depending on the location of the lesion. CT scan, MRI, and arteriography identify and localize the mass. Treatment is with intravenous antibiotics and, usually, surgical drainage of the abscess.

Meningitis

Infection of the meninges, with neurologic and systemic effects.
Causes: Infection with bacteria (staphylococcus, pneumococcus, meningococcus, *Haemophilus influenzae, Escherichia coli, Mycobacterium tuberculosis*), viruses (mumps virus, coxsackievirus, herpes simplex virus), fungi, or protozoans. Causative organisms may be introduced by a penetrating head wound, spread locally from infections of the ears or sinuses, or reach the meninges through the bloodstream from remote sites (pneumonia, endocarditis). Symptoms vary considerably with the etiologic agent; signs and symptoms are milder in viral than in bacterial meningitis, and the prognosis more favorable. Meningitis due to meningococcus (*Neisseria meningitidis*) is a rapidly progressive and highly lethal disease, particularly because the meningococcus causes a severe toxemia that can lead to shock and death, even in the absence of signs of meningitis.

History: Abrupt onset of fever, headache, and vomiting. Painful stiffness of the neck and back muscles, visual disturbances, and irritability, twitching, or seizures. Clouding of the sensorium, delirium, and coma may follow rapidly.

Physical Examination: Fever, depressed level of consciousness. **Nuchal rigidity**, painful stiffness of other muscles, hyperreflexia. **Kernig sign** (inability to extend the knee when the thigh is flexed). **Brudzinski sign** (passive flexion of the neck causes active flexion of the hip and knee). In an infant, bulging of the fontanelles.

Diagnostic Tests: Lumbar puncture shows elevated pressure. The CSF may be purulent. White blood cells and protein are elevated. In bacterial meningitis, CSF glucose is low. Smear and culture of the fluid identify bacterial agents. In viral (aseptic) meningitis the fluid is clear and the glucose is normal; viral culture may identify the cause.

Course: Without treatment, viral meningitis nearly always resolves without sequelae, and bacterial meningitis nearly always proves fatal, particularly in children and the elderly. Meningococcemia, an accompanying meningococcal meningitis, causes a petechial rash and profound and fulminant systemic abnormalities, including widespread hemorrhages and vascular collapse, sometimes due to adrenal hemorrhage (Waterhouse-Friderichsen syndrome). Patients who have recovered from meningitis may have residual mental retardation, paralysis, or seizures.

Treatment: Meningitis is an emergency. Hospitalization and administration of intravenous antibiotics are routine. Antibiotics are started even before reports of CSF studies are available, and discontinued or changed on the basis of these studies. Antibiotics are usually continued for three weeks or longer. Supportive care, including physical therapy, attention to nutrition and hydration, artificial ventilation, and measures to control fever, reverse shock, and reduce intracranial pressure, is vitally important.

Headache

Chronic or recurrent **headaches** can result from numerous causes, most of them not directly related to the nervous system. The most common type of headache is due to spasm in the muscles of the scalp, brow, and neck, most commonly induced by emotional stress or fatigue (**"tension headache"**). Two forms of headache originating in intracranial structures will be described here.

Migraine

Recurring severe unilateral headache with neurologic concomitants. **Cause**: Unknown. Head pain is apparently related to constriction, dilatation, and throbbing of meningeal and other vessels. Chemical factors (release of vasodilator substances, depletion of plasma serotonin) probably play a part. The disease runs in families and is more common in young women, affecting about 15% of adult women in the U.S. Oral contraceptives may bring on headaches in susceptible women.

History: Recurring episodes of severe unilateral throbbing headache accompanied by nausea, vomiting, photophobia, intolerance to noise, and sometimes neurologic symptoms (diplopia, transient local anesthesia or paralysis). In **classic migraine** the patient experiences a warning symptom (aura) before the headache begins. Most often this consists of seeing flashes or zigzags of light in both eyes, usually with transitory visual field defects (scintillating scotomas). In **common migraine** the aura does not occur, and headache may be less severe and more generalized. Headaches typically last for many hours and may be severely incapacitating. Often complete relief is not obtained until after sleep. In susceptible persons, a migraine headache may be triggered by emotional stress, fatigue, menstruation, skipping a meal, certain foods (chocolate, prepared foods containing nitrates), alcohol.

Physical Examination: Essentially normal during attacks, and entirely so between attacks.

Diagnostic Tests: Chiefly of use in ruling out more serious disorders; no specific findings.

Course: The disorder often begins in childhood and continues for many years. Depending on the presence of triggering factors, headaches may occur daily or only once a year.

Treatment: Mild analgesics sometimes help; nonsteroidal antiinflammatory drugs (ibuprofen, naproxen) and metoclopramide are often useful. Sumatriptan orally or by injection can abort a headache at any stage of its development. Ergotamine (orally, rectally, by injection or inhalation), with or without caffeine, frequently aborts an attack if taken immediately on the appearance of an aura. For patients who do not experience an aura, cannot take ergotamine or analgesics, or have extremely frequent headaches (one or more a week), prophylactic treatment usually provides good control. Prophylactic drugs include beta-adrenergic blocking agents (propranolol, atenolol) and others (amitriptyline).

Cluster Headache

Recurrent, brief episodes of severe unilateral orbital pain, of unknown cause. Attacks may come once or more daily for several weeks and then abruptly cease, perhaps recurring after an interval of weeks or months. Individual headaches may be triggered by alcohol or certain foods. The disorder is most often seen in middle-aged men. Headaches often occur at night, and are accompanied by redness and watering of the eye and by nasal congestion or rhinorrhea on the affected side. Each attack lasts about 20 minutes. There are no specific findings on examination or testing. Treatment of an acute attack with ergotamine or oxygen inhalation is sometimes effective. Prophylaxis against recurring headache may be achieved with ergotamine, lithium, adrenocortical steroids, methysergide, or the drugs used for prophylaxis of migraine headache.

Epilepsy

A neurologic disorder in which the patient experiences recurrent seizures consisting of transient disturbances of cerebral function due to paroxysmal neuronal discharge.

Causes: Seizure disorders, especially those first causing symptoms in childhood, are often idiopathic. Seizures can be induced by cerebral trauma, infection, vascular disease, neoplasms, degenerative diseases (Alzheimer disease), drugs and chemical poisons, metabolic disorders (renal failure, hypoglycemia), and, in children, high fever. In persons with idiopathic epilepsy, seizures may be triggered by physical or emotional stress, lack of sleep, fever, drugs, alcohol, alcohol withdrawal, menstruation, or flashing lights.

Symptoms: Seizures are classified on the basis of overt presentation:

Partial (only part of one cerebral cortex is involved).

Simple (no unconsciousness): local twitching or jerking; perception of flashing lights or other abnormal sensory phenomena.

Complex (impaired alertness or unconsciousness): sometimes with psychic symptoms or automatisms.

Generalized (entire cerebral cortex involved).

Absence (petit mal): brief loss of attention and perception.

Grand Mal (tonic-clonic): **Tonic phase**: victim becomes rigid, often cries out, loses consciousness, falls, stops breathing. **Clonic phase**:

generalized muscular jerking, may bite tongue or lips, may be incontinent of urine or stool. **Postictal state**: after awakening, subject is drowsy and amnesic for a variable period.

Myoclonic seizures: repeated shocklike, often violent contractions in one or more muscle groups.

Status epilepticus: series of grand mal seizures without waking intervals.

Physical Examination: Between seizures there is no detectable abnormality. Signs of neurologic disease may be found in secondary epilepsy.

Diagnostic Tests: The electroencephalogram generally shows focal abnormalities in the rate, rhythm, or relative intensity of cerebral cortical rhythms, allowing diagnosis and classification of epilepsy. Laboratory studies and CT scan or MRI may be performed to rule out treatable causes of epilepsy.

Treatment: In idiopathic epilepsy, long-term treatment with anticonvulsant medicine (phenytoin, carbamazepine, valproic acid, phenobarbital, ethosuximide, and others) provides excellent control for most patients. Blood levels of medicine may require monitoring to ensure optimum dosage. Avoidance of triggering factors is important. For intractable cases, surgical treatment is sometimes successful.

Transient Ischemic Attack and Stroke

Transient Ischemic Attack (TIA)

Sudden onset of neurologic symptoms that resolve completely within 24 hours.

Cause: Transient interruption of blood supply to some part of the brain. Common causes include blockage by emboli (from infected heart valves, mural thrombi, sloughed arteriosclerotic plaques) and reduction in blood supply due to the combined effects of arterial disease (arteritis, SLE) and reduced flow (hypotension, subclavian steal syndrome).

History: Sudden onset of focal neurologic symptoms (weakness, numbness, unilateral loss of vision, vertigo, ataxia, diplopia, drop attacks) depending on site of circulatory impairment, resolving in less than 24 hours (usually in less than 4 hours).

Physical Examination: Flaccid weakness or paralysis, hyperreflexia, hypesthesia or anesthesia, depending on site of lesion. All signs resolve within 24 hours.

Diagnostic Tests: CT scan may be done to rule out hemorrhage. Arteriography, MR angiography, or carotid duplex ultrasonography may be used to assess the cerebral circulation. X-ray, laboratory, and electrocardiography or echocardiography may trace the underlying cause.

Course: By definition a TIA has no complications. Many patients, however, will go on eventually to have one or more strokes.

Treatment: No treatment is needed for the acute episode, which has often resolved, before the patient is seen by a physician. Depending on the reason for the attacks, treatment directed against future attacks may include carotid endarterectomy, control of cardiac or systemic disease, and use of anticoagulant medicines. Long-term prophylactic administration of drugs that inhibit platelet aggregation (aspirin, ticlopidine) reduces the risk of further attacks. Heparin and coumadin may be needed if there is a major problem with thrombotic disease.

Stroke (Brain Attack, Cerebrovascular Accident, CVA)

Sudden onset of neurologic symptoms due to interruption of blood supply to some part of the brain. Stroke ranks third as a cause of death in the U.S.

Cause: Blockage of a cerebral artery by a clot (thrombosis) or embolus, or local hemorrhage from a cerebral vessel. Most cases are due to underlying vascular disease (arteriosclerosis, cerebral aneurysm, hypertension, diabetes mellitus, valvular heart disease).

History: Sudden onset of weakness, numbness or paralysis, usually on one side of the body, or other neurologic deficit (loss of vision, dizziness, difficulty speaking, confusion, loss of consciousness), depending on part of brain affected. Severe headache, vomiting, or seizures may also occur. Usually there is a history of cardiovascular disease, sometimes of preceding TIAs. Neurologic deficit may progress to coma and death.

Physical Examination: Evidence of neurologic deficit, depending on location and extent of brain tissue involved, and duration of circulatory impairment. Muscle weakness or paralysis, which may initially be flaccid but eventually becomes spastic, with rigidity, hyperreflexia, Babinski and other pathologic reflexes. Aphasia, confusion, delirium, coma.

Diagnostic Tests: CT scan of the head can show areas of hemorrhage or infarction. Magnetic resonance imaging may also be used, without contrast material. Lumbar puncture helps to distinguish thrombosis from hemorrhage (blood in fluid, elevated opening pressure). Blood studies, electrocardiography, and other diagnostic procedures may be used to identify underlying disease.

Course: Many cases of stroke resolve without any residual symptoms. Paralysis, weakness, or dementia may worsen. Stroke may progress rapidly to a fatal termination when the damage is extensive.

Treatment: If neurologic impairment is progressive and hemorrhage has been ruled out, anticoagulants (IV heparin followed by oral coumadin) are used during the acute phase. In selected cases, tissue plasminogen activator (tPA) may be administered to dissolve a freshly formed thrombus. Vigorous supportive treatment (oxygen, parenteral nutrition, prevention of respiratory and urinary tract infection, prevention of bedsores) must be instituted early. Physical therapy is important to maintain mobility and achieve maximum rehabilitation as neurologic function returns. Braces or splints may be necessary to promote mobility despite weakness of certain muscle groups.

Altered Consciousness

Depression of the level of consciousness or alertness can result from a wide variety of causes, some intracranial (trauma, hemorrhage, infection, neoplasm, vascular obstruction, increased intracranial pressure) and some systemic (anoxia, hypercapnia, shock, drugs, chemical poisons, electrolyte imbalance, hepatic or renal failure). Various grades of impaired consciousness are roughly distinguished as **clouding** or **blunting** (**obtusion**) of the sensorium, drowsiness (**somnolence**), stupor, semicoma, and (deep) coma. Coma demands vigorous diagnostic efforts (thorough history and physical examination with emphasis on neurologic findings, funduscopic examination, blood and urine studies, lumbar puncture, EEG, and head imaging). A widely used measure of the level of consciousness is the **Glasgow Coma Scale** (see box). Treatment of coma includes attention to airway, respiratory function, and circulation, and vigorous efforts to reverse or eliminate identifiable causes. Delirium and dementia are discussed as mental disorders in the next chapter.

Glasgow Coma Scale		
Best motor response (upper extremity)	6	Obeys command
	5	Localizes pain
	4	Withdraws from stimulus
	3	Abnormal flexing
	2	Extensor response
	1	None
Best verbal response	5	Oriented (makes sentences)
	4	Confused speech (words)
	3	Gibberish (vocal sounds)
	2	Incomprehensible sounds
	1	None
Eye opening	4	Spontaneous
	3	To speech
	2	To pain
	1	None

Peripheral Neuropathy

Disease or damage affecting one or more peripheral nerves, with resultant impairment of sensory or motor function or both. **Mononeuritis** is impairment of function in a single peripheral nerve. Polyneuritis is peripheral neuritis involving more than one nerve.

Mononeuritis

Causes: Trauma, local compression or entrapment (carpal tunnel syndrome, Bell palsy, both discussed below), local disease or infection (sarcoidosis, amyloidosis, Lyme disease, leprosy), or systemic disease (see systemic causes under *polyneuritis* below).

History: Hypesthesia, anesthesia, paresthesia, causalgia, weakness, wasting of muscles.

Physical Examination: Reflexes diminished or absent, muscular atrophy.

Diagnostic Tests: Electromyography and nerve conduction velocity tests confirm neural malfunction. Other studies may be undertaken to find the basic cause.

Treatment: Treatment of the underlying cause, when possible. Surgery, physical therapy.

Two common types of mononeuritis due to nerve entrapment are discussed here in more detail.

Carpal Tunnel Syndrome

Pain, tingling, and hypesthesia or anesthesia in the **thenar** (part of the palm proximal to the thumb and index finger), with weakness and eventual atrophy in muscles of the thenar supplied by the **median nerve**, as a result of compression of this nerve on the volar aspect of the wrist where it passes through the carpal tunnel, formed by wrist bones and the non-yielding carpal ligament. Many cases are induced by repetitive wrist flexion, as in jobs or hobbies. The incidence is increased during pregnancy and among persons with certain systemic diseases (diabetes mellitus, hyperthyroidism, rheumatoid arthritis).

Pain and tingling sometimes wake the patient at night, and elicit the response of shaking the hand to restore normal feeling. **Tinel sign** (shocklike pain when the volar aspect of the wrist is tapped) and **Phalen sign** (reproduction of pain or paresthesia when both wrists are flexed with the hands firmly pressing one another back to back for 60 seconds) are positive. Electromyography and nerve conduction velocity studies can confirm the site of nerve compression. Treatment is by removal of known underlying causes; splinting, at least at night; physical therapy; local injection of corticosteroid; and often surgical division of the carpal ligament.

Bell Palsy

Weakness or paralysis of muscles on one side of the face caused by inflammation or compression of the seventh cranial nerve (facial nerve) as it passes through the bony facial canal and emerges at the stylomastoid foramen behind the ear. The cause is unknown, but exposure to cold and herpes simplex virus infection have been suggested. Onset of symptoms is often accompanied by pain below or behind the ear. Onset of facial weakness is characteristically abrupt, producing a characteristic asymmetry of the face and diminished ability or inability to close the eyes, smile, or purse the lips. Speech and eating may be slightly disturbed. There may be impairment of hearing and taste on the tip of the tongue. The diagnosis is clinically evident, but electromyography and nerve conduction velocity studies may give indications of prognosis. More than half of cases resolve spontaneously in a few days to a few weeks, but residual weakness and asymmetry of the face, occasionally severe, may be permanent. For mild cases no treatment is necessary; systemic corticosteroids are prescribed if the paralysis is complete when first seen by the physician.

Polyneuritis

Causes: Hereditary (Charcot-Marie-Tooth disease, Dejerine-Sottas disease, Friedreich's ataxia), metabolic (diabetes mellitus, uremia), vitamin deficiency, alcoholism, drugs (INH, phenytoin), chemical poisons (lead, arsenic), autoimmunity (Guillain-Barré syndrome).

History: Essentially as for mononeuritis (see above), but involving nerves throughout the body, often in an irregular and shifting pattern.

Physical Examination: As in mononeuritis.

Diagnostic Tests: As in mononeuritis. Emphasis is on finding a systemic cause (diabetes mellitus, other metabolic diseases, lead poisoning).

Treatment: Removal or treatment of underlying cause, if possible. Otherwise as for mononeuritis.

Topics for Study or Discussion

1. Which cranial nerves exert their influence below the level of the head?

2. List five parts of the cranial nerve examination and five parts of the spinal nerve examination that cannot be performed on an unconscious patient.

3. Define or explain: ataxia, axon, Babinski reflex, lumbar puncture, polyneuritis, myelin, neuron, traumatic tap.

4. Distinguish between upper motor neuron lesions and lower motor neuron lesions.

5. Name three neurologic disorders that are inherited; three that are caused by systemic disease; and three that are usually lethal.

Chapter 19

Mental Disorders

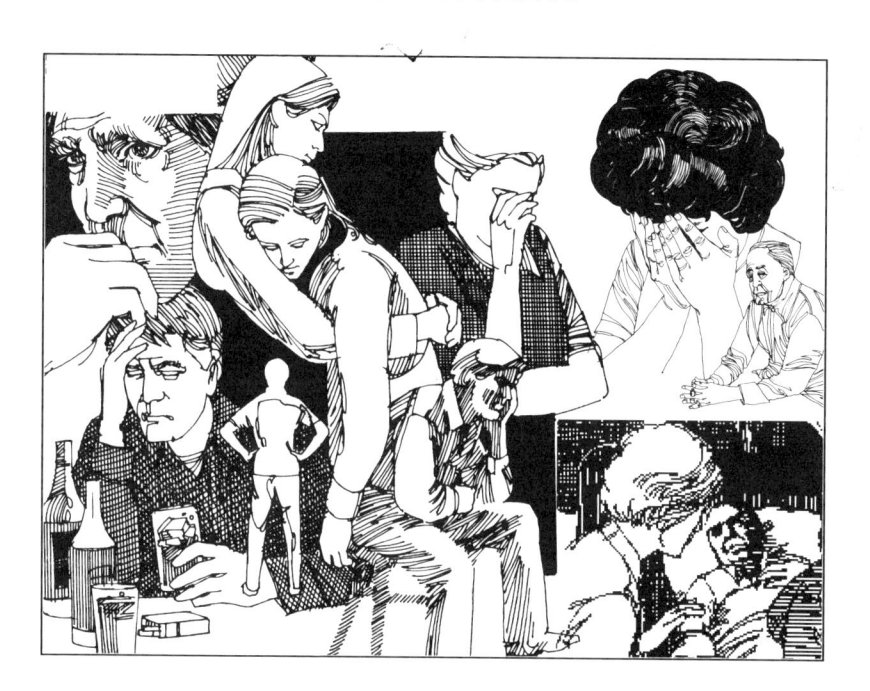

Learning Objectives

Upon completion of this chapter, the student should

- have a general understanding of current concepts as to the nature and causes of mental disorders;

- know the major categories of mental disorders, and distinguishing features of some of the commoner ones;

- have basic information about the treatment of mental disorders.

Introductory Remarks

Disorders of perception, mood, and behavior have always been placed in a separate category from other illnesses, by both physicians and laity. Except for a few conditions obviously caused by organic disease or injury of the central nervous system (alcoholic dementia, inability to speak after head injury or a stroke), mental illnesses were long thought to result from failure of normal personality development, inadequate adaptation to life stresses, acquired distortions of thought processes, and other vague and intangible factors. The specialty of **psychiatry** came into being as a field concentrating on disturbances of mood and thought for which no organic basis could be found.

Within the past few decades, psychiatric theory has undergone remarkable changes in orientation. With important exceptions, most modern psychologists and psychiatrists believe that *all* mental disorders are due to **structural**, **chemical**, or **electrical abnormalities** in the brain. This idea is supported by abundant evidence from diverse sources. Genetic studies show that many mental disorders run in families, and some have actually been traced to specific chromosomal abnormalities.

Biochemical research has established a correlation between the distribution of neurotransmitters such as **serotonin, dopamine**, and **norepinephrine** in the central nervous system and certain disorders of **cognition, mood**, and **behavior**. A chemical basis has been found for the way in which many drugs help in mental disorders, and new drugs designed with specific chemical goals have attained their object of providing improved control of anxiety, depression, and other common disorders. Although **drug therapy** may still be considered an adjunct to counseling and other forms of psychotherapy, for many disorders it is currently the most rapid, effective, and predictable mode of treatment.

Mental illnesses have been precisely defined and classified by the American Psychiatric Association in a publication called the *Diagnostic and Statistical Manual of Mental Disorders (DSM)*. The fourth edition of this book (*DSM-IV*), published in 1994, is based on and correlated with the classification, nomenclature, and code numbering of the *International Classification of Diseases*, ninth edition (*ICD-9*). It categorizes mental disorders and defines them according to precise and stringent diagnostic criteria. Ideally, all professional use of terminology regarding mental disorders should conform to the standards of *DSM-IV*. Access to a copy of this book is indispensable for the allied health professional who works with records pertaining to mental illness.

The following definition of mental disorder is abridged slightly from *DSM-IV*: a clinically significant behavioral or psychological syndrome or pattern that occurs in an individual and is associated with present distress or disability, or with a significant risk of suffering, death, pain, disability, or loss of freedom.

The principal diagnostic method used by psychiatrists in identifying or classifying mental illness is the formal **mental status examination**. This is a group of diagnostic assessments based on observation, history as related by the patient and others, and analysis of data gathered through interviewing the patient. The mental status examination may be performed in a single session, or may be gradually completed through several sessions. Some parts may not be able to be completed at all if the patient is entirely out of touch with reality, or is unable to respond to questions or commands.

The formal **mental status examination** consists of the following parts:

Appearance: Dress, grooming, makeup, hair care, jewelry or other adornments; slovenly, unkempt, bizarre, mismatched, or incongruous garments or adornments.

Sensorium: Responsiveness to visual, auditory, and tactile stimuli; alertness, attention span; ability to recognize and classify objects.

Activity and Behavior: Gait, posture, level of motor activity, speech; bizarre or compulsive actions, mannerisms, posturings, automatisms, mimicry.

Mood (Affect): Basic emotional state, and emotional content of responses to examiner (apathetic, blunted, depressed, elated, euphoric, flat, inappropriate, labile).

Thought Content: Unconventional thoughts, fantasies, phobias, obsessive ideas, delusions, hallucinations, poverty of imagination.

Intellectual Function: Speed, coherence, and relevance of abstract reasoning; mental arithmetic, interpretation of idioms ("time on your hands") and proverbs ("a rolling stone gathers no moss").

Orientation: Awareness of time ("What day, month, year is it?"), place ("Where are we? What city is this?"), person (ability to identify self, relatives, friends).

Memory: Recall of recent and remote events; general information ("How many cents in a quarter? Who is the president?"); confabulation.

Judgment: Competence in analyzing situations, solving problems, taking practical action ("What would you do if the house across the street caught fire?").

Insight: The patient's awareness of being ill or impaired, and awareness of the nature of the problem.

There is a certain overlapping of material between parts of the mental status examination. Some of the observations pertain to the field of neurology rather than psychiatry. In addition to the mental status examination outlined above, the patient may be asked to complete one or more formal, standardized tests of intelligence and personality.

The following pages contain information about some of the more common mental disorders. If you encounter unfamiliar terms, look them up in the glossary at the end of the chapter. The glossary contains a large number of terms not appearing in the text of this chapter.

Anxiety Disorders

A group of mental disorders characterized by chronic worry or fear. **Anxiety disorders** are the most common ones seen by psychiatrists; often anxiety accompanies other disorders (depression, schizophrenia).

Cause: Probably a malfunction in the part of the brain called the reticular formation. This system regulates sleep and wakefulness as well as many autonomic and endocrine functions. Persons with chronic anxiety have abnormal levels of certain neurotransmitters (norepinephrine, serotonin, gamma-aminobutyric acid) in brain tissue.

History: Persisting or recurring feelings of apprehension, uneasiness, worry, or fear (with or without a clearly defined object) that is out of proportion to any actual danger or threat. The sense of dread may become so absorbing as to distract the patient's attention from personal, social, and occupational activities. Anxiety may be triggered by a wide variety of settings and circumstances. Besides the mental condition of constant worry or dread, the patient usually experiences physical signs of autonomic and endocrine response: heightened muscle tension, rapid pulse, hyperventilation, sweating, insomnia, problems with appetite and sexual function. *DSM-IV* lists specific criteria for fourteen anxiety disorders. Five of these are described here.

Generalized Anxiety Disorder. An abiding state of excessive, distressing, and disabling worry about a number of issues, associated with restlessness, muscle tension, irritability, abnormal fatigue, and insomnia. The condition is twice as common in women, and often accompanies depression.

Social Phobia. The most common anxiety disorder. A phobia is an irrational fear of some object or situation, with resulting efforts to avoid it. While recognizing that the fear is unfounded or out of proportion to any actual danger, the victim of a phobia is unable to overcome it. The victim of social phobia experiences an exaggerated and persistent fear of embarrassment or humiliation in a social setting, or when appearing or performing in public. This can lead to severe social, educational, or occupational disability. Many persons with this disorder also suffer from depression or alcoholism.

Agoraphobia. An intense fear of being alone or being in a public place from which escape might be difficult, or help unavailable, in case of sudden incapacitation (such as passing out or having a heart attack). Victims of agoraphobia avoid open spaces, crowded enclosures such as stores or churches, tunnels, elevators, and public transportation.

Panic Disorder. Recurring sudden, spontaneous attacks of intense anxiety, lasting minutes or hours, and accompanied by marked physical symptoms such as chest pain, tachycardia, dyspnea or choking, sweating, faintness, tremors, and tingling in the extremities. Because of the type and severity of physical symptoms, panic disorder is sometimes mistaken for a heart attack or other life-threatening emergency by both the victim and others, including physicians. Although either agoraphobia or panic disorder can occur by itself, the two are often associated in the same patient.

Obsessive-Compulsive Disorder (OCD). A chronic anxiety disorder in which the patient suffers from both obsessions and compulsions. An obsession is a recurring or persisting idea, thought, or image that is perceived as intrusive, distracting, and repugnant, but that the victim is unable to ignore or suppress. Examples are recurring thoughts of harming oneself or others; fear of contamination or infections; and worry about losing or throwing away something that is or may later become important. A compulsion is an urge to repeat a ritualistic or stereotyped form of behavior that is recognized by the victim as irrational but that cannot be omitted without an increase of anxiety. Examples include excessive, repetitive handwashing; rigid attention to order or symmetry;

repeated checking of locks, switches, or clocks; and performance of everyday actions in a ritualized fashion.

Treatment: The treatment of an anxiety disorder depends on the exact nature of the disorder, its source, and its symptoms. Individual or group psychotherapy can provide emotional support, help the patient to gain insight into the nature of the problem, encourage psychic growth and maturation, and teach positive attitudes and goal-directed behavior. Most anxiety disorders respond well to short-term or long-term drug treatment. Agents that reduce the level of uneasiness and worry are called **anxiolytics**. Most of the anxiolytics in current use belong to the benzodiazepine class (alprazolam, oxazepam). Certain drugs used in the treatment of depression (fluoxetine, fluvoxamine) are useful in obsessive-compulsive disorder. Beta-adrenergic blocking agents such as propranolol can control the autonomic component of performance anxiety, social phobia, and panic disorder (tachycardia, sweaty palms, tremors).

Mood Disorders

Mood disorders include all emotional problems in which extreme variation from a normal sense of emotional comfort and well-being (varying from depression to mania) is the principal symptom. Major depression and bipolar disorder, the chief clinical presentations of mood disorder, are discussed in this section.

Major Depression (Clinical Depression)

Sustained or recurring periods of sadness and hopelessness.

Cause: Probably electrochemical malfunction in the limbic system of the brain, which is the principal focus of emotional activity and is intimately associated with memory areas and those concerned with autonomic and endocrine function. Disturbances in the levels, distribution, and metabolism of the neurotransmitters serotonin and dopamine appear to be responsible for emotional symptoms. In the form of depression known as **seasonal affective disorder** (SAD), patients experience low mood, increased desire for food and sleep, and a reduction in activity level as a consequence of the weather (colder, darker, shorter days of winter, with limited opportunities for recreation, especially outdoors). Depression in its various forms is second only to anxiety in incidence, and it often occurs in conjunction with anxiety. It is two to three times more common in women and tends to run in families. There is strong evidence of a genetic predisposition to depressive illness. It is more common in persons who have problems with drugs or alcohol, chronic physical illness, stressful life events, social isolation, or a history of being sexually abused. The first episode typically occurs before age 40. Recurrences are common.

History: Depressed, dejected, or blue mood accompanied by marked reduction of interest or pleasure in virtually all activities, gain or loss of weight, increased or decreased sleep, increased or decreased level of psychomotor activity, fatigue, feelings of guilt or worthlessness, diminished ability to concentrate, hopelessness, and recurring thoughts of death or suicide.

Treatment: A number of highly effective drugs are available to treat depression. These include the older **tricyclic compounds** (amitriptyline, imipramine), the **selective serotonin reuptake inhibitors (SSRIs)** (fluoxetine, sertraline), **monoamine oxidase inhibitors** (pargyline, phenelzine), and other agents (nefazodone, sertraline). Most patients experience troublesome side effects (drowsiness, headaches, dry mouth, disturbances of gastrointestinal or sexual function), but these tend to reduce or disappear with continued use. Typically it takes four to six weeks for antidepressant action to be noted. Counseling and other forms of psychotherapy may be useful in hastening remission and reducing the risk of relapse. Seasonal affective disorder often responds to exposure to bright light several hours a day during the winter. For severe depression that does not respond to drug therapy, electroshock therapy is controversial but sometimes beneficial.

Bipolar Disorder (Manic-Depressive Disorder)

A type of depressive illness in which the patient's mood oscillates between depression and mania.

Cause: Apparently a malfunction of the limbic system. Susceptibility to this disorder has been traced to a gene on chromosome 18. Half of patients have at least one parent with an affective disorder.

History: Alternations of mood between **mania** and **clinical depression**, with variable intervals of normal mood in between. A manic episode is a period of abnormal elevation of mood, irritability, or restlessness that lasts at least one week and is accompanied by some or all of the following: inflated self-esteem, hyperactivity, **flight of ideas**, abnormal talkativeness or **pressured speech** (rapid, strained speech as if the subject's mouth can't keep up with the flow of thoughts), reduced need for sleep, short attention span, and reckless behavior. Unlike anxiety and simple depression, bipolar disorder may include a loss of touch with reality; that is, it may be a true psychosis. During either the manic or the depressive phase, the patient may experience delusions or hallucinations, or may display grossly bizarre behavior.

Treatment: Drug therapy with lithium salts, carbamazepine, or valproic acid usually controls the manic phase of bipolar disorder and helps to prevent recurrences of mania. **Tranquilizers** and **antidepressants** may also be used. Mania generally causes severe impairment of social and occupational functioning and may require hospitalization.

Attention-Deficit Hyperactivity Disorder (ADHD)

A chronic behavioral disorder, most striking in children, involving hyperactivity, short attention span, and impulsiveness.

Cause: The disease runs in families, and about 25% of patients have at least one parent who is similarly affected. It is 3-8 times more common in boys. Magnetic resonance imaging has shown abnormalities in the corpus callosum, the band of fibers connecting the two cerebral hemispheres. The theory that sugar and food colorings or other additives trigger hyperactivity is entirely without scientific support.

History: Often there is evidence of behavioral disturbance in infancy, and the full-blown disorder is typically recognizable by the age of 6. The three cardinal features of ADHD are **inattentiveness** (short attention span, distractability, inability to complete tasks undertaken, difficulty in following directions, tendency to lose personal articles, disregard for personal safety), **impulsiveness** (blurting out one's thoughts without adequate reflection, butting in front of others in waiting lines), and **hyperactivity** (restlessness, fidgeting, or squirming instead of sitting or standing still, excessive talking). Children with this disorder have a high incidence of academic failure, conflict with parents, teachers, and law enforcement officials, antisocial behavior, and substance abuse.

Treatment: Central nervous system stimulants (dextroamphetamine, methylphenidate, and pemoline) are usually successful in enhancing learning ability and improving social functioning. These medicines are taken early in the day so as to avoid nighttime insomnia. When improvement in academic achievement is the chief goal of treatment, the patient may be given "drug holidays" on weekends and during school vacations.

Schizophrenia

A chronic or recurring **psychosis** due to a disorder of thought processes.

Cause: Susceptibility to schizophrenia is probably inherited as a complex of variations affecting several genes. Neurophysiologic studies have shown abnormally small size of the part of the brain called the thalamus, and changes in signal intensity in adjacent white matter.

History: Gradual onset, usually before age 40, of cognitive malfunctions—disturbances of perception and thinking characterized by **delusions**, **hallucinations**, gross distortion of mental function, or all of these. These basic features of schizophrenia are usually accompanied by reduced energy level, flat or depressed **affect**, **anhedonia** (inability to experience pleasure from normally pleasurable activities), and **abulia** (diminished ability to make decisions). Virtually all patients display impoverished thought content, social withdrawal, and impairment of occupational functioning. Even with intensive psychotherapy and drug treatment, about 25% of persons with schizophrenia require custodial or institutional care. Schizophrenia is divided, on the basis of dominant clinical manifestations, into the following types:

disorganized (hebephrenic) schizophrenia: severe breakdown of mental function and incongruous or silly behavior.

paranoid schizophrenia: prominent delusions of persecution or grandeur, often reinforced by hallucinations.

catatonic schizophrenia: statue-like posturing, rigidity, or stupor.

undifferentiated schizophrenia: without defining features.

residual schizophrenia: history of schizophrenia but only mild, non-psychotic residual impairment of mental function.

Treatment: Psychotherapy is inconsistently effective in helping patients overcome disordered thinking and improving social functioning. The modern treatment of schizophrenia depends heavily on the use of drugs known as **neuroleptics** or **antipsychotics**. The older members of this class belong to the group known chemically as **phenothiazines** (chlorpromazine, fluphenazine, trifluoperazine). Patients treated with these drugs frequently develop **parkinsonian symptoms**, including tremors, rigidity, and **akathisia** (extreme restlessness, inability to remain seated). These may be adequately controlled with drugs used to treat parkinsonism (benztropine, trihexyphenidyl). A few suffer from **tardive dyskinesia**, an irreversible neurologic disorder causing twitching and writhing movements, particularly in the lips and tongue. Neuroleptics in other classes (clozapine, haloperidol, risperidone) are useful alternatives but have their own side-effects. Fluphenazine and haloperidol can be given as long-acting injections to patients who have trouble complying with daily oral medicine regimens.

Delirium and Dementia

Transitory or irreversible impairment of cognitive functions due to organic changes in the cerebral cortex.

Delirium
An acute, often reversible disturbance of brain function characterized by confusion and impairment of consciousness, memory, attention, and mood.

Cause: Usually systemic: intoxication by alcohol or drugs, including prescribed medicines; withdrawal from alcohol (**delirium tremens**) or drugs; acute infection; endocrine disease (adrenal, pancreatic, pituitary, thyroid); disturbances of electrolyte balance, cardiopulmonary function, or nutrition; degenerative or neoplastic disease of the brain; and head trauma. Deficiency of thiamin in chronic alcoholism can cause either or both of two psychotic disorders: **Korsakoff syndrome** (amnesia with confabulation) and **Wernicke encephalopathy** (confusion with neurologic symptoms such as ataxia and ocular paresis).

History: Disorientation and mental confusion, typically of sudden onset, with other evidences of brain malfunction in varying degrees and proportions: impairment of alertness, inability to concentrate, delusions, hallucinations, loss of impulse control, loss of short-term memory, restlessness, and depression.

Treatment: Depends on the cause. Often the only treatment needed is discontinuing medicines with central nervous system side effects. Alcoholic psychoses may respond to intravenous thiamin.

Dementia

Chronic, progressive deterioration of mental function.

Cause: Dementia can be caused by any disease process or agent that destroys or damages cells in the cerebral cortex or association areas of the brain. More than half of all cases of dementia are due to **Alzheimer disease**, a genetically determined degenerative disease of cortical neurons that typically begins in late middle life. Atherosclerotic obstruction of blood flow to the cerebral cortex (**multi-infarct dementia**) accounts for another 20%. Among other causes of dementia may be mentioned **Creutzfeldt-Jakob disease**, **Huntington chorea**, and disorders related to **chronic alcoholism**. Some cases of dementia are due to **systemic disease** or **chemical intoxication**, often from prescribed medicines.

History: Usually gradual onset of steadily progressive deterioration of certain mental functions: short-term memory loss, inability to understand spoken or written language and to express oneself in speech and writing, diminished or distorted sensory perception, inability to perform purposeful actions, personality changes with irritability and depression, deterioration of impulse control.

Course: Depends on the cause of the disorder. Most dementias are irreversible and progressive. Alzheimer disease and arteriosclerotic dementias typically culminate in death within 5-10 years.

Treatment: Most forms of dementia respond poorly to medical treatment. In some patients, tacrine produces improvement in cognitive function. **Anxiolytics**, **neuroleptics**, and **antidepressants** may be used to control disorders of mood and behavior. **Behavioral therapy** is sometimes successful in reinforcing acceptable behavior and extinguishing unacceptable behavior. A comfortable, secure environment (preferably home, unless the patient is too disruptive or the burden of care too taxing for the family), with familiar faces and a simple, steady routine, provide a setting in which the patient's impairments are least distressing and disabling. Support and counsel for the family are of major importance in Alzheimer disease and other dementias in which long-term home care is appropriate.

Glossary

As mentioned earlier, this glossary contains many terms that do not appear in the text of the chapter. Please continue reading in order to learn new material and reinforce material already learned.

affect: one's prevailing mood or emotional state, pleasant or unpleasant, particularly as perceived by the examiner.

amnesia: loss of memory.

aversion therapy: a form of behavior therapy that associates an objectionable or undesirable pattern of behavior with an unpleasant experience or consequence, so as to reduce or extinguish the behavior.

behavior (behavioral) therapy: any type of psychotherapy that focuses on the alteration or correction of undesirable behavior, including such responses to external stimuli as anxiety, depression, and physical symptoms of emotion (tachycardia, muscle tension, sweating). Behavior therapy uses conditioning, muscle relaxation techniques, meditation, breathing retraining, biofeedback, guided learning, and other methods.

client: the recipient of psychotherapy; a term preferred to "patient" when the therapist is not a physician.

client-centered therapy: a form of psychotherapy in which the client is encouraged, with a minimum of direction by the therapist, to discover the sources of distressing mental symptoms and means of resolving them.

cognitive therapy: a form of psychotherapy based on promoting the client's rational understanding of the source of distressing emotions, thought patterns, and undesirable behaviors, and correction of these by adoption of more mature, balanced, and realistic attitudes.

compensation (overcompensation): a mechanism by which one covers up a defect or weakness by exaggerating or overdeveloping some other property or faculty.

confabulation: invention of stories about one's past, often bizarre and complex, to fill in gaps left by amnesia; a typical feature of Korsakoff syndrome in chronic alcoholics.

cyclothymia: abnormal lability of mood, which varies between excitement and depression without becoming severe enough to be called bipolar disorder.

delusion: a distorted belief or perception, such as thinking that one is a famous historical figure (Jesus, Napoleon) or that one is the object of persecution.

denial: a mechanism by which one refuses to believe, remember, or accept an unpleasant fact or circumstance, such as a past painful experience or the fact of being ill.

dysphoria: a general feeling of mental or emotional discomfort.

dysthymia: a depressed mood, usually chronic or recurrent, that is not severe enough to be called major depression.

electroconvulsive (electroshock) therapy: delivery of controlled electric shocks to the brain to alter electrochemical function, primarily in depression. The treatment, administered only by a physician, causes convulsions and loss of consciousness; the patient awakens in a state of disorientation. Several treatment sessions may be necessary before improvement is noted.

encephalopathy: any organic disease or damage of the brain, particularly the cerebral cortex, that causes impairment of mental or physical functioning; often due to degenerative diseases (Alzheimer disease, Creutzfeldt-Jakob disease) or chemical intoxications (alcohol, lead).

family therapy: psychotherapy that treats the family as a unit and seeks to promote understanding and correction of pathologic attitudes and relationships among members of the unit.

guilt: a sense of having done wrong, of having failed to meet one's own or others' expectations or standards, or of being inferior or inadequate; as used in psychiatry and psychoanalysis, guilt is a distinct concept from legal or moral guilt, which arises from deliberate violation of moral or civil rules.

group therapy: psychotherapy administered to several persons at once, making use of sharing of perceptions, experiences, and feelings, group dynamics, and mutual understanding and support.

hallucination: a sensory experience, usually auditory or visual, without any physical basis—for example, seeing snakes floating in the air, or hearing voices urging one to do something.

hypnosis: a technique in which the therapist places the client into a sleeplike trance in which outside stimuli are reduced to a minimum, the subconscious is more directly accessible, and the client is more susceptible to the influence of the therapist's suggestions and advice.

identification: a mental process whereby one takes on the properties or actions of another with whom an emotional tie exists (a boy walking and talking like his father; a woman dressing and behaving like a movie idol);

libido: sexual desire or drive; often, more generally, the totality of pleasure-directed energy or activity.

mechanism (also defense mechanism, ego-defensive mechanism, mental mechanism, unconscious mechanism): an automatic, unconscious mental process whereby repressed emotions (painful feelings, sexual urges) generate new beliefs or attitudes to protect the ego from a sense of guilt, inadequacy, or other negative feelings; see compensation, identification, projection, rationalization, repression, sublimation.

narcissism: extreme self-love; excessive preoccupation with oneself and one's own concerns and needs, to the exclusion of normal emotional ties with others.

neurosis: a mental disorder in which the patient experiences, and gives evidence of, emotional distress, but remains in touch with reality at all times.

neurotransmitter: a normal chemical substance produced in minute quantities by nerve tissue and involved in the transmission of electrical impulses from one nerve cell to another; the effect of a neurotransmitter may be to stimulate or inhibit the nerve cell on which it acts; well-known neurotransmitters include acetylcholine, dopamine, epinephrine, gamma-aminobutyric acid (GABA), norepinephrine, and serotonin.

pharmacotherapy: treatment with drugs, generally prescription drugs; only physicians (but not necessarily physicians specializing in psychiatry) are permitted by law to prescribe drugs.

play therapy: a form of psychotherapy used with children, in which structured or unstructured play settings with dolls and other toys enable the therapist to identify and correct false or unhealthy attitudes and behavior patterns.

projection: a mechanism whereby one unconsciously attributes one's own thoughts and attitudes (usually negative or unpleasant) to others as a means of dealing with a sense of guilt or inadequacy.

psyche: a vague term roughly equivalent to "mind."

psychiatry: the branch of medicine concerned with the diagnosis and treatment of mental disorders; all psychiatrists are physicians.

psychoanalysis: a school of clinical psychology founded by Sigmund Freud (see box) and based on lengthy, searching analysis of the patient's mental life, including particularly the content of the subconscious, which can be made manifest by hypnosis, dream interpretation, free association (nondirected reflections voiced by the patient), and other methods; many

The founder of both psychoanalysis and modern psychiatry was **Sigmund Freud** (1856-1939), a Viennese physician specializing in neurology. Early in his career he became interested in cases of physical impairment (paralysis, blindness) in which there was no evidence of an organic lesion and which sometimes resolved after the correction of a medical disorder.

Freud went on to formulate the theory, universally accepted today, that much of a person's mental life is subconscious—not accessible to reflection or memory, yet exerting a potent influence on attitudes, behavior, emotional state, mood, and general physical well-being.

Freud used hypnotism, dream interpretation, and prolonged analytic sessions with the patient to unlock hidden sources of mental and physical illness in the subconscious. The system he developed, known as **psychoanalysis**, was both diagnostic and therapeutic: through interaction with the therapist and gradual attainment of insight into subconscious thoughts, associations, wishes, and fears, the patient gains understanding of the problems and finds ways of solving them.

According to Freud's view, the human personality consists of three parts: the **ego**, each person's conscious view of reality and personal identity; the **id**, an unconscious reservoir of self-preserving and pleasure-seeking, particularly sexual, instincts and drives; and the **superego**, or conscience, a largely unconscious product of both ego and id, which monitors the ego.

Freud posited the existence of many ego-defensive mechanisms, including repression, compensation, and rationalization, by which we attempt to preserve equanimity and self-esteem despite personal failings, life stresses, and the rejection or hostility of others.

Freud lived to see his discoveries and theories accepted throughout the world. Many of his disciples went on to found their own schools of psychoanalysis. Although few modern students of mental illness accept all of Freud's original theories, he is universally honored as the discoverer of the subconscious and of ways to discover its ills and heal them.

psychiatrists are psychoanalysts, but not all psychoanalysts are psychiatrists (physicians).

psychodrama: a type of group therapy in which clients resolve conflicts and distressing emotional states by acting out their fantasies and fears in the setting of a dramatic performance, before an audience of fellow clients.

psychology: broadly, the study of all mental processes and functions (perception, memory, judgment, learning ability, mood, social interaction, communication, and others). Clinical psychology is a professional discipline concerned with the nonmedical treatment of mental disorders; a clinical psychologist ordinarily does not hold a medical degree.

psychosis: a mental disorder in which, in addition to emotional distress, the patient experiences a break with reality, manifested by delusions, hallucinations, and grossly bizarre or socially inappropriate behavior.

psychotherapy: any method or technique, except the administration of medicines, used in the treatment of mental disorders.

rational therapy: a form of treatment in which mental disorders, which are thought to result from misinformation, wrong belief systems, and distorted logic, are improved by the therapist's use of direct, positive teaching and advice.

rationalization: a mental process of justifying some act or omission through logical reasoning or argumentation, usually as a means of reducing feelings of guilt or inadequacy.

reality testing: the ability of an individual to perceive reality as it is, not as distorted by abnormal thought processes, disorders of perception, delusions, or hallucinations.

repression: the mental process of thrusting out of consciousness impulses or desires that are perceived as incompatible with one's own standards or sense of fitness, and that therefore generate unpleasant emotions; repressed material occupies a large part of the subconscious.

subconscious (mind): elements of one's personality (feelings, attitudes, prejudices, desires, behavior patterns) of which one is unaware; a general and somewhat vague term including but not always identical to what Freud called the unconscious (*Unbewusstsein*).

therapist: one who treats; in mental health, anyone administering psychotherapy.

suicidal ideation: thoughts of committing suicide as a relief from mental distress, without actual attempts at suicide.

sublimation: diversion of sexual energy or impulses into higher or more socially acceptable activities.

transference: the development, on the part of the client, of an emotional bond (positive or negative) with the therapist.

Topics for Discussion

1. Distinguish between neurosis and psychosis and give an example of each.

2. Name four types of therapy used in the treatment of mental disorders. Which of these is the most promptly and predictably effective?

3. Define or explain: anxiolytic, compulsion, delusion, hallucination, neuroleptic, obsession, phobia.

4. Insanity is a legal term referring to the inability of a person (usually an accused criminal) to distinguish between right and wrong and to make appropriate decisions about the rightness of personal actions. Which of the mental disorders discussed in this chapter might make a person legally insane?

5. How might the demonstration of genetic and neurochemical causes for most or even all mental disorders affect philosophy, laws, morality, religion, and other fundamental social institutions in the future?

Index

A, a
A cell 241
abdominal injury 92
aberration, chromosomal 22
ablation 120
abrasion 90
abscess 37, 108
  peritonsillar 158
  subphrenic 187
  tubo-ovarian 211
abuse, child 93
achlorhydria 251
acid-fast stain 42
acne rosacea 116
acne vulgaris 114
acquired 5
acquired immunodeficiency syndrome (AIDS) 60
acromegaly 233
ACTH (adrenocorticotropic hormone) 232
activated partial thromboplastin time 249
acute 5
acute bacterial endocarditis 131
acute glomerulonephritis 201
acute intermittent porphyria 29
acute lymphocytic leukemia (ALL) 256
acute lymphoblastic leukemia 256
acute renal failure 200
acute rheumatic fever 67
Addison disease 239
adenocarcinoma, colon and rectum 82
adenoma 83
adenohypophysis 232
adrenal glands 238

adrenocorticotropic hormone (ACTH) 232
adult respiratory distress syndrome (ARDS) 168
adynamic ileus 185
agammaglobulinemia 59
aggressive 13
AIDS (acquired immunodeficiency syndrome) 60
airborne infection 38
albumin, urinary 199
aldosterone 239
allergic rhinitis 155
allergy 63
alopecia 69, 119
alpha cell 241
alveolus, pulmonary 162
Alzheimer disease 329
amenorrhea 32, 214
amino acid 230
anal fissure 186
analysis
  chromosomal 24
  DNA 24
anaplasia 75, 83
androgen, adrenal 239
anemia 26, 250
  acquired hemolytic 253
  aplastic 255
  hemolytic 251
  iron deficiency 250
  pernicious 251
  sickle cell 252
aneuploidy 23
aneurysm 142, 159
  dissecting 142
  ventricular 136
angina pectoris 134
angiomatosis, bacillary 61
angle, costovertebral (CVA) 198
anisocytosis 251
anorexia 83, 176

anovulation 215
anthracosis 170
anti-oncogene 33
antibiotic 43
antibody 40, 56
  heterophile 47
antidiuretic hormone 232
antigen 56
antiviral drug 46
anuria 199
aortic stenosis 131
aplastic anemia 255
aponeurosis 265
appendicitis 181
arrhythmia 124
  cardiac 132
arterial blood gases 163
arteriosclerotic heart disease (ASHD) 133
arthritis 273
  degenerative 273
  rheumatoid 64
articular cartilage 265
asbestosis 170
ascites 124, 191
ASHD (arteriosclerotic heart disease) 133
aspartame 28
asterixis 191
asthma 166
asymptomatic 5
atelectasis 26, 83
atherosclerosis 142
atopic dermatitis 105
atrial septal defect 128
atypical lymphocyte 47
audiography 149
auscultation 9
  cardiac 124
autoimmunity 64
autosome 20
avascular necrosis 88, 267
azotemia 200

337

B, b

B cell 241
B lymphocyte 56
bacillary angiomatosis 61
bacteremia 40
bacteria 36
Baker cyst 268
baldness 119
barium enema 177
barium swallow 177
barrel chest 166
Barrett esophagus 178
basal body temperature 216
basal cell carcinoma 118
basilar 26
basophil 247
battered child syndrome 93
Bence Jones protein 260
benign (neoplasm) 72
benign neglect 13
benign prostatic hyperplasia (BPH) 207
Berger disease 201
beta cell 241
bilirubin, indirect-reacting 249
biopsy 75
    bone marrow 249
    needle 75
bleb 102
bleeding, dysfunctional uterine 215
blepharitis 120
block, heart 132
blood 246
bloodborne infection 38
body, inclusion 52
bone 264
bone marrow 246, 264
borborygmus 177
bradyarrhythmia 125
bradycardia 125
breast 227
breast cancer 79
breast examination 216
Broders classification 75
bronchiectasis 26, 165
bronchitis 164
bronchoalveolar lavage (BAL) 164
bronchogenic carcinoma 78
bronchoscopy 163
Brushfield spots 32
bulla 102, 159
burns, thermal 95
bursa 265, 268
bursitis 268

C, c

calcitonin 237
calorie 231
calorimeter 231
cancer 73
    breast 79
    prostate 81
Candida 158
candidosis 61
capacity, iron-binding 249
carbohydrate 230
carboxyhemoglobin 249
carbuncle 108
carcinogen 72
carcinoma,
    basal cell 118
    bronchogenic 78
    squamous cell 119
cardiomegaly 69
cardiorrhexis 136
carrier 38
cartilage 269
    articular 265
casts, urinary 199
catheterization, bladder 199
CD4+ lymphocyte count 60
cell
    A 241
    alpha 241
    B 241
    beta 241
    multinucleated giant 53
    myeloid 246
    red blood 246

cell *(cont.)*
    stem 258
    target 250
    white blood 246
cell-mediated immunity 57
cellulitis 37, 108
cerebral concussion 91
cerumen 148
cervical intraepithelial neoplasia (CIN) 225
cervix, carcinoma of 225
chancre 209
Chédiak-Higashi disease 59
chemotherapy of cancer 77
chest
    barrel 166
    flail 92
chickenpox 50
child abuse 93
chlamydia infection 211
cholecystitis 192
cholelithiasis 192
cholera 180
cholesteatoma 151
chondromalacia patellae 270
chorea 68
chromosomal analysis 24
chromosome 20
    Philadelphia 257
chronic 6
chronic lymphocytic leukemia 258
chronic myelogenous leukemia (CML) 257
Chvostek sign 238
cicatrix 103
CIN (cervical intraepithelial neoplasia) 225
cirrhosis
    hepatic 190
    Laënnec 190
    portal 190
classification, Broders 75
claudication, intermittent 142

cleft lip 31
cleft palate 31
clone 83
clotting time 249
clubbing, digital 26, 163
CMV (cytomegalovirus) 61
coarctation of the aorta 127
cochlea 148
cold injury 95
colic, ureteral 198
colitis, ulcerative 183
colon carcinoma 82
colostomy 83
colposcopy 216
comedo 103, 114
comminuted fracture 87
communicable disease 38
comorbidity 16
complete blood count (CBC) 247
complication 12
compound fracture 87
concentration, mean corpuscular hemoglobin 248
concussion, cerebral 91
condyloma acuminatum 112
condyloma lata 209
congenital 6, 20
congenital adrenal hyperplasia 241
congenital heart disease 127
congestive heart failure 138
conservative 13
constipation 176
contact dermatitis 106
contagious 38
contusion 87
contusion, cerebral 91
Coombs test
   direct 253
   indirect 253
cor pulmonale 26
coronary artery disease 133
corpus luteum 220

cortex, adrenal 238
corticosteroid 26
cortisol 238
coryza 154
cosmetic 13
count
   CD+ lymphocyte 60
   complete blood 247
   differential, of white blood cells 248
   platelet 248
   red blood cell 247
   reticulocyte 249
   white blood cell 248
counterstain 42
crepitus 268
cretinism 234
crisis
   addisonian 239
   adrenal 239
   blastic 258
Crohn disease 182
crust 103
cryoprobe 120
cryotherapy 120
cuffing, peribronchial 26
cul-de-sac 218, 222
culdoscopy 218
culture 10, 42
cumulative trauma disorder (CTD) 94
cure 13
Cushing disease 240
Cushing syndrome 240
CVA (costovertebral angle) pain 198
cyanosis 163
cyst 103
   Baker 268
   chocolate 222
   endometrial, of ovary 222
cystic fibrosis 25
cystic mastitis 227
cystitis 204
cystosarcoma phyllodes 228

cystoscopy 200
cystourethrogram, voiding 200
cytogenetics 24
cytology 11
cytomegalovirus (CMV) 61

D, d
D&C 217
debridement 90
debulking 77
decibel 159
defect
   atrial septal 128
   cardiac conduction 132
   ventricular septal 129
deficiency 7
degenerative 7
degenerative joint disease (DJD) 273
deletion, chromosomal 23
dementia 69
DeQuervain disease 237
dermatitis 105, 120
   atopic 105
   contact 106
   seborrheic 105
dermatome 52
dermatophytid 109
dermatosis 120
dermis 102
dermographism 120
developmental 7
device, intrauterine contraceptive (IUD) 222
diabetes insipidus 234
diabetes mellitus 242
   insulin-dependent 242
   non-insulin-dependent 243
Diagnostic and Statistical Manual 4
diaphoresis 125
diaphysis 264
diascopy 104
diastole 124

differential diagnosis 15
DiGeorge syndrome 59
dilatation and curettage
  (D&C) 217
dilatation, cardiac 125
disabling 6
disc
  herniated 269
  intervertebral 269
discharge, vaginal 215
discoid 69
discoid lupus 66
disease
  Addison 239
  Berger 201
  Chédiak-Higashi 59
  communicable 38
  congenital heart 127
  coronary artery 133
  Crohn 182
  Cushing 240
  degenerative joint 273
  DeQuervain 237
  fibrocystic, of breast
    227
  gastroesophageal reflux
    178
  Glanzmann 261
  Graves 235
  Hashimoto 236
  hemolytic, of the new-
    born 254
  Hodgkin 259
  Legg-Calvé-Perthes 267
  Lyme 48
  Ménière 152
  Osgood-Schlatter 267
  Paget 271
  pelvic inflammatory
    (PID) 210, 224
  Raynaud 143
  reactive airways (RAD)
    166
  severe combined
    immunodeficiency 59
  sexually transmitted 208
  sexually transmitted 39

disease *(cont.)*
  tropical 39
  valvular heart 129
  venereal 39
disinfectant 43
dislocation 89
disorder, cumulative trauma
  (CTD) 94
displaced fracture 87
diverticulitis, colonic 184
diverticulum 184
DNA analysis 24
DNA probe 24
dominant gene 21
Down syndrome 23, 31
droplet spread 38
drowning 94
DSM-IV 4
dysentery, bacillary 180
dysfunctional uterine bleeding 215
dysmenorrhea 214, 221
dyspareunia 211, 214
dysphagia 176
dyspnea 27, 83, 125
dyspnea, paroxysmal
  nocturnal 125
dystrophy, muscular 266
dysuria 199, 214

E, e
ear, swimmer's 150
eburnation 273
ecchymosis 87, 103
ectopia 30
eczema 28, 105
edema 125
  acute pulmonary 139
  dependent 125
  peripheral 125
  pitting 125
effluvium, telogen 119
effusion 69, 83
  pleural 83, 172
elective 13
electric shock 96

electrophoresis, hemoglobin
  249
elliptocytosis 251
embolism 143
  pulmonary 171
emphysema, pulmonary
  166
encephalitis 52
end-stage 6
endocarditis 131
endocrine glands 230
endolymph 159
endometriosis 222
endometritis 224
endometrium 219
  carcinoma of 226
endorectal 83
endoscopy 11
enema, barium 177
enteritis, regional 182
entcrocolitis 69
  pseudomembranous 180
eosinophil 247
epidemiology 38
epidermis 102
epididymitis 206
epididymo-orchitis 206
epiphysis 264
epistaxis 156
Epstein-Barr virus 47
erosion 103
erysipelas 108
erythema chronicum
  migrans 48
erythematous 69
erythroblastosis fetalis 253
erythrocyte 246
erythrocyte sedimentation
  rate (ESR) 52, 249
erythropoiesis 246
eschar 103
esophageal hiatus hernia
  178
esophagitis 178
esophagus, Barrett 178
essential 7

Index • 341

esterase, leukocyte 199
estrogen 218
etiology 6
exacerbation 120
examination
　breast 216
　pelvic 215
exanthem 52
excoriation 104
exocrine 27
extradural hemorrhage 91
extramedullary
　hematopoiesis 256
exudate, pleural 172

F, f
failure, acute renal 200
familial 7
fat 230
febrile 52
femoral hernia 188
ferritin, serum 249
fever
　acute rheumatic 67
　scarlet 49, 158
　typhoid 180
fibrinogen 246
fibroadenoma of breast 227
fibrocystic disease of breast 227
fibroid, uterine 223
fibromyalgia syndrome 268
fibromyoma, uterine 223
film, lateral decubitus 172
fissure 104
　anal 186
Fitz-Hugh–Curtis
　syndrome 211, 224
flail chest 92
flatulence 27, 177
flora 52
follicle
　graafian 218
　ovarian 218
follicle-stimulating hormone (FSH) 218, 232
folliculitis 107

fomite 38
fracture 87
　comminuted 87
　compound 87
　displaced 87
　hairline 88
　impacted 88
　stress 88
fremitus, tactile 172
friable 121
frozen section 75
FTA-ABS 209
fulminant 6
functional 7
fungi 36
furuncle 108

G, g
GABHS (group A beta-hemolytic streptococci) 49
gallbladder 189, 192
gallop rhythm 125
gallstones 192
gases, arterial blood 163
gastroenteritis 52, 180
gastroesophageal reflux disease (GERD) 178
gene 20
genotype 21
GERD (gastroesophageal reflux disease) 178
gigantism 233
Glanzmann disease 261
Gleason grading 81
globulin
　immune 56
　thyroid binding (TBG) 234
glomerulonephritis, acute 201
glucagon 241
glucocorticoid 238
glucose-6-phosphate dehydrogenase deficiency 252
gonadotropin, human chorionic (hCG) 220

gonadotropin-releasing hormone (GnRH) 218
gonorrhea 210
gout 274
grade 12
grading (of cancer) 75
grading, Gleason 81
Gram-negative 42
Gram-positive 42
Gram stain 42
granulocyte 246
Graves disease 235
Grey Turner sign 194
Group A beta-hemolytic streptococci (GABHS) 49
gunshot wound 90
gynecology 214
gynecomastia 32

H, h
habitus 30
hairline fracture 88
Hashimoto disease 236
hay fever 155
hearing loss 153
heart block 132
Heberden node 273
Helicobacter pylori 179
hemarthrosis 262
hematemesis 176
hematochezia 176
hematocrit 248
hematoma 87
hematopoiesis,
　extramedullary 256
hematuria 199
hemoglobin 246, 248
　mean corpuscular 248
hemoglobin electrophoresis 249
hemoglobin S 252
hemolytic anemia 251
hemolytic disease of the newborn 254
hemoperitoneum 92
hemophilia 261

342 • Human Diseases

hemoptysis 83, 125
hemorrhage
  extradural 91
  intracranial 91
  subarachnoid 91
  subdural 91
hemorrhoids 186
hemothorax 92
hepatic 83
hepatitis
  chronic active 190
  chronic persistent 190
hepatitis A 189
hepatitis B 189
hepatitis C 190
hepatitis D 190
hepatojugular reflex 125
hepatomegaly 125
hereditary 7, 20
heredofamilial 7
hernia
  abdominal 187
  esophageal hiatus 178
  femoral 188
  inguinal
    direct 188
    indirect 188
  umbilical 188
herniated nucleus pulposus 269
heroic 13
herpes simplex 61, 110
herpes zoster 51, 62
heterophile antibody 47
heterozygous 21
Hippocrates 27
hirsutism 120
histiocyte 247
histology 11
histoplasmosis 61
HIV 60
hives 116
Hodgkin disease 259
Homans sign 145
homologous genes 21
homozygous 21

hormone 83, 230
  adrenocorticotropic 232
  antidiuretic 232
  follicle-stimulating (FSH) 218, 232
  gonadotropin-releasing (GnRH) 218
  luteinizing (LH) 218, 232
  parathyroid 237
  releasing 230
  thyroid stimulating 232
  tropic 230
host 39
HPV (human papillomavirus) 33, 111
human chorionic gonadotropin (hCG) 220
human immunodeficiency virus (HIV) 60
human papillomavirus (HPV) 33, 111, 225
humoral 52
humoral immunity 56
hyperactivity 29
hyperacute 6
hypermenorrhea 215
hyperparathyroidism 238
hyperplasia 83
  benign prostatic (BPH) 207
  congenital adrenal 241
hyperprolactinemia 221
hypertension 140
  portal 191
hyperthyroidism 235
hypertrophic 120
hypertrophy, cardiac 125
hypoalbuminemia 27
hypocalcemia 194
hypochromic 250
hypomenorrhea 215
hypoparathyroidism 237
hypophysis 232
hypotension 69, 139
hypothyroidism 234
hypotonia 32
Hz (hertz) 159

I, i
id reaction 109
IDDM (insulin dependent diabetes mellitus) 242
idiopathic 7
idiopathic thrombocytopenic purpura (ITP) 260
ileus 27
  adynamic 185
IM (infectious mononucleosis) 47
imaging (diagnostic) 11
immune globulin 56
immunity 40, 56
  cell-mediated 57
  humoral 56
immunodeficiency 59
impacted fracture 88
impaction 159
impetigo 52, 107
inborn error of metabolism 24
incarceration of hernia 188
incised wound 90
inclusion body 52
incontinence 199
  urinary 205
incubation 42
incubation period 40
incus 148
infantile 6
infarction 125
  myocardial 135
  pulmonary 171
infection 36
  opportunistic 59
  opportunistic, in AIDS 61
infectious 7
infectious mononucleosis (IM) 47
infective endocarditis 131
infestation 36
infiltrate 27
inflammation 37
injury
  abdominal 92
  cold 95

Index • 343

injury *(cont.)*
 radiation 96
 spinal 91
 inoculation 42
 inoperable 13
 inspection 9
 insulin-dependent diabetes mellitus (IDDM) 242
 interferon 46
 intermittent 6
 intermittent claudication 142
International Classification of Diseases 4
 intestinal obstruction 185
 intima 127
 intrauterine contraceptive device (IUD) 222
 intravenous pyelogram (IVP) 200
 intussusception 185
 invasive 11
 inversion, chromosomal 23
 iron deficiency anemia 250
 iron-binding capacity 249
 iron, serum 249
 irritable bowel syndrome 182
 ischemia 125
 islets of Langerhans 241
 IUD (intrauterine contraceptive device) 222

J, j
 jaundice 189
 Job syndrome 59
 joint 265
 junction
  squamocolumnar 217
  ureteropelvic (UPJ) 202
  ureterovesical (UVJ) 202
 juvenile 6

K, k
 Kaposi sarcoma 62
 karyotype 23

 karyotyping 24
 Keith-Wagener changes 125, 141
 keloid 104
 keratitis 121
  dendritis 121
 Kerley B lines 139
 kidney, polycystic 200
 kidney stone 202
 kilocalorie 231
 Klinefelter syndrome 32
 Koebner phenomenon 117
 kyphosis 271

L, l
 laceration 90
  cerebral 91
 laminectomy 270
 Langerhans, islets of 241
 laparoscopy 177, 218
 laparotomy 177
 larynx 159
 lateral decubitus film 172
 lavage, bronchoalveolar (BAL) 164
 Legg-Calvé-Perthes disease 267
 lesion 52
 leukemia 256
  chronic lymphocytic 258
  chronic myelogenous 257
 leukocyte 246
  polymorphonuclear 247
 leukocyte esterase 199
 leukoplakia, oral hairy 62
 lichenification 104
 lientery 176
 life-threatening 6, 12
 ligament 88, 265
 light, Wood 104
 lines, Kerley B 139
 lipid 230
 lithotripsy, extracorporeal shock wave 203
 liver 188
 locus 21

 lues 208
 lumen 126
 lupus, discoid 66
 lupus erythematosus 65
 luteinizing hormone (LH) 218, 232
 Lyme disease 48
 lymphadenopathy 69
 lymphoblast 257
 lymphocyte 53, 56, 60, 247
  atypical 47
  B 56
  killer T 57
  T 56
 lymphoma 259
  non-Hodgkin 259

M, m
 macrocytosis 251
 macular 69
 macule 103
 malaise 159
 malar 69
 malignant 6, 72
 malignant melanoma 83, 119
 malleus 148
 maneuver, Valsalva 159
 Marfan syndrome 30
 marrow, bone 246, 264
 masterly inactivity 14
 mastitis, cystic 227
 mastoiditis 151
 McBurney point 181
 McMurray test 270
 mean corpuscular hemoglobin (MCH) 248
 mean corpuscular hemoglobin concentration (MCHC) 248
 mean corpuscular volume (MCV) 248
 meconium 27
 meconium ileus 25
 mediastinal 83
 medium, culture 42
 medulla, adrenal 238
 megakaryocyte 247

344 • Human Diseases

meiosis 21
melanoma 83
 malignant 119
menarche 218
Mendel, Gregor 22
Ménière disease 152
meniscus, torn 270
menopause 218
menorrhagia 215
menstruation, normal 218
mesothelioma, pleural 170
metabolism 230
metaphysis 264
metastasis 72
microbiology 11
microcytic 250
microorganism 42, 53
mineral, dietary 231
mineralocorticoid 239
mitosis 21
mitral stenosis 130
mitral valve prolapse 31, 131
molecular disease 8
mongolism 31
monocyte 246
monodrug therapy 14
mononucleosis, infectious 47
monosomy 23
mosaicism 23, 32
motor nerve 264
multinucleated giant cell 53
multiple endocrine neoplasia 244
multiple myeloma 259
multiple trauma 96
mural thrombus 137
murmur, cardiac 126
muscular dystrophy 266
mutation, genetic 22
mycobacteria 42
Mycobacterium tuberculosis 169
myeloma, multiple 259
myocardial infarction 135

myocarditis 136
myoclonus 29
myoma, uterine 223
myopia 31
myringotomy 152
myxedema 234

N, n
necrosis 83
 avascular 88, 267
negative 16
Neisseria gonorrhoeae 210
neonatal 6
neoplasia 72
 cervical intraepithelial 225
 multiple endocrine 244
neoplasm 72
nephritis 69
nephrotic syndrome 202
nerve, motor 264
neuritic (pain) 53
neurohypophysis 232
neutrophil 247
nevus 121
NIDDM (non-insulin-dependent diabetes mellitus) 243
nitrite, urinary 199
nocturia 83, 127
node, Heberden 273
nodule 103
non-Hodgkin lymphoma 259
noncontributory 9
nondisjunction, chromosomal 23
noninvasive 11
nonmendelian inheritance 23
nonunion 88
normal 16
nosebleed 156
nucleus pulposus, herniated 269
nutrition 230

nutritional 8
nystagmus 159

O, o
obesity 232
obstruction, intestinal 185
occult 120
oligomenorrhea 215
oliguria 199
oncogene 33
oncology 73
onset 12
opportunistic infection 59
 in AIDS 61
oral hairy leukoplakia 62
organic 8
Osgood-Schlatter disease 267
osmotic fragility test 249
osteoarthritis 273
osteomyelitis 272
osteophyte 273
osteoporosis 271
otitis externa 150
otitis media 151
otorhinolaryngologist 148
otoscope 148
overweight 232
ovulation 219
oxytocin 232

P, p
Paget disease 271
palliative 14
palliative treatment 83
palpable 83
palpation 9
palpitation 126
pancreas 193
 endocrine function of 241
pancreatitis
 acute 193
 chronic 194
Pap (Papanicolaou) smear 216

Index • 345

papillomavirus, human (HPV) 111, 225
papule 103
paralysis 29
paraneoplastic syndrome 83
parasite 36
parathyroid glands 237
parathyroid hormone (PTH) 237
paroxysmal 6
paroxysmal nocturnal dyspnea 125
patent ductus arteriosus 129
pathogen 36
PCR 24
pectus excavatum 31
pediculosis 113
pelvic examination 215
pelvic inflammatory disease (PID) 210, 224
peptic esophagitis 178
peptic ulcer 179
percussion 9
perfusion 126
pericardiocentesis 139
pericarditis 69, 136
   constrictive 138
pericardium 124
period, incubation 40
period of communicability 39
periosteum 264
peritoneum 186
peritonitis 187
peritonsillar abscess 158
pernicious anemia 251
petechia 103, 127
phagocyte 246
pharyngitis 157
phenomenon, Koebner 117
phenotype 21
phenylketonuria 28
Philadelphia chromosome 257
phthiriasis 113
phthisis 170

physical therapy 14
PID 210
pile, sentinel 186
pinna 149
pit 104
pituitary gland 232
pityriasis rosea 118
PKU 28
placenta 220
plantar 121
plaque 103
plasma 246
platelet 247
platelet count 248
pleura 162
pleural effusion 83, 172
pleural exudate 172
pleural friction rub 163
pleural mesothelioma 170
pleural transudate 172
pleurisy 69
Plummer-Vinson syndrome 250
PMI (point of maximal intensity) 127
PMS (premenstrual syndrome) 223
pneumoconiosis 170
Pneumocystis carinii pneumonia 62
pneumonia 168
   Pneumocystis carinii 62
pneumonitis 168
pneumothorax 92
   spontaneous 172
pneumotympanometry 150
point, McBurney 181
point of maximal intensity (PMI) 127
poisoning 97
pollakiuria 199
polycystic kidney 200
polycythemia vera 255
polydipsia 234
polyglandular deficiency syndrome 244

polymenorrhea 215
polymerase chain reaction 24
polymorphonuclear leukocyte 247
polyp 83
   nasal 155
polyuria 199, 234
porphyria, acute intermittent 29
portacaval shunt 191
portal hypertension 191
position, Trendelenburg 141
pouch of Douglas 218
powder burn lesion 223
precordial 127
premenstrual syndrome (PMS) 223
present 12
primary disease 9
proprioception 264
probe, DNA 24
prodrome 12
progesterone 220
prognosis 12
progressive 6
prolactin 220
prolapse, mitral valve 31, 130
prophylactic 27
prostate cancer 81
prostatitis 207
protein 230
   Bence Jones 260
prothrombin time 249
proto-oncogene 33
protocol 14
   chemotherapy 77
pseudomembranous enterocolitis 180
psoriasis 117
psychomotor retardation 29
pulmonary edema 140
pulmonary embolism 171
pulmonary emphysema 166
pulmonary function tests 163

346 • Human Diseases

pulmonary infarction 171
pulse 127
pulsus paradoxus 139
puncture 90
purpura 69, 103
  idiopathic thrombocytopenic 260
purulent 69, 159
pus 37
pustule 103
pyelonephritis 203
pyoderma 108

Q, q
quinsy (peritonsillar abscess) 158

R, r
radiation injury 96
radiation therapy 77
radical 14
radioallergosorbent test (RAST) 63
radiography 11
radiology 11
rale 27, 127, 163
  crepitant 127
rape 93
RAST (radioallergosorbent test) 63
rate
  erythrocyte sedimentation 52, 249
  sed 249
Raynaud disease 144
Raynaud phenomenon 144
reaction, id 109
reactive airways disease (RAD) 166
recessive gene 21
rectal carcinoma 82
recurrent 6
red blood cell (RBC) 246
red blood cell count 248
red herring 16
reflux, hepatojugular 125
regimen 14

regional enteritis 182
regurgitation 31
Reiter syndrome, 211
relapsing 6
relin 230
remissive 6
renal failure 200, 203
resection 83
  transurethral (TUR), of prostate 208
residual volume, urinary 199
resistance 39
retardation, psychomotor 29
reticulocyte 246
reticulocyte count 249
retinitis 69
Reye syndrome 53
rheumatic fever 67
rheumatoid arthritis 64
rhinitis 69, 159
  allergic 155
rhinophyma 116, 121
rhinoscopy 154
rhinoscope 159
rhonchus 126, 163
rhythm, gallop 125
ringworm 108, 109
Rinne test 150
Romberg test 153
rosacea 116
RPR 209
rub, pleural friction 163

S, s
salpingitis 210, 224
sarcoma, Kaposi 62
scab 104
scabies 113
scale 104
scan 11
  ventilation-perfusion 164, 171
scar 104
scarlatina 158
scarlet fever 49, 158
Schilling test 251

SCID (severe combined immunodeficiency disease) 59
scoliosis 31, 266
screen, strep 49, 157
screening, cancer 74
seborrheic dermatitis 105
secondary disease 9
section, frozen 75
sed rate 249
self-limiting 7
senile 7
sentinel pile 186
septicemia 40
sequela 13
serology 11
serous gland 159
serum 246
serum ferritin 249
serum hepatitis 189
serum iron 249
serum iron-binding capacity 249
severe combined immunodeficiency disease (SCID) 59
sex chromosome 20
sex-linked disorder 22
sexually transmitted disease 39
shingles (herpes zoster) 51
shock 140
  electric 96
  precordial 127
shunt, portacaval 191
sickle cell anemia 252
sickle cell trait 252
sickling 252
sickling test 249
sign 10
  Chvostek 238
  Grey Turner 194
  Homans 146
  string 182
  Trousseau 238
silent 7
silicosis 170

Index • 347

sinuses, paranasal 154
sinusitis 155
Sjögren syndrome 66
slipped disc 269
smear 12, 41
  microbiologic 41
  nasal 154
  Pap (Papanicolaou) 216
  Tzanck 53
somatostatin 233
sound
  first heart (S1) 124
  second heart (S2) 124
spectrum, antimicrobial 45
speculum 159
  vaginal 216
spermatozoon 206
spherocytosis 251
spinal injury 91
spinnbarkeit 216
splenomegaly 69
spontaneous pneumothorax 172
spots, Brushfield 32
sprain 88
squamocolumnar junction 217
squamous cell carcinoma 119
stage 13
staging (of cancer) 76
stain
  acid-fast 42
  Gram 42
stapes 148
status asthmaticus 167
steatorrhea 27, 194
stem cell 258
stenosis 159
  aortic 132
  mitral 130
sterility 32
stigma 32, 127
stone, kidney 202
strain 89
strangulation, of hernia 188
strep screen 49, 157

strep throat 49, 157
streptococcus, group A beta-hemolytic 49
stress fracture 88
striae 240
string sign 182
subacute 7
subacute bacterial endocarditis 132
subarachnoid hemorrhage 91
subclinical 7
subdural hemorrhage 91
subluxation 89
subphrenic abscess 187
suffocation 94
sulfonamide 43
sunburn 96
supportive 14
suppuration 37
surgical 14
swimmer's ear 150
symptom 9
symptomatic 14
syncope 127
syndrome
  acquired immunodeficiency (AIDS) 60
  acute urethral 211
  adult respiratory distress (ARDS) 168
  battered child 93
  Cushing 240
  DiGeorge 59
  Down 23, 31
  fibromyalgia 268
  Fitz-Hugh–Curtis 211, 224
  irritable bowel 182
  Job 59
  Klinefelter 32
  Marfan 30
  nephrotic 202
  paraneoplastic 83
  Plummer-Vinson 250
  polyglandular deficiency 244
  premenstrual (PMS) 223

syndrome *(cont.)*
  Reiter 211
  Reye 53
  Sjögren 66
  Turner 23, 32
  Wiskott-Aldrich 59
  Zollinger-Ellison 179
synergism 14
synthesis 53
syphilis 208
systole 124

T, t
T lymphocyte 56
T-N-M classification 13, 76
tachyarrhythmia 127
tachycardia 127
tactile fremitus 172
target cell 250
telangiectasis 103, 121
telogen effluvium 119
temperature, basal body 216
tendinitis 267
tendon 265
tenosynovitis 267
tentative diagnosis 16
terminal 7
test
  direct Coombs 253
  fluorescent treponemal antibody absorption (FTA-ABS) 209
  indirect Coombs 253
  McMurray 270
  osmotic fragility 249
  pulmonary function 163
  Rinne 150
  Romberg 153
  Schilling 251
  sickling 249
  tilt 141
  Weber 149
testicular torsion 207
therapeutic trial 14
therapy, radiation 77
thoracic injury 92

348 • Human Diseases

thoracotomy 173
thrill 127
thrombasthenia 261
thrombophlebitis 145
thrombosis 144
thrombus 144
　mural 137
thrush 53, 158
thyroid binding globulin
　(TBG) 234
thyroiditis
　chronic lymphocytic 236
　giant cell 237
　granulomatous 237
　subacute 237
thyrotoxicosis 235
tilt test 141
time
　activated partial
　　thromboplastin 249
　clotting 249
　prothrombin 249
tinea capitis 109
tinea circinata 108
tinea corporis 108
tinnitus 152
tophus 274
topical 159
torsion, testicular 207
toxemia 40
toxin 37
toxoid 57
toxoplasmosis 62
trait, sickle cell 252
translocation, chromosomal
　23
transmissible 39
transrectal 83
transudate, pleural 172
transurethral resection
　(TUR) of prostate 208
trauma, multiple 86, 96
traumatic 8
Trendelenburg position 141

Treponema pallidum 208
triage 97
trisomy 23, 31
tropical disease 39
Trousseau sign 238
TSH (thyroid stimulating
　hormone) 232
tuberculosis 169
tubo-ovarian abscess 211
tumor 72
tumor suppressor gene 33
turgor, skin 180
Turner syndrome 23, 32
tympanites 180
tympanocentesis 150
tympanoplasty 152
typhoid fever 180
Tzanck smear 53

U, u
ulcer 104
　peptic 179
ulcerative colitis 183
uremia 200
ureteral colic 198
urinalysis 199
urolithiasis 202
uropathy, obstructive 208
urticaria 116

V, v
vaccine 57
vacuolization 53
vaginitis 226
vaginosis, bacterial 227
Valsalva maneuver 159
valvular heart disease 130
varicella 50, 62
vascular 127
vasculitis 69
vasoconstrictor 159
vasopressin 232
VDRL 209
vector 39, 121

venereal disease 39
venipuncture 128
ventilation-perfusion scan
　164, 171
ventricular aneurysm 137
ventricular septal defect
　130
verruca 111
vertigo 152
vesicle 53, 103
virilization 120
virulence 39
virus 36
　Epstein-Barr 47
　HIV 60
vitamin 231
vitiligo 117
voiding cystourethrogram
　200
volume
　mean corpuscular 248
　residual urinary 199
volvulus 185
vulvovaginitis 226

W, w
warts 111
Weber test 149
wheal 69, 103
white blood cell (WBC)
　246
Wiskott-Aldrich syndrome
　59
Wood light 104
working diagnosis 16
wound
　gunshot 90
　incised 90

Z, z
Zollinger-Ellison syndrome
　179
zoster 51, 62